"*Empty Plate* is a refreshingly original and insightful approach to true "Holistic" health. An enjoyable, thought-provoking blend of history, tradition, and science .... A must-read for those with a serious interest in integrative approaches to health."

~Terry Wahls, MD
researcher, educator, and author of the *Wahls Protocol*

"*Empty Plate* is a little gem, not only in the world of nutrition – it also reminds us of our interconnectedness with the natural world and its influence on our well-being. It creatively connects food with mindfulness and sustainability, offers key principles to support healthy living, and is peppered with thoughtful personal reflections. Kudos to the authors - well done!"

~Veda L. Andrus EdD, MSN, RN, HN-BC®
Vice President, Education and Program Development
The BirchTree Center for Healthcare Transformation

"Every nurse should be required to read *Empty Plate* for their benefit and that of their patients."

~Mary Hagood, FNP-C

"Tammera Karr and Kathleen Bell feed body, mind, and spirit in *Empty Plate.* They teach us how to begin anew to fill our plate with food that nourishes, a mind that is calm, a world that encourages sustainability and a profound connection to nature. *Empty Plate* is personal with writings and poetry. It provides a historical and traditional perspective that you won't find elsewhere. It's also based on current research and provides practical tools throughout. This book will shift your attention and, ultimately, your actions. Gift yourself with a guiltless treat by reading *Empty Plate."*

~Elizabeth Lipski, PhD, CNS, FACN
nutritionist, professor, author of *Digestive Wellness.*
Faculty Maryland University of Integrative Health

"Hippocrates stated long ago that *food is medicine*. On many levels, *color is medicine*, especially the colors of food. Tammera and Kathleen have captured the impact of color on our physical, mental, and spiritual wellbeing. I am excited to see how they explored their perceptions of color and meal plates to reflect our holistic wellbeing. *Empty Plate* is a colorful dance exploring and inviting us to discover how various aspects of our lives are interconnected."

~ Deanna Minich, PhD

nutritionist, educator, author of the *Whole Detox* and the *Rainbow Diet,* and President of the American College of Nutrition

"The *Empty Plate* is much more than a book about food and nutrition. It reflects the integrated wisdom of heart-centered experts Tammera Karr and Kathleen Bell. Supported by extensive scientific evidence and in a true holistic approach, food and nutrition are presented from a perspective that brings a much wider understanding to the idea of food and sustenance than most of us have considered. Every chapter offers insight into a different aspect of taking nourishment into our bodies that, when employed consciously and intentionally, increases our cells' ability to receive nourishment from what we eat. The historical awareness shared describes the threads to our own and other cultures that influence our food choices, habits relating to food, and how we consume our food. Every topic in The *Empty Plate* is woven together masterfully, proposing a paradigm shift in our approach to food that promises greater enjoyment while consuming food and leads to improved health of the Whole."

~ Deonne Wright RN, HN-BC ®
Oregon Holistic Nurses Association Founding Board Member
author, spiritual counselor, clinical aromatherapist

"Once again, Dr. Karr has penned a must-read for the Integrated Clinician and Scientist. "*Empty Plate*" is chock full of wonderful holistic pearls that will serve both patients as well as practitioners.

5 Stars for a true pioneer of our day in the quest to further improve the quality of life for ALL!!"

~ ***Amalia Fantasia, PhD***
Clinical Director/Founder
Integrated Medical Associates, NJ
author of *"God's" Ingredients (My Thirty-Year Journey in IV Nutritional Medicine)*

"Who would guess that an "*Empty Plate*" could be so full! Tammera Karr and Kathleen Bell have written a solidly referenced, compelling book that is enjoyable to read and overflowing with keen observations drawn from history, culture, nature and mindfulness teachings. They have produced a food-based *holistic* guide to an intentional lifestyle for practitioners and individuals alike. It will expand and enrich your relationship with every aspect of nourishment. Make this book a permanent part of your wellness library today!"

~ ***Miriam G Zacharias, MS, NTP, BCHN®***
nutrition professional, educator,
and author of *The PEACE Process*

"Books about nutrition can be educational, generally informative, and helpful; rarely is such a book thought-provoking. Tammera Karr and Kathleen Bell's "*Empty Plate*" is all of that and more. This may be one of the most meaningful, impactful books on food that I have ever read. Proving once and for all that even the most heavily cited and researched book can be moving, I knew I was in for a pivotal moment when I read Tammera's poem in the beginning of the text, "Thunder and Rain."

With decades between them of anecdotes and experiences; this book is rooted in facts, statistics, quotations, and history. The authors have created an indispensable guide for the health/nutrition practitioner in navigating the obstacles and solutions for clients; and a "must-read" for individuals searching for the wisdom, fortitude, and guidance in how to eat to support good health and longevity."

~Barbara Rodgers – NC, BCHN®
President, National Association of Nutrition Professionals (NANP)
Author of "*Baby Maker --A complete guide to holistic nutrition for fertility, conception, and pregnancy*"

"In her newest book, *Empty Plate*: Food, Sustainability, Mindfulness, Tammera Karr teams up with Kathleen Bell to provide a refreshing and unique approach to the interrelationship of food, sustainability, and mindfulness. The authors skillfully link our personal eating habits to the ecosystem, the history of food, sustainability, and mindfulness using science, personal anecdotes, and wisdom from the ancients. The book is extensively referenced throughout to substantiate the many unusual facts given, adding credibility to the information provided. Although there is a single chapter titled "Mindfulness," the entire book speaks to mindfulness in its many aspects.

Whether read from cover to cover or in sections, it provides keen insights into our connectedness with food and how it affects our personal health, happiness, peace of mind, behavior, and the role we play in the earth's sustainability and health. It demonstrates, sometimes in subtle ways, that our life experiences blend what we eat and what is eating us. How we fill our empty plate, literally or metaphorically, depends on what we pay attention to in our lives and how mindful we are. Like Tammera's other books, it contributes to our collective wisdom and understanding of food on multiple levels, leaving us to contemplate how much we are in control of our personal experience of life."

~ James Wilson, ND, DC, PhD
author, educator clinician, Co-founder of Canadian Memorial Chiropractic College and the Ontario College of Naturopathic Medicine (CCNM)

"While the landscape of life that we knew was being dismantled by mandated lockdowns in the name of the novel coronavirus, COVID-19, Tammera, and Kathleen were busy crafting nourishment for the nurturers. They were busy preserving the 'good stuff' of life and living. *Empty Plate* is another content-dense, satisfying read, true to Tammera Karr's style. As caregivers, we need these tools to keep ourselves well. As we are able to 'keep our cup full,' then we can offer wellness to ourselves from the position of 'fullness, and from overflow'... to those entrusted to our care and service. "

~Lorie Amitrano, FNP-C

"*Empty Plate* is a beautiful compilation of history, tradition, and science empowering wellness possibilities with an insightful approach to holistic wellbeing. Tammera's and Kathleen's passion for nutrition and wellness shines through in their mindful writing of this book as a guide to inform and support you in choosing the right healing journey for you. This is a supportive and informative resource to add to your wellness library."

~ Kerry McClure, NC, BCHN®
nutrition professional, educator, speaker, co-author of
Beyond Meditation: making mindfulness accessible for everyone

"*Empty Plate* by Tammera Karr and Kathleen Bell reaches out. It draws you in with beautiful illustrations, historical teachings, nutritional instructions, timely quotes from great minds, and a plateful of science explaining why you need to eat the right foods to maintain a positive attitude in these trying times. They teach you about modern-day farming, colors of food and their nutritional implications, and touch on how these positively affect our physical and mental health. To bring it all together, they write about mindfulness and how it can affect our wellbeing.

Food, eating, thinking, thankfulness – the authors gently encourage and remind us how to use our resources to lead us back to a stronger, healthier physical and mental state of being; that we should be teaching our children and grandchildren. Here's to positive reflections on our next empty plate tomorrow morning and the opportunity to fill it with goodness! Thank you, Tammera and Kathleen."

~David T. Zava, PhD
CEO and Chief Scientist ZRT Laboratories

"If there was ever a time to use the term "wholistic" for emphasis, *Empty Plate* is it. Their focus on creating and sustaining health takes you above and beyond the food you put on your empty plate, although their research in this area is highly extensive. They thoughtfully take a whole-person approach incorporating topics and techniques like eating a mindful meal and spending time in nature that truly nourishes the body, mind, and spirit.

Their recommendations around food and water alone are worth the price of the book. The chapter on color and sound is a fun and educational addition. And of course, a book by Tammera wouldn't be complete without a little food history sprinkled throughout. This is like an encyclopedia of holistic health… a keeper that you will find yourself referencing often."

~MaryAnn Marks, NC, MBA
Co-founder and CEO, LabSmarts

"In these pages Tammera Karr and Kathleen Bell offer a beautiful resource that helps us to understand and nourish not just the body but also the mind and the spirit. An encyclopedic reference for holistic health, mindfulness, and sustainability. This is a book to be savored."

~Mira Dessy, NE, BCHHP
The Ingredient Guru
nutrition educator, real food advocate, and
author of *The Pantry Principle*: how to read the label and
understand what's really in your food

To Jean

May your plate be found with hope, health and happiness!

Kathleen Bell

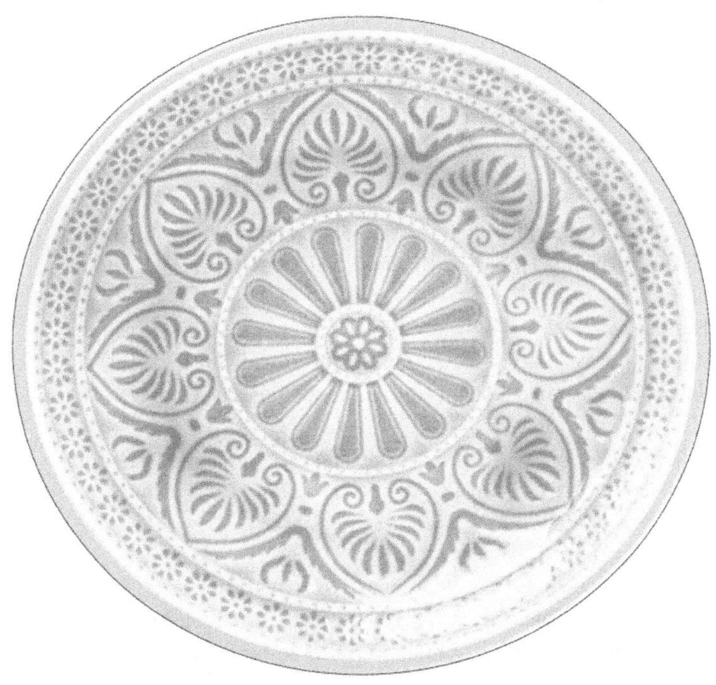

Empty Plate

Food ♣ Sustainability ♣ Mindfulness

Also, by Tammera J. Karr

Our Journey with Food
Our Journey with Food Cookery Book

Works by Kathleen Bell

- ❖ Preparing You for the Big Day: A Guide to Childbirth for the BIRTH PLACE at Nashua Memorial Hospital. Nashua, NH

- ❖ The Use of Whirlpool Tubs for Management of Pain in Active First Stage Labor: A Descriptive Study. Master's Research Thesis: University of Utah School of Nursing, Salt Lake City, Utah

- ❖ In Wynn, A. & Woo, T. Pharmacotherapeutics for Nurse Practitioner Prescribers (3rd ed), Ch. 48 - Women as Patients. F.A. Davis, Philadelphia, PA

- ❖ In Kaakinen, et al. Family Health Care Nursing (5th ed), Ch.12 – Nursing of Childbearing Families. F.A. Davis: Philadelphia, PA. Also authored accompanying online Instructor's Manual for this textbook.

- ❖ Veltri, L. et al. (2016) Controlled Postpartum – Newborn Simulation with Objective Evaluation Exchanged for Clinical Learning. Clinical Simulation in Nursing (12)

- ❖ Going Global: AHNA Expands Awareness of Holistic Nursing Internationally, Beginnings, 2/2017 (vol 37/1)

- ❖ Teaching Therapeutic Touch to Pediatric Nursing Students in Chronic Care, Beginnings, 10/2017 (vol 37/5

Empty Plate

Food ☘ Sustainability ☘ Mindfulness

By Tammera J. Karr
&
Kathleen Bell

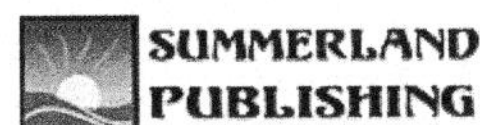

Cover Design and Empty Plate progression images
by JV Media Design

Image Source:
shutterstock.com, pexels.com, Library of Congress, M. Karr collection, Vintage Advertising Archive

Content Review Experts
Lorie Amitrano, FNP-C
Veda L. Andrus EdD, MSN, RN, HN-BC®
Chris Dennen, PhD
Elizabeth Lipski, PhD., CNS, FACN, IFMCP
James Wilson, ND, DC, PhD

Editing by Julie Thenell, MS Ed, BCHN®
Proofreading by Carol Rodriguez, BA

ISBN: 978-1-7329072-3-2
Library of Congress: 201955278

Disclaimer

This book is designed as a reference volume. It is made available to the public with the understanding that the authors and the publisher are not rendering medical or other professional advice tailored to individual needs and situations. You should not use information in this book as a substitute for a licensed healthcare professional's advice. Consult a healthcare professional to address any personal health concerns.

Because nutritional supplements can interact with medications or affect some medical conditions, you should always check with your prescribing healthcare professional before using food, nutraceutical, or herbal remedies described in this book.

The authors and publisher disclaim any liability whatsoever with respect to any loss, injury, or damage arising out of the use of this book.

Mention of specific products, companies, laboratories, or organizations does not imply that this book's publisher and authors endorse such products, companies, laboratories, or organizations.

Dedicated to the Holistic Nurses who have inspired and guided us in our understanding of healing through quantum and natural approaches.

For all those who educate and share the wisdom of traditional healthcare, foods, and knowledge.

In thanksgiving and gratitude for those who came before and showed us the way.

"If I have seen further than others, it is by standing upon the shoulders of giants."

~Isaac Newton

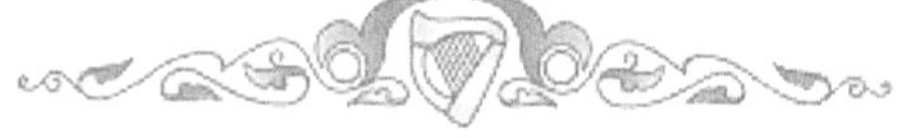

Thunder & Rain

As the thunder rumbled, the wind ran off the mountain, the tree boughs thrashed.

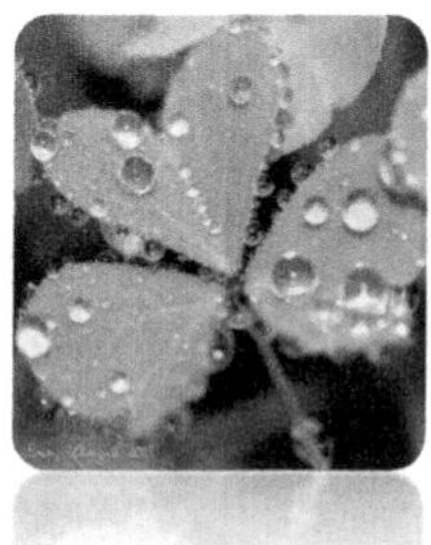

I shouted to the wind. Why should I care? No one is listening.

Then a soft touch on my cheek and a gentle voice in my ear replied.

The rumble and roar of the thunder and wind catch your attention, but it is the soft breeze that comforts and the rain that brings life from the dry earth.

It is the gentle ministering's, the cooling touch, the willing ear, and readiness to share that opens the heart. It is not the loud or the force with which we shout that changes the heart; it is the compassion, dedication, and willingness of spirit.

As the rain began to mist my face, it washed away my tears of frustration. It soothed and refreshed, and it was then that I understood, someone had heard me and cared.

~ Tammera J. Karr

Table of Contents

Forward

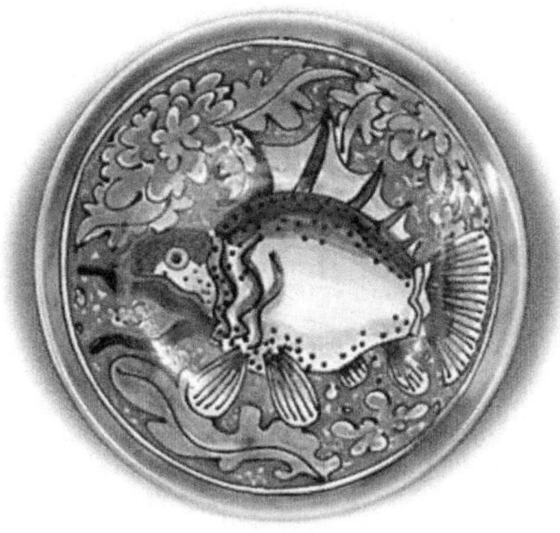

Consciousness sleeps in
minerals.
Dreams in
plants,
Awakes in
animals,
And becomes
visible in humans.

~Rumi

I first met Tammera Karr in Portland, Oregon, in 2013. She came to do a cooking demonstration for members of the Portland Chapter of the *American Holistic Nurses Association* (AHNA). After enlisting a few of us to haul in all the food and cooking paraphernalia, plus plates and utensils for us all to use to enjoy the fruits of her labor, she dived right into her favorite topic – whole foods for holistic health. Like one of the food-show stars on TV, she talked the entire time while she cooked, her running commentary highly animated, lively, funny, well-researched, and interspersed with stories from her personal practice as a holistic nutritionist.

Anyone who is a nurse knows that the way to a nurse's heart involves food (if you don't believe me, just look in on any nursing conference or convention!) and the telling of real-life stories about how providing care impacts peoples' lives. That day Tam's delightful combination of passion and scientific expertise about foods and her ability to share insightful, caring stories of her holistic practice experience captured my own heart, and our professional association and friendship began.

Fast forward to 2020, with all of us struggling with the various effects of a worldwide pandemic. When Tammera called me to propose collaboration on a book that would serve as an accompaniment to her online course about holistic nutrition, I accepted without hesitation. Because I believe there is no better time than the present for the essential messages herein.

"Take care of your body; it is the only place you have to live."

This anonymous quotation was given to me by a student in the Integrative Holistic Healing Arts Program, a continuing professional education offering of AHNA. As faculty in this program since its inception in 2018, I teach the subjects Nutrition and Philosophy of Spirituality and Healing. At the beginning of the Nutrition talk, I write the above quote on a flip chart and then modify it slightly into this:

"Take care of your body/mind/spirit, for these are the places where you live."

Holistically speaking, our minds and bodies are inseparable. Did you know that scientists have dedicated their entire careers to determine the exact location of the "mind" within the body? Virtually all have failed to do so.

Luminaries such as Dr. Bruce Lipton, Dr. Candace Pert, and Dr. Deepak Chopra agree that each one of the human body's 50 trillion cells has its own innate intelligence.[1, 2, 3] Their research has also shown that cells are "motivated" to cooperate with one another to form the complexity of multiple systems known as a human being to sustain biological life. They further teach that each unique human organism must be animated by its own unique spirit to be fully and individually alive.

Throughout my study of meditation and mindfulness, I have learned that holistic health systems such as Ayurveda, Traditional Chinese Medicine (TCM), or Indigenous practices are often based on the laws of *Nature* that do not change over time and apply everywhere and in all settings. Western thinking about health often focuses on treating disease because we define health as the absence of disease. But treating disease is different than creating health.

Tammera and I share the understanding of sustainability via holistic nutrition in this way: the idea is to nourish the body/mind/spirit in ways that keep all the complex systems in the body in balance to prevent disease and create health. We consider the body/mind/spirit to be an ACTIVITY that is a verb, not a noun. Dr. Deepak Chopra is fond of saying, "Your body is a process, not a structure."

> *"When diet is wrong, medicine is of no use. When diet is correct, medicine is of no need."*
>
> ~Ancient Ayurvedic proverb

What we feed our bodies/minds/spirits changes our responses in each moment; it also has the capacity to leave behind a "vibrational footprint" that can affect our resilience. Everything that happens in the mind plays out with effects on the body.

Our every thought and feeling's energetic signals create chemical changes at a cellular level. Our cells control the "healthy" expression of our genes primarily governed by our choices (conscious and unconscious). We are not at the mercy of genetics alone as the scientific discipline of epigenetics continues to demonstrate. [4,5] Our basic essence is consciousness (or spirit), and to sustain health and growth, a person must maintain a connection to their essence through mindfulness.

We know that both health and disease depend on our ability to digest and assimilate the food we eat, as well as our ability to digest and assimilate our experiences and emotions. In other words; our food metabolizes, creates, and sustains us!

> *"Let food be thy medicine, and medicine be thy food."*
> Attributed to Hippocrates, considered by many as the father of modern medicine.

Shall we take a look at what is on our Empty Plate in the pages to come?

~ Kathleen Bell, RN, MSN, CNM, AHN-BC®

---

1. Lipton, B. (2016) The Biology of Belief 10th Anniversary Edition: Unleashing The Power Of Consciousness, Matter & Miracles. Hay House.

2. Chopra, D. & Tanzi, R. (2018) The Healing Self: A Revolutionary New Plan To Supercharge Your Immunity And Stay Well For Life. Penguin/Random House.

3. Pert, C. (1997). Molecules Of Emotion: The Science Behind Mind/Body Medicine. Simon & Schuster.

4. Lipton, B. (2016) The Biology Of Belief 10th Anniversary Edition: Unleashing The Power Of Consciousness, Matter & Miracles. Hay House.

5. Chopra, D. & Tanzi, R. (2018) The Healing Self: A Revolutionary New Plan To Supercharge Your Immunity And Stay Well For Life. Penguin/Random House.

Forward

Introduction

Perspective is always an excellent place to begin a conversation, especially when that conversation may challenge deeply held beliefs.

> perspective
> *1) point of view and*
> *2) the proper relative position of objects or phenomena one perceives.*
> Webster's College Dictionary Third Edition

In his famous soliloquy about perspective, Hamlet said it best: "Ay, there's the rub!" Because perspective is always personal, part of any conversation involves learning a little about the people offering up their thoughts. We'd like to introduce ourselves to you.

Let us begin with Tammera, a board-certified holistic nutritionist with family connections to sustainable forestry, ranching, and agriculture. She has repeatedly seen the efforts made by loggers, ranchers, and farmers to mitigate soil erosion, water pollution and protect wildlife. These actions are anchored in a love for nature, way of life and traditional values from varied cultural backgrounds. Our modern world does not always understand what is happening *on the ground* when it comes to these generational vocations or *ways of life.*

> *<u>Vocation</u>:* a person's employment or main occupation, especially regarded as particularly worthy and requiring great dedication. [1]

Media, through multiple sources, presents images often without context when it comes to food and health. The viewer may have limited or no knowledge of life for those who produce the food we eat.

When an individual's livelihood and life involve being surrounded by nature, livestock, and wildlife; there is a sense of awe and gratitude that resides deep within a being's soul. Decades of living in remote areas and travels to eighteen countries and thirty states illustrated to Tammera the value of traditional foods; their connectivity to the environment, people, and culture. This reinforced childhood memories of wonderful traditional foods made by Basque, Irish, German, Hispanic, and Scandinavian community members. These combined factors ignited a passion, one that fuels much of what follows in this book.

Kathleen knew she was a nurse at six years old because the kids on the school playground (older and younger) came to her to soothe the bumps, bruises, cuts, and excreta. That happened daily. And not only physical care was sought; a victim of childhood sexual abuse herself, Kathleen listened compassionately to stories of other children who were being abused in multiple ways and learned how to advocate for those who were injured in body/mind/spirit.

Raised by first-generation American parents, with immigrant grandparents on both sides of her immediate family, Kathleen learned to love cooking and baking traditional cultural foods along with *old-world values*. Even when working multiple jobs, she gathered her family to eat home-cooked meals together.

As her career evolved from caring for infants and children to becoming a certified nurse-midwife and women's health care nurse practitioner, Kathleen continued her dedication to lifelong learning. Working in higher education has served as a platform for global travel to practice her arts. Attending thousands of births and deaths, each experience unique, she gained wisdom and perspective about what matters most on the planet. In midlife, both parents' sudden deaths within the same month propelled her onto a new spiritual path; she studied meditation, became a certified Meditation Specialist, and received advanced practice certification in Holistic Nursing. Kathleen's passion for healing, knowledge, and the desire to share that gained wisdom with others is evident in the pages that follow.

How Empty Plate came to be ~ by Tammera J. Karr

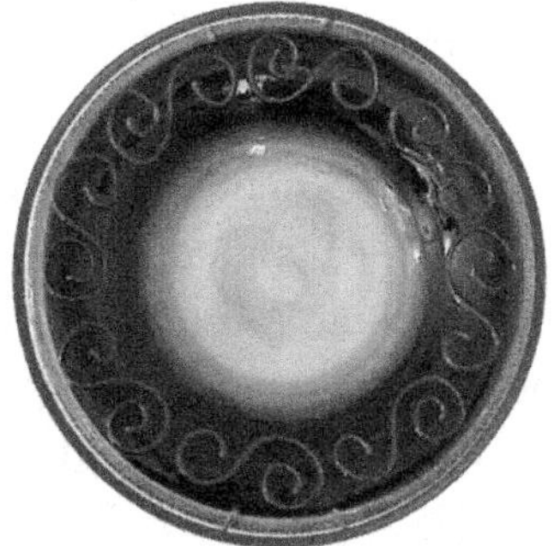

I am drawn to plates and glass, the way they catch the light, the feel of the surface, the shape, color, and of course, the history. There is so much to see when we look at an empty plate.

The empty plate recently became a meditative point for

me as I unwrapped a plate tucked away in a box. I had forgotten how much I enjoyed this plate; it was a favorite hung on the wall in my office at one time. I traced the rings of colors, savored the areas where the glazed paints had mingled and blended. I wondered about all these nuances and my thoughts traveled to the history, culture, and lessons of the plate.

There is a sturdiness and sustainability to the plates used by some, a translucent fragility to others. Yet, the perception of fragility can be misleading, just as our assumptions about food, sustainability, and mindfulness can be.

The empty plate equally serves as an example of our lives; how we fill, overfill, and scrape away our health. As children, we are told to *be careful* when handed a plate, and each mouthful of food can be a new experience. As teens, we pile our plates full to the brim with enthusiasm; powering our fearless run toward the future. As adults, we find our plates filled with foods that may not satisfy, or weigh us down; and as we age, the plate holds less and less until it is scraped clean and put away for the next user.

The empty plate also holds promise and possibilities when we consider it as a vessel for the future and health. Our health may have fine cracks in it, like the intricacy of the hair-thin cracks in the bone china glaze. But those cracks are only a small imperfection on the surface, and they do not run deep, cause a chip or permanent break. But if a plate, no matter how perfect is abused — handled without care, or put under strain, it will break. It takes specialized knowledge and training to repair broken ceramics, pottery, glass, and porcelain. It requires specialized skill, that is difficult to find in this modern toss-away age. [2, 3]

> *"We are all connected:*
> *from cell to community to cosmos."*
>
> ~Deanna Minich, PhD author of *The Rainbow Diet*

The artistry of the hand-painted stoneware, the texture and depth of the wooden trencher; all leads the imagination to distant times and far off worlds. These plates that spark our imagination can represent plans for the future, hopes and dreams that make a portion of our life sustainable. Food served on an unassuming plate made from banana leaves is no less of a marvel, as the surface emerges from beneath the food. The banana leaf plate opens the mind to the simpler ways of life; one with connection and less noise. Here the banana leaf plate reflects mindfulness, calm and grounding for health with sounds, colors, and nature. The empty plate of life and history has so much more to teach us — let the journey continue!

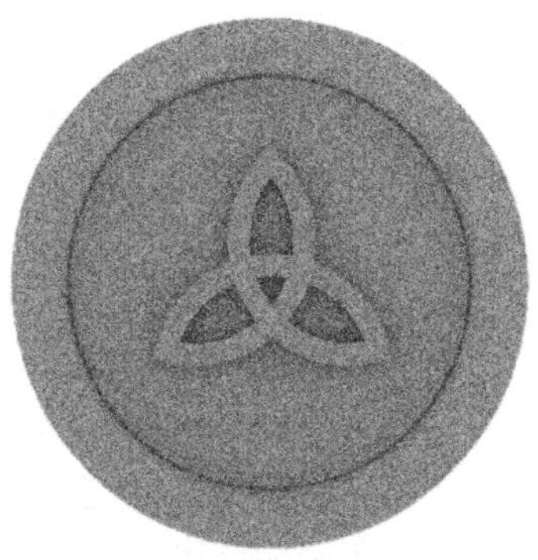

Perspective from History

The history of the plate and all things made from clay and wood dates back to ancient times. [4,5] During the *Jōmon* period, the paleo culture of Japan's *Ainu* produced clay pottery by baking the earthen objects in open fire pits. Anthropologists surmise this culture first arose in Japan at least 12,000 years ago, and perhaps as early as 16,000 years ago. Pottery is one of the enduring characteristics of this ancient culture, developed as a result of being well-nourished and sedentary. Life, it seems, was far easier for *Ainu* hunter-gatherers than we might think. Food was abundant and weather temperate, allowing for time to develop tools beyond those made from stone. For the *Ainu*, having an ease of access to food meant time on their hands to develop skills, art, language, and society.

In 1877 Edward S. Morse, American zoologist, and orientalist, first used the name *cord-marked* to *sherds* of pottery and later translated it into Japanese as *Jōmon*. [6,7,8,9] The style of pottery from the first phases of paleolithic *Jōmon* culture was decorated by impressing cords into the surface of wet clay and are the oldest examples of pottery in the world. [10] Among the finds are: deep bowls used for making stews, shallow bowls that resemble plates, drinking and spouted vessels, figurines, incense burners, and lamps. [11]

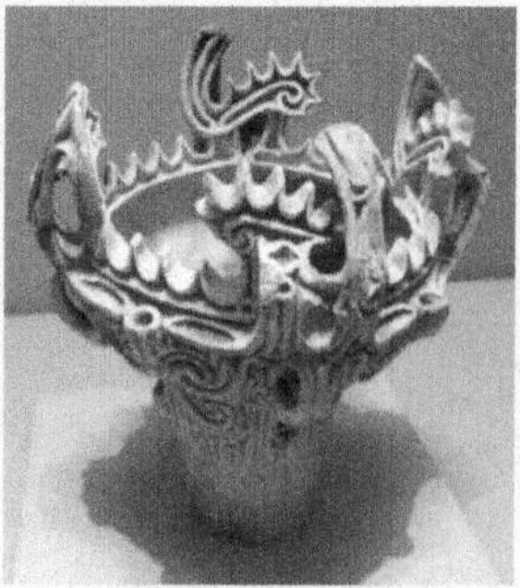

Jōmon 'fire-flame' Vessel
By Daderot (Public Domain)

---

1. Merriam Websters Dictionary Second Edition
2. Kintsugi: The Centuries-Old Art Of Repairing Broken Pottery With Gold, By Kelly Richman-Abdou On September 5, 2019: Https://Mymodernmet.Com/Kintsugi-Kintsukuroi/
3. The Art Of Repairing Broken Ceramics Creates A New Kind Of Beauty, Pottery Is Fixed For Practical Purposes—And Aesthetic Ones As Well. By Evan Nicole Brown February 15, 2019: Https://Www.Atlasobscura.Com/Articles/Repairing-Broken-Ceramics
4. Pottery Page 472 Encyclopedia Of Kitchen History, 2004 Fitzroy Dearborn NY
5. Plate (Dishware) Https://En.Wikipedia.Org/Wiki/Plate_(Dishware)
6. Mason, Penelope E., With Donald Dinwiddie, History Of Japanese Art, 2nd Edn 2005, Pearson Prentice Hall, ISBN 0-13-117602-1, 9780131176027
7. Koyama, Shuzo, And David Hurst Thomas (Eds.). (1979). Affluent Foragers: Pacific Coasts East And West. Senri Ethnological Studies No. 9. Osaka: National Museum Of Ethnology.
8. Kobayashi, Tatsuo. (2004). Jomon Reflections: Forager Life And Culture In The Prehistoric Japanese Archipelago. Ed. Simon Kaner With Oki Nakamura. Oxford, England: Oxbow Books. (Main Text 186 Pages, All On Jomon) ISBN 978-1-84217-088-5
9. Google Arts And Culture, Jomon Period Https://Artsandculture.Google.Com/Entity/M0165pb
10. Ancient History Encyclopedia, Jomon Pottery. Https://Www.Ancient.Eu/Jomon_Pottery/
11. World's Oldest Pottery Used To Cook Fish In Japan | JOMON FOOD | Facts And Details: Http://Factsanddetails.Com/Japan/Cat16/Sub105/Entry-5279.Html#Chapter-5

Chapter One
Food that Nourishes & Connects Us

"To the hunting-and-gathering Andaman Islanders of India, fire is 'the first thing they think of carrying when they go on a journey,' 'the center round which social life moves,' and the possession that distinguishes humans from animals. Animals need food, water, and shelter. We humans need all those things, but we need fire too." [1]

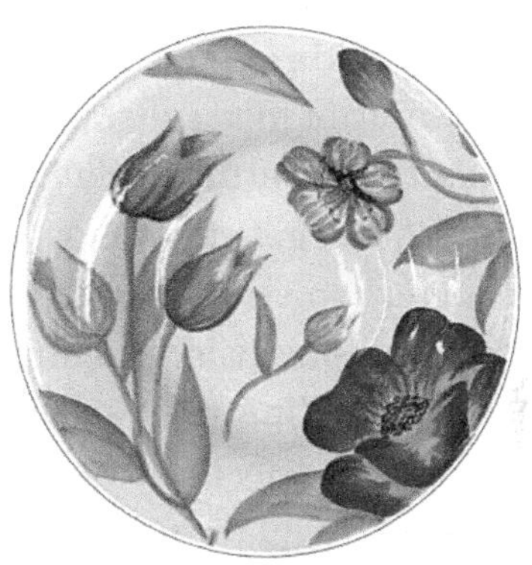

~Richard Wrangham,
Catching Fire: How Cooking Made Us Human

Perspective influences our views on everything: history, food, health, sustainability, and mindfulness. There are multiple layers to these topics, just as there is in forming a plate from clay, water, pigment, and fire. Our world has changed in countless ways since the paleolithic period of Europe, Asia, and North America. Many of those changes make it difficult, if not impossible, for us to live today as paleo-people lived. Additionally, we tend to romanticize and underestimate societies of the past. In reality, modern individuals have lost far more in ability and knowledge than we have gained. [2, 3, 4, 5]

Self-reliance and awareness of the environment, the cycles of life, ritual time and quiet, plant knowledge for medicine and food. The creative problem-solving by earlier cultures allowed them to flow with life's challenges, adapt to *change*, and think outside the box. When we look at ancient artifacts, the box appears later in history. [6] The graceful curve of the pot and the basket are, by contrast, still visibly in use today. The natural world lends itself to curves. These ancient paleo-peoples literally invented the wheel that we continue today to stress over and strive to reinvent almost daily.

Ancient cultures appear to have intuitively understood the synergistic combining of food substances with heat in order to activate their potential. The attuned skill of observation, through trial and error was passed from generation to generation. The use of fire and cooking by ancient peoples made undigestable, tough tuberous roots, nuts, seeds, and meats into palatable nutrient-dense foods. Their cooking methods utilized grinding, roasting, drying, brazing, searing, boiling, or baking. Cooking not only increased the nutrient content and digestibility of foods, but regular consumption of such superior foods over time changed our brains and bodies into the genus scientists now call *Homo sapiens sapiens*. [7,8]

Nourishment versus calories

In today's world, food is no longer hunted and gathered from the local area or region, nor does it remain distinct to a geographic country as it once was. Our food is global, and nowadays, even in remote parts of the world, people are enjoying foods from far-off lands. Often these are newly found traditional foods packed with both nutrition and simplicity. Importantly, these traditional foods are why we are here today. Without the synergistic combination of chemical structures found in food and chelated through natural processes of sunshine, fermenting and cooking — ancient humans' ability to grow, adapt, and manipulate the world around them would not have happened.

Our health is dependent on the nutrients absorbed from foods far more than from calories. [9] Nutrients like vitamin A, found in organ meat, are necessary to absorb vitamin D, maintain immune function and eye health. Vitamin C, an essential vitamin for health, is also found in plant foods and, surprisingly, in the adrenal glands and liver, from larger animals like moose and caribou of northern climates. Vitamin C is necessary for immune function, heart health, cellular integrity, and eye health and can only be gained through foods. Wild grass, seeds, and rice provided rich sources of B vitamins. Wild foods abound with antioxidants, polyphenols, and minerals. Indigenous peoples learned from their ancestors (Paleo) the time and seasons to harvest mushrooms, how to tap pine trees for sap: used for wounds and chewing gum. Early humans, learned how to use fire as an agricultural tool for keeping grasslands and valuable starch root and nut crops healthy.

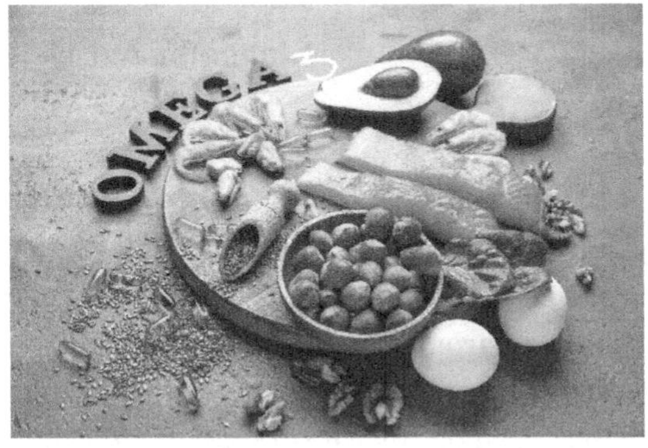

There are some nutrients found predominately in plants and others in animal meats. Each year nutrition science reveals more about nutrients found in traditional whole foods and their indispensable role in health.

Principle 1: To achieve sustainable health, which allows us to enjoy our lives fully, we need to consume nutrient-dense whole foods prepared in traditional ways.

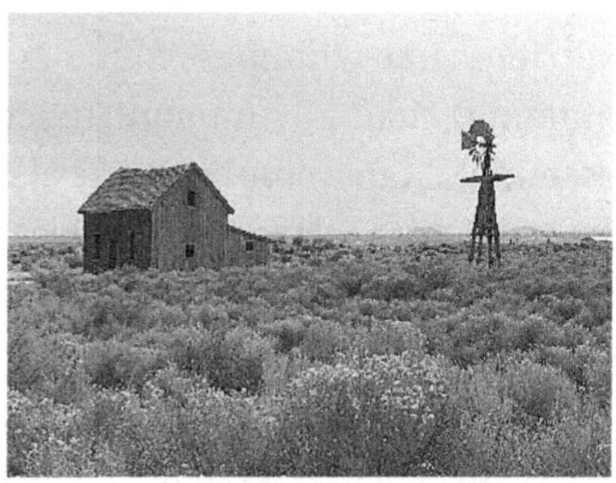

Expanding our view

Because humans are so diverse in their heritage and genetics, looking at only one approach to health care provides an incomplete picture. Scientific advances and research have opened our eyes to: the microbiome, virome, complex hormone pathways, and refined understanding of human physiology and biology. Many questions have been answered on the role of polyphenols, herbs, nutrient uptake by cells, and the role of human DNA. Modern science has also expanded our knowledge of the individuality of human physiology and biology. Illustrating the differences in how the male and female body works due to chemical exposures affecting hormones, disrupted sleep patterns from artificial light, differences in cognitive function between ages, and susceptibilities to viral illnesses.

Research has even shed light on how blood types are indicators of disparities in health. [10, 11, 12, 13, 14] In 2012, *Nature Genetics* published findings on two new blood types found in only a very small number of individuals. University of Vermont biologist Bryan Ballif and colleagues report on two proteins found on red blood cells responsible for these lesser-known blood types. "Beyond the ABO blood type and the Rhesus (Rh) blood type, the International Blood Transfusion Society recognizes twenty-eight additional blood types with names like Duffy, Kidd, Diego, and Lutheran. But Langereis and Junior have not been on this list. Although the antigens for the Junior and Langereis (or Lan) blood types were identified decades ago in pregnant women having difficulties carrying babies with incompatible blood types, the genetic basis of these antigens has been unknown until now." [15]

Over the past twelve years, researchers have developed methods to determine blood types using DNA technology rather than by examining just red blood cells. Modern technology is essential for clients who receive large amounts of blood or need blood often, as blood becomes a mixture of their own and several different donors. The mixing of blood from so many different individuals makes it challenging to determine the client's unique blood type variances. Researchers have found that the genetic cause of each blood type system must be known for DNA tests to work. [16]

More and more researchers are learning how different individuals, actually are while appearing the same. Just as the hand-painted patterns on an empty plate may look the same at a glance, a more in-depth inspection reveals variances and subtle differences.

So now let's think of an image of a spoked wagon wheel; the center hub (DNA) cannot support the wagon (health) without the spokes (nutrient-dense foods) or the form and structure of the outer rims (sustainability and mindfulness). All three elements must be present for the wheel to function properly. Without balance through nutrition, sustainability, and mindfulness; health soon looks like an old cracked and dry-rotted wagon wheel, unable to support the wagon load called *life*.

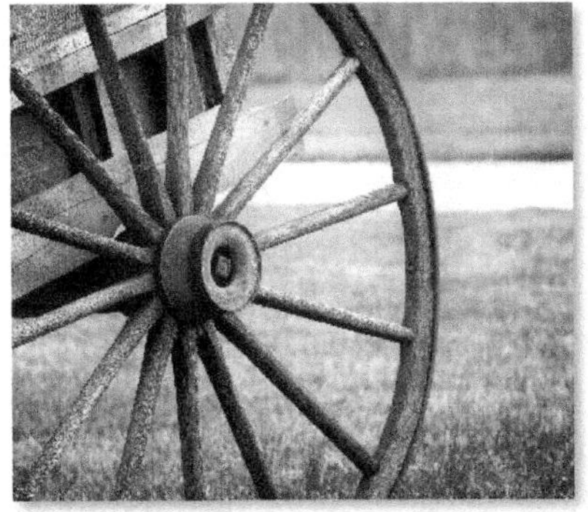

This book was written because the authors believe our journey with food is incomplete if we do not also look at sustainability and mindfulness. We cannot maintain energy, reproduction, cognitive function, and physical stamina without food and the nutrition it releases through digestion. In a very *real* sense, the food we eat *sustains* us.

The concepts of *sustenance*, as referred to in the above paragraph, and sustainability — meaning solutions to present issues related to how food is grown, produced, transported, consumed, and wasted — are intricately related. They are inextricably woven throughout the entire contents of this book.

A beginning definition of mindfulness is simple awareness. As we progress with filling our empty plate throughout the following chapters, many illustrations of the value of mindfulness will be shared.

The modern food problem

The authors are distinguishing between *processed foods*, which, by definition, are any foods not in their natural state; (i.e., chopped, peeled, cooked, dried, frozen, fermented, or canned) and *industrial-ultra-processed-foods,* are those made in factories with chemicals and highly refined ingredients.

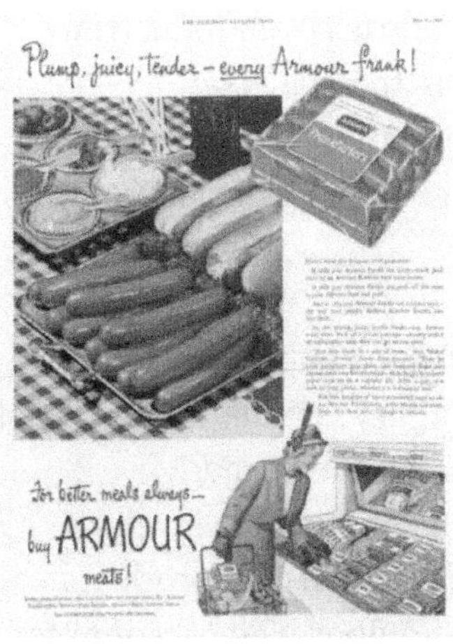

Saturday Evening Post 1950

Modern foods are linked to a growing number of escalating chronic health problems in the United States. The same can be found in other countries as well. A 2016 study on food purchased by consumers in New Zealand looked at foods from eight categories, consumption of which affects the risk of obesity and diet-related chronic diseases. Food products were selected from the 2014 Nutritrack database. The Internationally Standardized International Network for Food and Obesity/Non-Communicable Diseases Research, Monitoring and Action Support (INFORMAS) taxonomy was used to classify packages' claims.

The findings: Out of 7,058 individual health and nutrition claims found on labels cereals displayed the most significant proportion of claims, of which one-third were on *less-healthy* cereals. Clearly, these health and nutrition claims found on packages work to mislead consumers' perceptions of the nutritional quality of foods. [17]

In the United States, the Federation of American Societies for Experimental Biology (FASEB) published findings on consumer buying habits in 2015. "A nation-wide analysis of U.S. grocery purchases revealed highly processed foods make up more than 60% of the calories in the food Americans buy. These industrial food products tend to have more fat, sugar, and salt than lower-processed foods." [18] Researchers at the U.S. Centers for Disease Control and Prevention (CDC) found for every 5% increase in calories from industrial-ultra-processed foods a person ate; there was a corresponding decrease in overall health. [19]

Adults who ate approximately 70% of their calories from industrial-ultra-processed foods. They were half as likely to have *ideal* cardiovascular health, as defined by the American Heart Association, compared with people who ate 40% or fewer of their calories from industrial-ultra-processed foods. [20, 21, 22]

Industrial-ultra-processed foods include packaged baked goods and snacks, chips, candies, fizzy/energy drinks, sugary cereals, instant meals containing food additives, dehydrated vegetable soups, and reconstituted meat and fish products — often contain high levels of added ultra-refined sugar, fat, and salt. [23] These food-like products were found lacking in all essential vitamins and fiber. They account for around 25–60% of daily energy intake in first-order countries. [24]

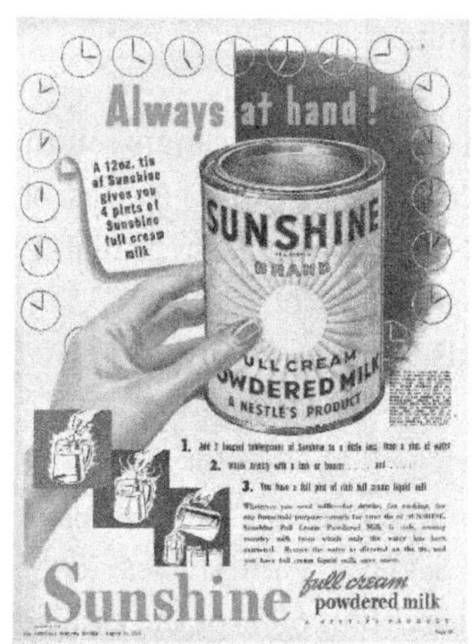

The Australian Women's Weekly -1946

Older studies linked industrial-ultra-processed foods to higher obesity risks, high blood pressure, high cholesterol, diabetes, and cancers. Researchers based in France and Brazil assessed potential associations between industrial-ultra-processed foods and increased risk of cardiovascular and cerebrovascular disease (conditions affecting blood supply to the heart and brain). [25]

Results: an absolute 10% increase in the proportion of industrial-ultra-processed food in the diet was associated with significantly higher overall cardiovascular disease rates, coronary heart disease, and cerebrovascular disease (an increase of 12%, 13%, and 11%, respectively). In contrast, the researchers found a significant association between whole unprocessed or minimally processed foods and lower risks of all reported diseases. [26]

Researchers found strong associations between industrial-ultra-processed food intake and all-cause mortality in a corresponding second study based in Spain. Foods were grouped according to the degree of processing, and fatalities were measured over an average of 10 years. [27] The results disclosed that higher consumption of industrial-ultra-processed foods (more than four servings per day) was associated with a 62% increased risk of all-cause mortality compared with a lower consumption (less than two servings per day). For each additional daily serving of industrial-ultra-processed food, mortality risk increased by 18%. [28]

Our elasticity and adaptability depend on more than food

In an equally real sense, researchers know that elasticity and adaptability during challenging events like pandemics, and life transitions; are a combination of how well-nourished the brain and body are — through mindful choices about nutrition and other behaviors. The conscious decisions to eat healthy foods, get quality sleep, spend time in nature, limit the ingestion of disrupting or harmful media/substances, or to take a moment of pause for gratitude — all constitute nourishment for our bodies, minds, and spirits.

> *Principle 2*: If we are following merely the course of least resistance with food and behavioral choices in our lifestyle, our good health and wellbeing will not be sustainable.

Whole-brain perspective leads to renewed skills

Critical and whole-brain thinking, along with *common sense*, are often referred to as being *not so common*. [29] The reality is that our modern education can be sorely lacking when it comes to past generations' skills. Often, we are out of practice in using skills of *common sense*. Although we can look at history for clues on how ancient peoples survived and thrived, it doesn't give us their expertise, nor the luxury to take the time to live as they did.

As we begin a new decade, our world is entirely different than ever before. Even if we might have the skill, time, and environment that supports a romanticized lifestyle of bygone days — we have to ask ourselves. *Do we really want to work that hard? Can we give up the many facets of our modern world that define us now*?

The incorporation of mindfulness and sustainability into the broader idea of nourishment for modern lives isn't about turning back the calendar, politics, environmental agendas, or religious beliefs. It is about owning the choices we make and being the best version of ourselves, along with helping the next generation view their empty plate with open eyes of wonder and possibilities.

Bringing calm to chaos

By expanding ones perspective through the combined lenses of mindfulness; tradition, and science, it can allow for the best of all views to guide; and bring a balance between modern and traditional approaches to health, lifestyle, and nourishment.

Mindfulness is not solely limited to the practice of meditation; mindfulness also includes the ability to discern and make choices based on knowledge, facts, and intuition. Mindfulness is that moment of pause to recognize and acknowledge the present moment before moving forward, which may allow us to see both obstacles and the possibilities before us.

Think of it this way: Mindfulness is our empty plate; food and sustainability form our health; that is the savory meal resting on the surface.

It is easy in the modern world to view ancient cultures and people with either idealism or disdain; believing modern society is somehow more advanced and superior to past cultures without pizza delivery, electronics, and central air. However, biases are not limited to only those of the past. There are times we pooh-pooh someone who lives in a metropolitan area for eating industrial fast-food instead of selections labeled organic; or roll the eyes over a modern homesteader making cheese and canning. How we view food in particular, and the way people eat, is all about perspective.

The same is true about where diet and food fall into one's thoughts about health. Clients may feel reading labels and buying *health food* is a waste of time and all a scam. Equally, clients can become so obsessed with the *health and cleanness* of their food they are practically paralyzed in the market; worse yet, it becomes almost impossible to enjoy a meal with them. This last part is so important because, as a species, we have shared a meal with others since the beginnings of evolution. [30, 31] This need to commune with others while eating plays a role in why restaurants are popular, especially for singles; eating with others allows for sharing ancient memories tucked deep in cellular mitochondria.[32, 33, 34, 35]

Principle 3: If we fail to view our diet, health, and lifestyle through the lens of mindfulness, all that is most precious in our lives will not be sustainable.

First, let's be honest; the American food culture has been pretty messed up for over eighty years. There are real reasons to be concerned about food and water (more on water), especially where safety and quality are concerned. Part of the difference between the current generation and one's great-grandparents began with the Industrial Revolution of the 1800s. By the 19th century with the assembly line's initiation, canned and frozen foods began taking society from the farm or backyard to the Piggly Wiggly.[36] It wasn't until the end of World War II and the *Agricultural Chemical Revolution* that mega-corporations opened Pandora's box of newly available chemicals for food crops and food manufacturing.[37, 38, 39]

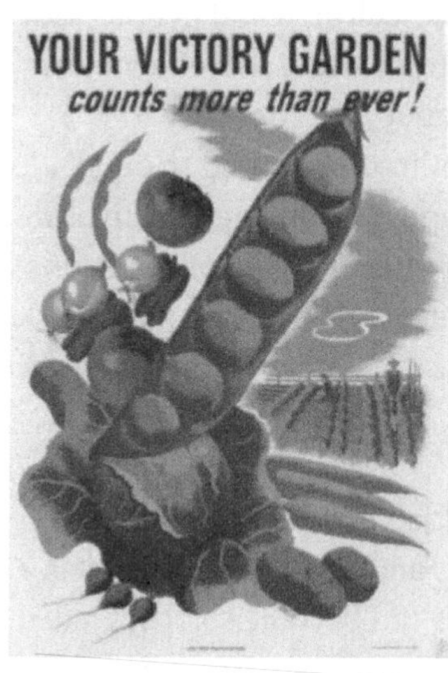

The late 20th century brought first-world countries (as defined by the UN following World War II) to a *roundabout* in healthcare approaches. The 21st century views on health care are a blended version of allopathic, integrative, traditional, and holistic models.[40, 41] These varied approaches can be at odds with each other, adding to consumer confusion and frustration. However, the silver lining of this moment-in-time is a growing acknowledgment and understanding of the priceless value that food from traditional and cultural sources provides.

To review the facts: The lifestyle of ancient peoples was grueling and fraught with danger. Life expectancy was forty to forty-five years of age on average, and evidence supports it was infrequent for more than two generations to be co-present. [42, 43, 44, 45]

Twenty years into the new millennium means four to five generations of individuals simultaneously alive today on the planet; some of whom have been taught to believe the *Doctor Knows Best, Science is Good, Traditional Medicine is Quackery,* and *Better Living Through Chemistry.* [46, 47] Additionally, the tech-industry is influencing food trends in ways that resemble bad science fiction. Bland or flavorless meal replacements like Soylent® are being touted as foods to prevent climate change — and better for the environment than eating livestock. Neither of these claims can stand up to fact-checking. The pandemic of 2020 revealed that airplanes, many industries, and fossil-fuel-powered vehicles were far more at odds with global climate conditions than cattle.

Thankfully, the younger generation of Millennials is embracing traditional agriculture, homesteading, gardening, and animal husbandry: along with artisanal and traditional food preparation. The authors cannot know for a certainty that generations following the Millennials will embrace and value sustainable lifestyles in the same manner — but we hope they do.

The pandemic of 2020 also brought about a return to the kitchen. With stay-at-home orders in place for months on end, individuals reacquainted themselves with the once mysterious room and unfamiliar activities of the kitchen. The developments of 2020 gives hope that the growing challenges of food insecurity in the United States (due to affordability, availability, mobility, and multi-national food manufacturers controlling the type of foods available in many areas) can be ameliorated.[48] A study released in 2018 on food insecurity in older adults found *food insecurity* was significantly associated with economic factors. The findings showed higher values for the prevalence of chronic diseases, poor management of chronic diseases, and decreased health-related quality of life in older adults living in communities.[49, 50] The cycle of food insecurity and chronic disease begins when an individual or family cannot afford enough nutritious food. The combination of stress and poor nutrition can make health management increasingly challenging.[51]

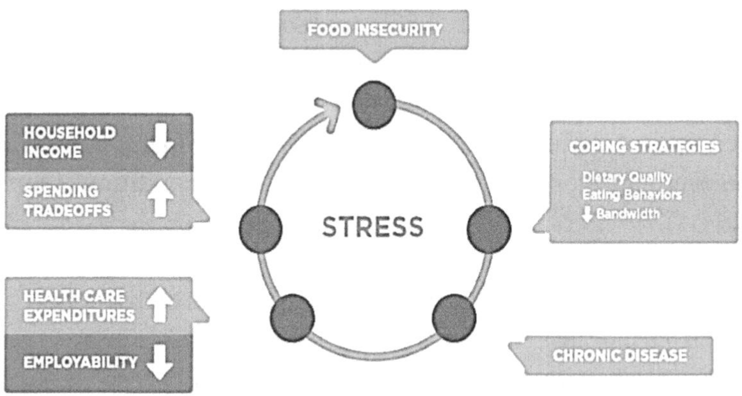

Additionally, the time and money needed to cope with these health conditions strain the household budget, leaving little money for essential nutrition and medical care. This causes the cycle to continue, increasing the risk of worsening existing conditions.[52] When food insecurity is present, sustainable health and mindful living are unattainable.

In the fall of 2020, the *Wall Street Journal* reported on the growing food insecurity in Latin American countries. It is easy to compartmentalize our thinking about food into what we see in the local market and be blind to the multitude of areas where food is affected by seemingly unrelated events in global economies. One area involves fossil fuels and transportation, as the *Wall Street Journal* article titled "Venezuela's Food Chain is Breaking, and Millions Go Hungry" outlines. When gas, diesel, or canola oil-based fuels are unavailable or production is limited or halted, farmers are unable to fuel tractors or farm equipment to plant and harvest. When transportation of food falters due to fuel shortages, millions of tons of food spoil in depots, fields, and aboard cargo ships. What increasingly becomes available to consumers in countries like Venezuela are "junk" foods and non-edible items. Ana Nunes, a sixty-two-year-old retired municipal worker in western Venezuela, shared in the *Journal* article her meals consisting of a few corn-flour *arepas* (pancakes), and continued to say "instead of quality foods, the markets sell garbage like animal hides and rotten cheese." 53

Top 10 worst food crises in 2019 by number of people in crisis or worse

Country	People in crisis or worse
Yemen	15.9 million
Dem. Rep. of Congo	15.6
Afghanistan	11.3
Venezuela	9.3
Ethiopia	8
South Sudan	7
Syria	6.6
Sudan	5.9
Northern Nigeria	5
Haiti	3.7

Global Network Against Crises and the Food Security Information Network

When individuals have access to community gardens or live close to food production; accessibility allows people to harvest and store foods while the nutrient content is at its highest. The availability and use of fresh foods provide quality nutrition, not empty calories. Historically, it has always been true that when humans have access to abundant food supplies; advances in culture, intelligence, and adaptability happen.

When changes in local area economies involving increased availability of fresh foods occur, the population has a high capacity to produce positive, healthy changes that influence sustainability. This is a key component of humanity's sustainability that involves the greater or lesser availability of fresh food. When vacant lots are revitalized into community gardens in large cities, people come together; and food insecurity in the elderly and in impoverished areas lessens, with the addition of countless other benefits. [54, 55, 56]

During clinical practice, Tammera has had many clients who were children during the Great Depression of the 1930s and World War II. A recurring comment from these elders pertains to food and hunger; "we knew we were poor, but we never went hungry; there was always a garden and food to eat."

Something to think about.

Perspective from history

The seemingly ever-present Bovine domestication dates back 10,500 years. These animals provided durable clothing and shelter, necessary fats for energy, vitamins, minerals, and collagens — a nutrient-rich protein source for brain function and health, long before pre-pottery Neolithic cultures emerged. [57, 58]

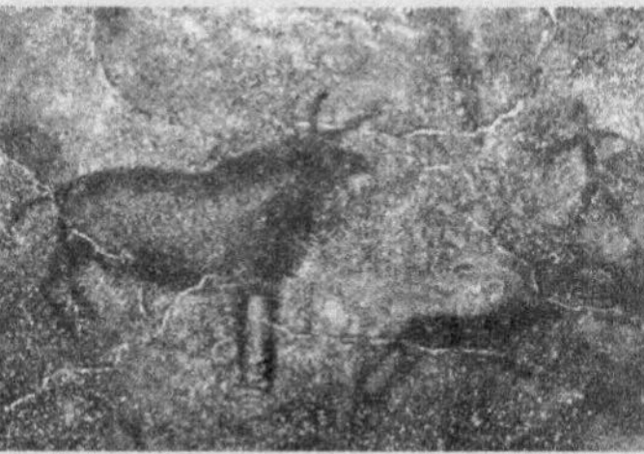

What science has to say about our diets

When looking at the information on how food is affecting the health of countries, it is important to understand the difference between malnourishment of the 1900s and the escalating secondary *nutritional deficiencies* of the 21st century. [59] Today those in industrialized *first-world* or *first-order* countries are not merely overfed; they are overfed and undernourished. The bulk of the foods eaten are devoid of vitamins, minerals, and cofactors that enable the human digestive system to capture and transport nutrition into the bloodstream and beyond through cell membranes to nourish the mitochondria. [60]

Between 2013 and 2016, about 37% of US adults consumed fast food daily. The National Center for Health Statistics 2018 report went on to reveal:

> That fast food consumption varied by age, income level, race, and sex. Overall, 31.7% of lower-income, 36.4% of middle-income, and 42% of higher-income adults said they had eaten fast food. More men (48.3%) than women, (39.1%) said they ate fast food during lunch. However, more women, (25.7%) than men (19.5%), said they had it as a snack. [61]

In a highly industrialized processed food world, it is easy to believe that pizza, pasta, and frozen vegetables are providing all of an individual's nutritional needs; even more so when they are labeled *organic, natural,* and *GMO-free*. More often than not, the information on the label is purely marketing. [62, 63, 64] Even though 67% of consumers read and examine food labels, they often misinterpret the information when making purchasing decisions. [65, 66, 67] A study released by Tufts University in 2020 featured the following: Of 1,030 U.S. adults who responded to a survey with photos of both hypothetical and real whole-grain food products. The photos showed various whole grain labels on

the package, along with the nutrition facts and ingredients list. Participants were asked to identify the healthier option. [68]
Findings: For the hypothetical products, 29–47% of respondents answered incorrectly. For real products that were not mostly composed of whole grains, 43–51% of respondents *overstated* the whole grain content (specifically, 41% overstated for multigrain crackers, 43% for honey wheat bread, and 51% for 12-grain bread). [69]

> Our study results show that many consumers cannot correctly identify the amount of whole grains or select a healthier whole-grain product," said first author Parke Wilde, a food economist and professor at the Friedman School. [70]

How a person applies nutrition labeling information to their decisions remains a stumbling block. For the most part, the data is difficult to understand, read, and make applicable, daily. [71]

> *"Food is not just nutrition.*
> *It's art. It's beauty. It's connection."*
>
> ~Deanna Minich, PhD author of *The Whole Detox*

What is the right diet?

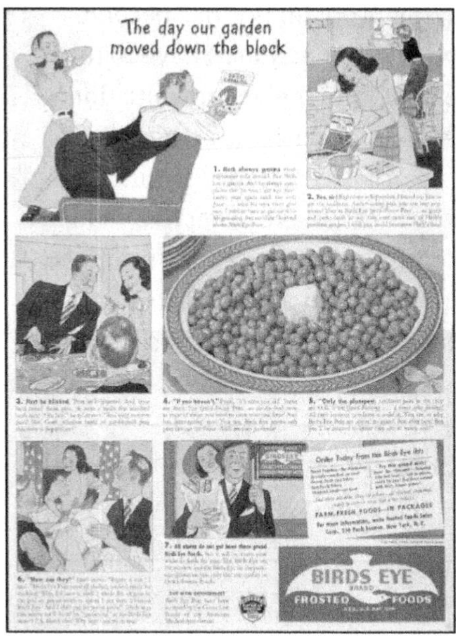

Life Magazine 1940

The debate over which food model is the healthiest is likely to continue for decades, but the two models miles ahead of any other are the traditional Mediterranean and the Paleo diets — followed by a flexible vegetarian model. All three food approaches have in common: increasing consumption of *real* whole foods, especially vegetables. Additionally, the Mediterranean and Paleo diets place increased focus on including quality traditional fats, more varieties of vegetables, herbs, fruit, seafood, and quality proteins from herbivores, and poultry. These traditional approaches to foods also include fermenting and cooking for digestibility, followed by significant reductions in eating industrial ultra-refined processed fats, sugar, grains, and foods.

Who is right when it comes to opinions on diet? Even though accepted dietetic nutrition views can appear to be stuck in the 1970s, there is a growing awareness of integrative and holistic nutrition science. Nutrition Science is evolving faster than the debaters' opinions, and this causes resistance from allopathic viewpoints. Added to the conflicting views is a flood of information on social media. While the internet makes cutting edge science available to the masses, it can also be like playing the game of Twister®; useful and clinically relevant information is often jumbled together with nonsense. Which only adds to the confusion when consumers and clinicians are trying to make informed choices. Should a person only trust their doctor or healthcare provider? Most healthcare providers are doing their best to stay informed on what approaches are safe for their patients; the problem is it has become physically impossible for them to *Know it All*. Consumers have to take responsibility for their health and seek out knowledgeable nutrition experts; this is crucial to sustainable health. [72] With the availability of information from research scientists, health care databases, nutrition, and food blogs on the internet; individuals can make proactive changes to food selections, regardless of the trends and in academic or popular views. These changes transform individuals from a passive to an active role in personal health care; in a sustainable and mindful manner.

Principle 4: No one can care more than you — it is vital individuals play an active, responsible role in their own health.

What the current research is supporting

Flexitarian is the new 21st century word when describing food approaches. [73] This word's value allows one to attain a balance between flesh and plant with less guilt or stigma. This flexible approach to food is not a free pass to eating industrial-ultra-processed foods, but it can allow one to enjoy traditionally made foods from quality natural sources. Yes, that means if you are willing to make a pizza from scratch using the best and freshest possible ingredients once or twice a month: Go for it! Flexitarian approaches also adapt to gluten-free, grain-free, dairy-free, allergen-free, and more. Being flexible opens the path for cultural foods, *Keto*, *Paleo*, and the *Pegan diet;* coined by Dr. Terry Wahls and described by Dr. Mark Hyman as a kind of hybridized version of paleo and vegan food models. [74, 75]

Dr. Wahls is Assistant Chief of Staff at Iowa City Veterans Administration Medical Center and Clinical Professor of Medicine at the University of Iowa. And she is changing the paradigm on diet's importance in chronic autoimmune conditions. In asserting that a comprehensive lifestyle protocol centered on Paleo/Keto diet models can alter the course of multiple sclerosis (MS) Dr. Wahls is challenging medical axioms: that MS is irreversible; that motor or cognitive function once lost is lost forever; that diets are at best, *adjunctive*, but never truly therapeutic. Dr. Wahls's ongoing research is soundly overturning these deeply held *medical* opinions. Results of Wahls research and findings are nothing less than miraculous. Showing that a diet of fresh whole foods, including animal (fish and poultry included) proteins. And that whole foods have higher nutrition value, when prepared in traditional methods such as fermenting, raw, and cooked. Dr. Wahls's integrative and flexible approach to diet, nutraceuticals, detoxification, and exercise has achieved outcomes unattainable with conventional MS drugs for many of her clients. [76] Just as the pattern on a plate is exposed when consuming a meal, the Dr. Wahls research is revealing a broader and irrefutable view of food's value to regaining and maintaining health. [77]

Dr. Mark Hyman is a family physician and the head of Strategy and Innovation at the Cleveland Clinic Center for Functional Medicine, and Board President for Clinical Affairs for The Institute for Functional Medicine. Dr. Hyman writes this on his blog; he believes that we all deserve a life of vitality — that we have the potential to create it for ourselves. With the release of his newest book, *The Pegan Diet*, Dr. Hyman, like Dr. Terry Wahls, is shining a full-on, first-order Fresnel lens lighthouse beam on the value of food when it comes to health.

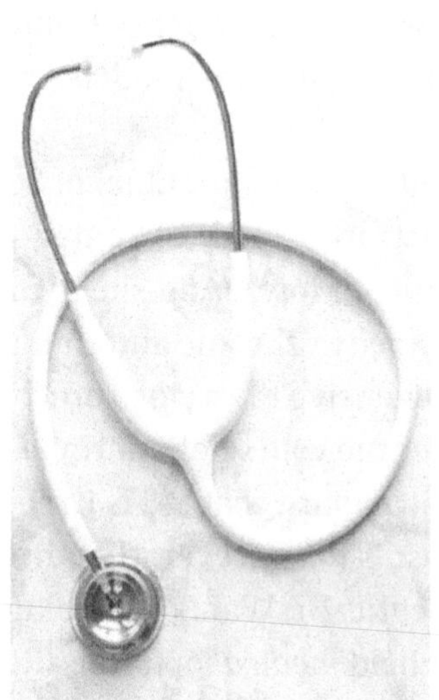

As a doctor, it is my job to figure out the best way to keep my patients healthy. We now know that food is medicine, perhaps the most powerful drug on the planet with the power to cause or cure most diseases. If food is more than just calories, if food is information that controls every aspect of our biology and health, then I better know what to advise people to prevent, treat and even reverse chronic disease. writes Dr. Hyman on his blog. [78]

Dr. Hyman goes on to list the cost of chronic disease to the global economy, caused mainly by what many are eating: 47 trillion dollars over the next twenty years and causing over 50 million preventable deaths a year. [79]

In a conversation with Tammera, Dr. Wahls explained why *The Wahls Protocol* is more flexible than other diets. [80]

"We have to be flexible when it comes to food and our patients if we expect them to succeed," Dr. Wahls continued, "but eating nine servings of colorful vegetables daily is still the goal when it comes to symptom remission."

Eating whole phytonutrient-rich fruits, vegetables, and organic meats, including organ meat, is central to providing the body with the nutrients necessary for deep cellular regeneration.

The dietary models supported by knowledgeable physicians like Terry Wahls and Mark Hyman are rich in plant-based foods and are easy to adapt to our traditional food cultures. The key is the inclusion of vegetables; something that has been largely missing from the industrialized diet from day one in American history. The addition of vegetables has only been popular in Europe for about two hundred years. [81] However, according to the World Health Organization (WHO), fruit and vegetable consumption vary significantly between northern and southern countries. Even though Europeans eat more fresh foods than Americans, they still fall short of the WHO recommendations for vegetable and fruit consumption. [82, 83]

The food and the water consumed daily, is an area in life, over which adults have total control — *everyone has the power of choice*. With the addition of mindfulness to food-related behavior, individuals may well be able to turn back the clock on age-related illnesses and cognitive decline. [84, 85, 86] This proactive next step moves individuals from simply sustaining health to *regenerating health,* which we will look at in Chapter Six, *Sweet Rewards.*

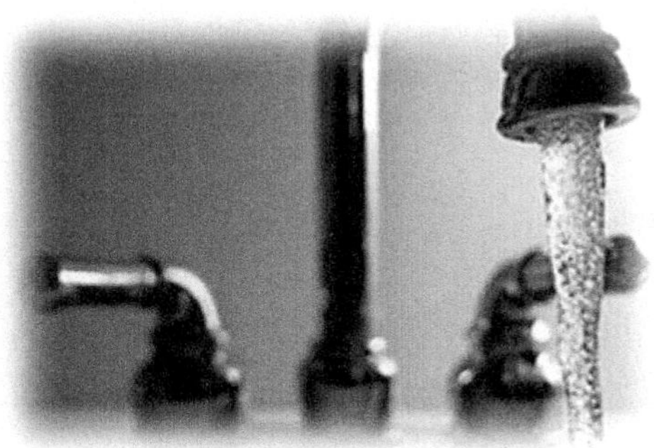

Water, water and not a drop to drink

How much time have you spent thinking about water?
Warning: The following is not for the faint of heart.

Turbulent waters from natural and human-made events often carry chemicals that are far from friendly to health. In regions with mining; cadmium, mercury, and arsenic levels are often well above safe levels. Naturally-occurring sulfur, iron, copper, phosphorus, sodium, zinc and uranium are also present in runoff water used for municipal drinking water. [87]

In an effort to keep or regain health, individuals can fall short of the goal if they neglect to address water contamination. The human body is made up of 60% water, the brain and heart are composed of 73% water, and the lungs about 83% water. Health depends on clean water — water clear of prescription drugs, petroleum, agricultural runoff, and heavy metals. [88]

Most of us turn on the water tap, and the flow rushes forth in hot, cold, or between, based on our manual adjustment of the knobs. The convenience of free-flowing, clear, clean water in our homes and businesses is an overlooked and undervalued resource that makes life possible. Many of the eastern U.S. water systems date to the time of the Civil War and have largely been

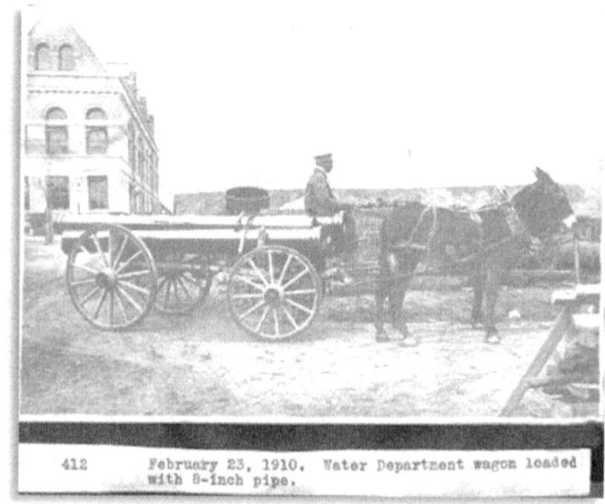

412 February 23, 1910. Water Department wagon loaded with 8-inch pipe.

ignored by politicians and residents accustomed to paying almost nothing for water delivery and sewage removal. Each year, hundreds of thousands of ruptures damage streets and homes and cause dangerous pollutants to seep into drinking water supplies. [89] Municipal water systems are not new; most of the ones in service for large metropolitan areas like Washington DC are over 100-years old and were planned for a 300-year life cycle. [90, 91]

Water systems are not only a problem in the United States. In the United Kingdom (UK), three billion liters of drinking water is lost daily through pipe failures. [92] The implications of pipe failure are significant and with an estimated 35% future increase in UK water demand by 2050. Researchers have found water pipe failures during the winter are typically found in iron and, to a lesser extent, steel and ductile iron pipes associated with cold temperatures prolonged or periods of frost. A higher number of pipe failures are typically found in asbestos cement and polyvinyl chloride pipes during the summer. [93]

Tap water provides valuable minerals into the diet. Minerals like calcium and magnesium are essential for health. Mineral content depends on where one lives, the age of the municipal water plant and the infrastructure the water flows through. [94] Also keep in mind if you are on well water — the water coming from the faucet is only as clean as the groundwater and the water pipes' quality in the home or building. The World Health Organization (WHO) report on "Essential Nutrients in Drinking Water." states in the Introduction: [95]

> Chemical composition of drinking water also depends on the industry's contaminating effects, human settlements, agricultural activities, and water treatment and distribution. [96]
>
> Leaching of minerals from metal components used in water treatment plants and plumbing materials occurs when the pH and hardness of water are not adjusted. Some of the primary

> sources of dissolved metals include: for cu- copper or brass plumbing system; fe- cast iron, steel, and galvanized plumbing system; zn- zinc galvanized pipes; ni- chromium-nickel stainless plumbing system; pb- derived from tin-lead or lead solder; and for cd- as an impurity in zinc galvanized pipes or cadmium containing solders."

Clear water, especially if there is a slight chlorine smell, induces individuals to believe the water is *clean* and free of contamination. Yet, the reality is far different. As the residents of many cities across America have learned; Flint, Michigan is just one of what is a growing list of towns with contaminated drinking water. Thousands of Nebraska residents are facing ongoing water contamination from the devastating floods of 2019. [97]

But I drink only bottled water

First, let's look at the *Raw Water* movement in some parts of the United States. Yes, you read that right. It isn't a typo. While researching for this book, the authors came across *The Strategist* site and an article by Maxine Builder titled, "Is There Anything Wrong with Tap Water (and What You Should Buy to Filter It)?" Until reading this article, we had been blissfully ignorant of the virtues and cost of raw water.

According to Maxine Builder: "The raw-water trend stems from a concern about chemicals in municipal tap-water supplies." As the founder of Live Water, the company bottling and marketing this untreated, unfiltered water, told the *New York Times*, "Tap water? You're drinking toilet water with birth control drugs in them — Chloramine, and on top of that, they're putting in fluoride. Call me a conspiracy theorist, but it's a mind-control drug that has no benefit to our dental health." And his fellow raw-water acolytes agree".

Ok here is the deal; there are countless parasites and pathogens found in water; *Giardia* (*Giardia intestinalis, Giardia lamblia*, or *Giardia duodenalis*), commonly called beaver fever, is found in mountain ponds, springs, streams, and depressions throughout the western United States. Animals like raccoons also add to the parasites found in water; *Baylisascaris procyonis* can infect humans, particularly children, and cause severe neurologic illness. [98] *Giardia*, along with cholera, typhoid fever, cryptosporidium, and bacillary dysentery are the fun-filled illnesses available to unsuspecting hikers who do not use suitable water treatment or filtration when collecting water. In response to the growing Raw Water trend, food-safety experts are flagging all the disturbing substances in the natural water supply, including, but not limited to, animal feces and the parasite giardia. [99]

Bottled water is far from perfect and contributes to the growing mountain of plastic refuse that is not recycled. Bottled water may also be a leading cause of chemical contamination from polychlorinated biphenyls, polybrominated diphenyl ethers (PBDEs), bisphenol A (BPA), and polyethylene terephthalate, associated with reproductive problems, including miscarriage, increased cancer risk, attention, and cognition problems. A growing awareness of harmful water constituents to health has led to a decline in consumption of tap water in North America, and bottled water use has increased. [100, 101, 102, 103]

Water filters

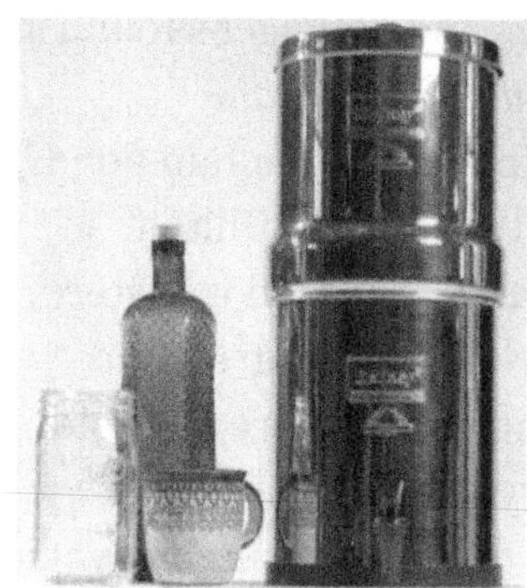

Berkey Home Water Filter

Water filter manufacturers advertise on their labels the sweet, clear water taste or the reduced chlorine contamination. If you've ever used a pitcher-style water filter, it probably adjusted the water's taste and odor, but did it remove the toxins you thought it would? The most noticeable chemical extracted is generally chlorine. On a review of several market places, it was easy for the authors to locate multiple varieties of water filter pitchers, bottles, straws, containers, and countertop units; most contain only one filtration medium — charcoal.

Activated charcoal (AC) removes chlorine, total trihalomethanes (TTHMs), and some pesticides. According to Purdue University, "AC filters primarily improve taste and odors in-home water treatment systems. Taste and odor, although undesirable, are generally not considered health risks." AC filters are increasingly used to remove some of the contaminants discovered in municipal water supplies. However, AC removes the largest molecules first, which then inhibits the filtering of smaller chemical molecules. Chlorine and fluoride are large molecules, so they are trapped at the greatest rate by AC medium.

AC effectively removes volatile organic compounds, pesticides, and benzene. It can also remove some metals and radon. AC systems are limited in the types of compounds they can effectively remove as single-stage filters.

The homeowner must determine which water contaminants are present before purchasing a system. Have your water analyzed by the local health department or a reputable laboratory. Here is a brief rundown on what different types of water filters do.

**For further recommendations, see the recommendations list located at the back.*

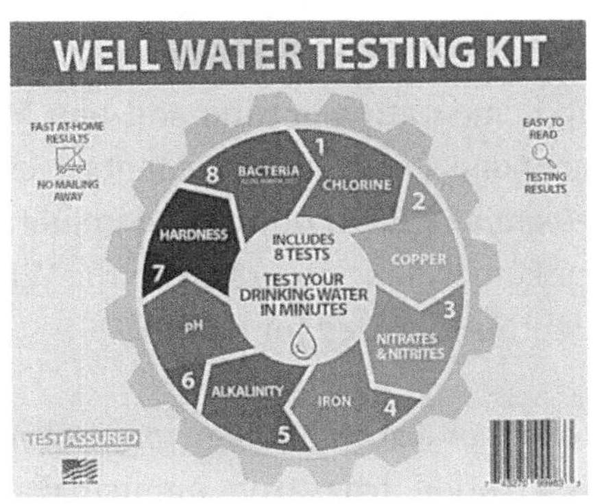

Affordable water test kits can be found online, through water suppliers and local hardware stores.

A standard drugstore water filter won't help you when you're trying to remove heavy metals and prescription medications from your water. Under the counter or multi-stage whole house filtration system provide the most effective option. Whole house systems provide filtered water to all household faucets; including toilets, laundry, and showers. This approach can reduce damage to appliances and plumbing in areas with hard water. The removal of chlorine, chloroform, inorganic arsenic, TTHMs, lead, polychlorinated biphenyls (PCBs), pesticides, herbicides, and mercury generally result from these type of filtration systems. That sounds great, but these filters will become loaded with whatever the largest molecules are first; that is chlorine, fluoride, and *fecal coliform.* Additionally, just like furnace filters, the water filter cartridges must be replaced on a quarterly or annual basis dependent on water type and use.

What are other options for those who may not have space or the ability to use such filters?

Reverse-osmosis systems (RO) are expensive and require installation under the sink. They work ONLY on the faucet they are attached to. Additionally, RO systems remove all minerals from the water. That means consumers need to replace these valuable minerals through supplementation or filter add-ons. Minerals commonly found in limestone and organic elements present in plant humus deposits determine the pH of water; demineralized water is "not considered ideal drinking water," according to the WHO, due to the loss of essential minerals required for health. [104, 105]

While modern technology may not be up to the task of removing prescription drugs from municipal and well water supplies — a quality home water filtration system will ensure a maximum reduction in chemical/toxin/pathogen exposure. It isn't what you can see in the water; it is what you can't see that may damage health.

> *Principle 5:* Use a quality water filter for all drinking and cooking water to reduce toxins.

The key to remember is fresh, local, and seasonal [106]

Over the last fifteen years, farmers' markets have been popping up in small communities and metropolitan areas. The USDA Agricultural Marketing Services website provides information on local farmers' markets along with local/state Farm Extension Services. [107] On review, one can find the quality of the produce at local farm markets *very, very* different from supermarkets and natural food outlets. First, the vibrancy of the colors, next the size. A head of bok choy from a mega-store is barely enough to make a serving for one. By contrast, a head of bok choy from local farms can be an incredible hulk in size, able to feed two or three people. Nutrient content has also been found to be higher in locally produced foods, which launched the term *farm to table.* [108]

If individuals are going to spend money and time preparing a meal from fresh ingredients, they want to know what they are getting. European studies have answered many of the questions on why individuals are willing to spend more on fresh foods. It all boils down to better nutrient availability, taste, quality, supporting local growers, and safer food. Therefore, the same mindful care should be employed when selecting produce and meats for individuals' home-cooked meals as a *Michelin Star* chef uses when buying for their restaurant.

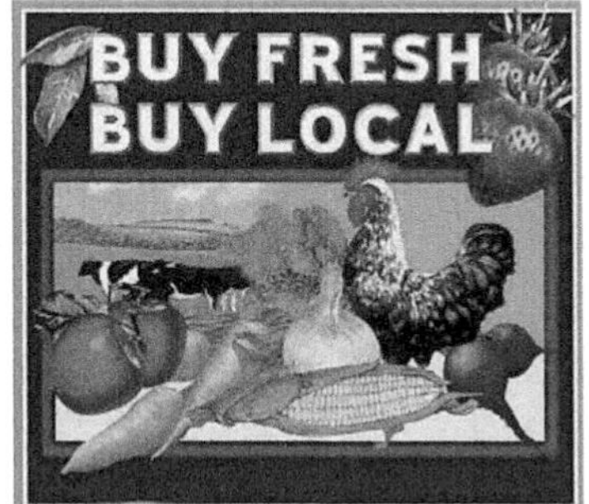

When modeling cultural diets like the Mediterranean, individuals need to do more than follow a glossy magazine recipe. One must look at the content of a true Mediterranean diet filled with all the cultural dishes, not just ingredients that fit trendy agendas. A broader food model to diet emerges when we look at all the ingredients, including herbs and spices, that allow for diversity and freedom with foods. [109, 110, 111]

Principle 6: Buy as much food as possible from local sources, especially fresh produce and meats.

Shedding light into our food cupboards

While anyone can spend hours reading labels and contemplating specialty ingredients, most folks leave this arduous task to nutrition professionals to research for them. One can find unusual produce, ingredients, specialty grains or pastas, and the utensils designed to serve them in any given store. Cookbooks today feature recipes from around the globe, and it is easy to collect specialty ingredients that may lay in cupboards unused for months or even years.

> ***Tip***: Save flavorful leftover broth in ice trays. Once frozen, the cubes can be placed in a storage container and frozen for fast and nourishing use.

To develop a functioning pantry, we have first to do some evaluation of what is worth keeping. We will look at this more in Chapter Two. So, just how many specialty foods are needed on hand? The answer to that question depends on culture, tastes, and willingness to play with food. Not everyone has the time or interest in preparing elaborate dishes. That is why the authors go back so often to traditional foods and combinations. A hearty stock can be used for soup and gravy or as a medium for braising meat and sautéing vegetables. Several quality products are available, including dried bouillon, for those who do not make broth or stock at home.

Individuals employ a grain-free lifestyle; just gained a lot of room in kitchen cupboards. But whenever space is made, eventually, it will fill with other things. Be mindful of storage space and its value. As much as the authors loathe food waste, they equally see no value in wasting storage space on inedible food products.

If those items are food, now is an excellent time to decide:

- Are the ingredients needed or outdated?
- Are the foods in the pantry versatile and enjoyable?

Enjoy simple food

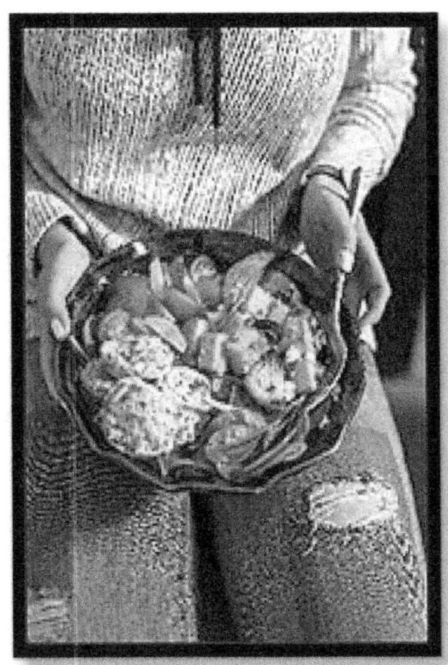

Food doesn't have to be elaborate; sometimes, all one needs is a can of tuna, some chopped fresh tomato with lime on rye crackers, or a cup of hot broth. In Europe, it is common to serve local cheeses with walnuts, fresh fruit, and honey. Tammera remembers the first time she ate goat cheese with cured meats, walnuts, and honey for a simple meal following a theatrical performance. The cheese's tartness was perfectly accented by the salty meat, the honey's sweetness, and the crunch of walnuts.

When folks eat, the meal can be met with apathy or elation due to past experiences, nutrient deficiencies, illness, or cognitive function. Food signals hormone and brain chemistry to prepare for food or as is the case with industrial-ultra-processed food; the chemicals enhance cravings and suppress satiation hormones. Many foods intensify memories and evoke strong emotional responses. Tammera saw this happen with a Vietnam veteran when an Italian dinner was served with parmesan cheese. The man bolted from the table as the smell of the cheese stimulated a combat flashback.

Food is powerful in every aspect. A well-timed simple meal shared with a friend or lover forms vivid memories of images, smells, tastes, sounds, and textures. The modern American expectation of a meal usually involves *super-size*; the bigger the burger, the better, or so people have been programmed by marketers to believe. The opposite is true in many countries, less influenced by the multi-national food franchise industry. [112] When Tammera was in Argentina and Chile the meals were about family and friends, conversation, and laughter. Even though the portion sizes looked small, it left the guests completely satisfied and not overstuffed.

Local food awareness programs in Canada and the U.S. are an attempt to increase nutrition education. The Centers for Disease Control and Prevention found that elementary school students in the United States receive, on average, just 3.4 hours of food and nutrition education each year. The US Federal Trade Commission found that the food industry spends nearly $2 billion per year marketing to children; 73% of that marketing promotes food and beverages high in sugars and fats yet low in recommended nutrients. [113] Organizations like Common Thread, Edible School Yard, Food Corps (a branch of AmeriCorps) and The Curriculum of Cuisine in Portland, Oregon work to connect children with whole foods and teach culinary skills. [114, 115, 116] With all food education programs, however, communities need to encourage and support their local schools in changing curriculum and meal programs for them to be productive. Other countries like Denmark and the United Kingdom are aggressively changing children's education programs and the national view on vegetables. [117]

A few tips

- Eat a breakfast that contains protein and complex carbohydrates like naturally fermented vegetables, oatmeal, nuts, and fruit. Remember, many cultures use soup, broth, or savory dishes for breakfast. Research published in the Endocrine Society's *Journal of Clinical Endocrinology & Metabolism* revealed the body expends energy when digesting food for the absorption, digestion, transport, and storage of nutrients. This process, known as diet-induced thermogenesis (DIT), is a measure of how well one's metabolism is working and can differ depending on each meal.

  > Our results show that a meal eaten for breakfast, regardless of the number of calories it contains, creates twice as high diet-induced thermogenesis as the same meal consumed for dinner, said the study's corresponding author, Juliane Richter, of the *University of Lübeck* in Germany. [118]

  It is time to change the view on breakfast and ditch the cereal, pastries, and sugar; especially for children. Above all, remember these are recommendations; some individuals have modified meal schedules for health or work reasons. Adaptability and flexibility with meals is one way to reduce stress and maintain sustainable health.

- Traditional Chinese Medicine (TCM) recommends body temperature or warm water to begin breaking the fasting period following sleep. Water is essential for health, and when we drink warm water, it promotes blood circulation in the stomach, allowing for better absorption and detoxification. Upon waking up, squeeze some fresh lemon juice into a glass, fill with warm water and drink. Warm lemon water has numerous health benefits, including supporting digestion, immune system, natural vitamins, minerals, and antioxidants. Warm lemon water stimulates peristalsis, reducing constipation. According to a study published in 2014 in *Clinical and Experimental Pharmacology and Physiology*, a compound found in lemons called naringenin calms liver inflammation. *Life Sciences* reported in 2003 the results of a study indicating that eriocitrin, a flavonoid in lemons, protect the liver against exercise-induced oxidative stress and may inhibit fatty liver disease. [119, 120, 121]

- Minimize dairy as it can be mucus-forming and lead to chest, nasal, gut congestion, and constipation. This is a contested approach in some medical circles; however, when reviewing historical methods to reduce mucus congestion in nursing texts, eliminating dairy is a common recommendation. Even raw, whole dairy can be problematic for individuals with asthma, allergies, and autoimmune illnesses like celiac and Crohn's diseases. [122, 123]

- Add fresh and dried herbs to your meals like parsley, basil, and fennel to improve digestion. Herbs like: garlic, oregano, thyme, citrus, and hibiscus aid in absorbing nutrients and natural compounds for strengthening immune function and reducing inflammation. Hibiscus tea has been used for centuries to control hypertension and improve immune function. [124, 125]

- Whole vegetables and fruits are valuable sources of fiber needed to maintain a healthy digestive system. Ideally, twenty to thirty grams of fiber from whole foods are recommended by the American Diabetic Association, but some individuals may require fiber supplements due to health challenges. [126] To keep bowels moving with a regular fiber supplement, try plain psyllium seed if there are no thyroid challenges. Start with one-fourth of the recommended amount on the product label. Over two weeks, slowly increase to the full recommended dosage. Psyllium, flax, hemp, and oat fiber require water in the bowels to work properly, some individuals have *very* dry or impaired bowel function due to medications or health conditions: hypothyroid, colon cancer, rectocele, nerve damage, pregnancy, dehydration. **For those with hypothyroidism**, the best fiber to use is organic acacia fiber. Acacia is a soluble plant fiber that can be added to foods or mixed in water. One of the beauties of acacia fiber is a transparent flavorless, soluble fiber with no goo, slime, or clumpy gelatin when it sits for a few minutes. **No matter what** fiber you use, understand adequate water consumption is essential. Often, individuals using psyllium, chia, or flax fiber experience gastrointestinal cramping. Starting with too much fiber and not enough water is generally the cause of cramping and discomfort.

- Make lunch the biggest meal. A small study published in the Endocrine Society's *Journal of Clinical Endocrinology & Metabolism* sheds new light on how eating a late dinner worsens glucose tolerance and reduces the amount of fat burned. "The effect of late eating varies greatly between people and depends on their usual bedtime," said the study's corresponding author Jonathan C. Jun, MD, of the Johns Hopkins University School of Medicine in Baltimore, Maryland. "This shows that some people might be more vulnerable to late eating than others. If the metabolic effects we observed with a single meal keep occurring chronically, then late eating could lead to consequences such as diabetes or obesity." [127]

- Take a break. [128] If it is taken at all, the lunch break is often used for a multitude of other things; from gym workouts and shopping to grading papers or patient charting. More often than not, women in particular, will go all day on coffee and a snack bar, saving their eating for dinner. The downside is the risk of overeating at dinner. Lunch breaks at one time were normal; everyone in a workplace, school, or town took a break at lunch for 1–1.5 hours. This allowed for a step away from the demands of *work* and gave people the opportunity to get off their feet or go outside. This break midday allowed for people to take a moment of pause, reset their minds, and recharge their energy stores. [129]

> Nurses' wellbeing is central to ensuring the best outcomes for patients," said study author Dr. Annamaria Bagnasco of the University of Genoa, Italy. "When wards have poor leadership and fragmented teams with no development prospects for nurses, this should raise an alarm that there is a risk of burnout." [130, 131]

- Begin each meal with a mindful moment of gratitude — take three deep breaths, and begin with cooked and raw vegetables, which stimulate a calming response from the parasympathetic nervous system; according to Traditional Chinese Medicine *(*TCM*)*.

- Share as many meals with others as possible, even if it is at the same diner or restaurant. Invite a friend to share meals by doing potlucks in the park, backyard, or beach. The loss of shared eating time has consequences that damage our health; humans have social natures and have spent more of their history eating meals with others than alone. A shared meal is one way families, communities, share cultures, express themselves and connect with each other.

The loss of mealtimes is part of a broader cultural crack in the plate of our lives. Nowhere is this more noticeable than in healthcare workers' schedules. In the 1970s, cafeteria meals and scheduled meal break times were a given for nurses; the lunch break allowed for a nourishing meal, conversation, and decompression from the rigors of caring for others. By contrast, many medical centers today utilize vending machines in place of staff cafeterias. These machines are a poor food replacement, providing highly processed foods with too much refined sugar, too many refined fat calories, and no substantive nutrition. Nurses and other healthcare workers are deprived of each other's company while they eat, and the very people who are working to help others are now themselves more likely to be overweight, burned out, and at risk of severe health problems. [132]

Survey findings of over 2,769 were published in the European Society of Cardiology in 2020. One area questionnaire respondent answered pertained to emotional exhaustion. Emotional exhaustion was investigated using the Maslach Burnout Inventory, which measures feelings about work. For example, feeling emotionally drained, used up, fatigued in the morning, burned out, frustrated, working too hard, stressed, or *at the end of my rope*. The researchers then analyzed the relationship between emotional exhaustion and the working environment. Improving the workplace environment was associated with an 81% fall in emotional exhaustion — even with the same skill mix and nurse-patient ratio. [133]

➢ Most of all, smile while eating, listen to enjoyable, calming, or upbeat music; mindfully savor the flavors, and fall in love with the meal as an essential aspect of your culture and well-being.

Changing the pattern

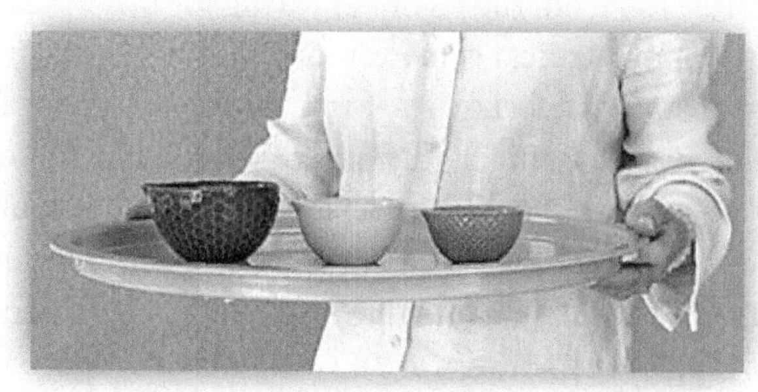

Our reliance on science to determine what to eat can lead to disaster. Mega-food corporations have billions of dollars to spend on convincing consumers that livestock ranching is causing irreparable damage to the planet. This has more to do with riding a profitable climate agenda trend than actual science. Multi-national food companies use established marketing and psychological campaigns to sway politicians through lobbying, healthcare providers through cherry-picked research, and advertising through media outlets to consumers. Without realizing it, individuals have swallowed the *hook, line, and sinker* and been reeled in on unpublicized agendas driven by economics.

The second example of special-interest agendas' power over food is synthesized lab created food, which, contrary to the publicized campaigns and assertions from celebrities, does not equate with the end of global hunger or climate change. *Lab-created* means food that is a hundred steps away from natural sources and away from food security for many. Reliance on lab-created foods can lead to food insecurity due to dependence on corporations, predominantly outside of an individual's regional area or national borders. While these foods may appear inexpensive, accessible, and convenient on the surface, they lack the nutrition and synergy of local natural foods and connection to others. Low-income individuals can participate in local fresh food programs through Community Supported Agriculture called CSAs, food pantries, and state extension gleaning trails. [134, 135] In exchange for time, fresh produce is provided to volunteers; freeing limited revenue for vital needs outside of food and connecting them with the community.

For over twenty-five years, Community Supported Agriculture (CSA) has become a popular way for consumers to buy local, seasonal food directly from a farmer. Here are the basics: a farmer offers a certain number of *shares* to the public. Typically, the share consists of a box of vegetables, but other farm products are also included. Interested consumers purchase a share (aka. a membership or a subscription) and, in return, receive a box (bag, basket) of seasonal produce each week throughout the farming season. This arrangement creates several rewards for both the farmer and the consumer.

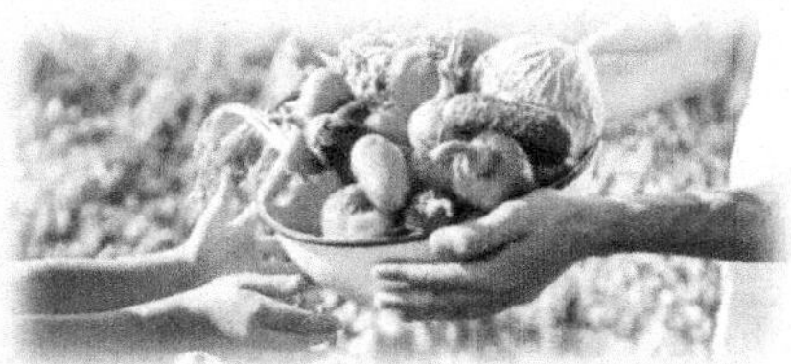

Industrialized-ultra-processed foods effects on global health

As an example of how mega-food (large scale manufactured food from multi-national companies) can dramatically affect a country's health, consumers need only look at the changes in the health of the populations in Mexico and Brazil. Once the North American Free Trade Agreement (NAFTA) went into effect in 1994. Nestlé, Pepsi, and Coca-Cola moved south of the border and launched aggressive marketing campaigns touting their products' safety and nutritional quality.

Bee Wilson writes in her book, *The Way We Eat Now*.

> Over just eleven years, from 1988 to 1999, the number of overweight and obese people in Mexico nearly doubled, from 33.4% of the population to 59.6%. From 1999 to 2004, 7-Eleven doubled its number of stores in Mexico. There are Mexican towns where running water is sporadic, and Coca-Cola is more readily available than bottled water.
>
> The prevalence of overweight and obesity among people in Mexico rose 78% from 1988 to 1998, and by 2006 more than 8% of Mexicans were type 2 diabetics." [136, 137, 138]

"Since the beginning of human time, people have passed knowledge about food, cultivation, and cooking methods down through generation after generation.

Ancient wisdom enhanced mineral and nutrient bioavailability. Food and medicine were interwoven. "

~Dr. Elizabeth Lipski, author of *Digestive Wellness*

After NAFTA and the moving of mega-food manufacturing to Central and Latin America, water was no longer the beverage used with meals;

now, sugary sodas almost exclusively became the norm. Gone too were locally produced corn tortillas; with their unique flavor, variety, diversity, and nutrient content reflective of the area where the centuries-old corn had been raised. [139]

Concurrent with the increase in industrial foods, the Mexican government ended subsidies for traditionally grown native corn, and the market was flooded with cheap yellow corn from the U.S. and Canada. These changes equaled a sharp decline in the nutrition available to the population.

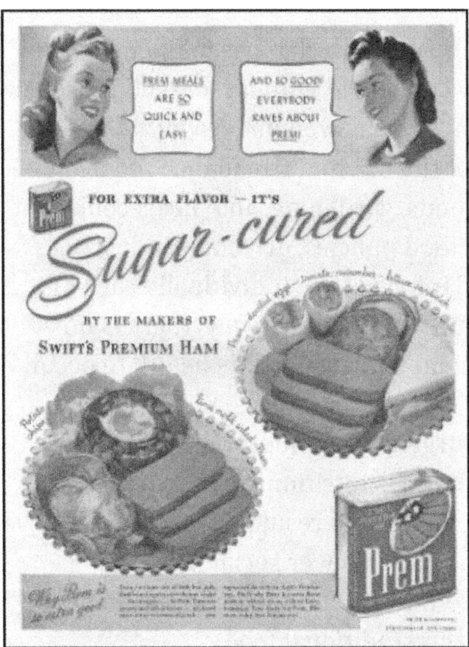

Swift & Company Life Magazine–1941

In Brazil, Nestlé boasted in 2012 of the nutritional quality and safety of their food products. Snack foods of chocolate pudding, yogurts, processed cereal, and sodas were made available through the use of seven thousand door-to-door salespersons, predominantly women. Nestlé claims they brought a valuable sense of independence and income to female salespersons. [140] The Brazilian population soon saw skyrocketing obesity, type 2 diabetes, anemia, and nutritional insufficiencies. And the plague of modern illnesses hit the Brazilian population even faster than Mexico. [141] These two Latin American populations did not have the advantage of adapting to a gradual increase in industrial foods in their daily diets over forty years, as occurred in the U.S..

> *Principle 7*: Fruits and veggies are Mother Nature's fast foods — most of them are highly portable and can be eaten with minimal processing or preparation.

For Canadians and Americans, national health changes happened over nine decades and were not directly connected with increased industrial food consumption until the 21st century was well underway. Correspondingly, the populations of the U.S. and Canada moved away from physical activity, traditional foods, gardening, and meals cooked at home. Marketing and government food policies, driven by industry, bombarded consumers with biased information. Individually each of these factors may not, seem like much; but cumulatively, there is no opportunity for adequate nourishment and sustainable health to occur.

The pandemic of 2020 forced a resurgence in home-prepared meals. It was no surprise to functional and holistic nutritionists that clients and the media reported health improvements as a result of cooking and eating at home. Sourdough bread posts took over social media as individuals filled time and sought comfort in the ancient movements of kneading, the smells, and tastes of this traditional food.

Overnight in 2020, FedEx and UPS became the grocery delivery persons of the 21st century of home meal kits for thousands of Americans. Fresh foods delivered right to the door is reminiscent of grocery, milk, and meat deliveries to the home in the 1950s in many metropolitan and larger populated regions. [142, 143] Home food delivery has benefits and shortfalls. Advantages include convenience and time savings for individuals. The downside is foods are seldom locally produced, affecting nutrient content and quality. And as with any large-scale processing, there is an increased risk of food poisoning or contamination.

Consumers are voting with their dollar every time they buy a product or food. Dr. Mark Hyman routinely reminds readers that "our most political act is what we put on our forks." An individual's shopping habits are letting marketing analysts know their interests and how they spend money. While the American government or medical associations may not support a return to traditional foods and healthier choices, individuals are free to make changes. One's perspective on foods, sustainability, and health, helps people align a *mindful* knowledge with consumer value.

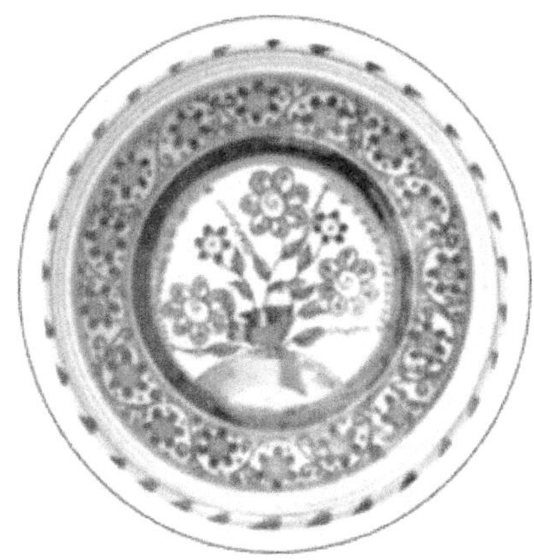

We have a realistic model to emulate when looking at the European perspective on food. Unlike Americans and those from the United Kingdom, European consumers trade the expense of whole natural food's and the time-consuming preparation of traditional dishes for the specific taste, quality, appearance, nutritional value, healthiness, and safety aspects. [144] A mindful approach to foods value can return it to a place of importance now and in the future. [145]

> *Principle 8:* Celebrate your heritage by eating foods once a week from your origins as a gift to your DNA.

Change of perspective

It is hard to be positively affected by the word *diet* for many women in America over thirty. Too often, individuals think of diet as *die with a t.* As seasonal marketing for weight loss resurges. These cyclic campaigns often trigger a mad rush to the gym combined with deprivation, starvation, or fad foods. Views on looks, performance, and health can be distorted in the current age. For some individuals; their perceived cultural perceptions, whether as athletes or desirability, can result in unhealthy eating patterns, especially for teens and younger adults. Eating disorders are at an all-time high, and males are just as susceptible to developing eating disorders as females, especially if they are athletes. [146, 147, 148]

> *"The most important thing about diet is not having a battle with food, but being at peace with it."*
>
> ~Dr. Elizabeth Lipski, author of *Digestive Wellness*

Now more than ever, it is time to change the perspective on diet. Dr. Elizabeth Lipski has one of the best views on the word *diet.* During a conversation with Tammera, she shared the origin of the word *diet* in the classical Greek sense and its translation to *way of living, manner of life,* and *regular (daily) work.* Definitions like these have been lost to the modern weight-loss industry. After looking at the meanings of this small word, one from the middle ages deserves further attention in this current age; from *old High German*, the translation of *diet* means *people.*

Now, when the word *diet* is spoken or read, one should think of a *way of life* and ourselves as members of traditional communities. No longer should one's perspective equate diet with deprivation of everything that tastes good. The modern world provides the luxury to savor foods from around the globe, adding a dash of traditional home flavor to the mix. Before the individuals of today, the meals have a measure of freedom: grand or simple, depending on how one feels and enjoyed without guilt.

That in itself is huge!

The hardest challenge to face

The hardest challenge before many individuals today is developing a love affair, or at least a friendship, with a diverse group of vegetables. By fostering this coming together on the plate, ingredients combine to enhance the savory flavor of meats, sweet freshness of vegetables, and richness of healthy fats. After all, vegetables provide color to stimulate the brain, activate the immune system, and nourish the microbiome. All of this adds to thriving health instead of one on the decline. Along with vegetables, a fiesta of colorful fruits brings a smile; they are sweet, juicy, and come with fond memories of favorite desserts. In their natural state, fruits create an orchestra of synergistic responses within DNA, up-regulating multiple sought-after health traits: cancer and heart disease reduction, improved cognitive function, reduced auto-immune conditions and allergies, and increased fertility, to name just a few. As our perception changes, our empty plate form comes into clarity and begins to hold more nourishment to sustains us.

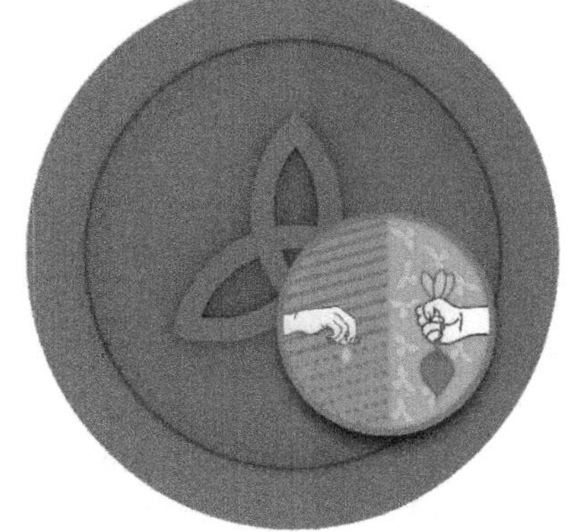

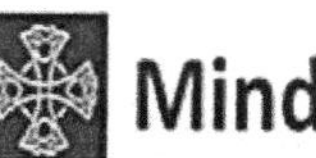

Mindful-Pantry Meal Builder

Our pantry and kitchen is filled with wonderful nutritious foods – BUT how do we turn these foods into fast and flexible meals? We begin by making a graph or list of what we have on hand, next we divide these foods into categories. Pick one or more from each category – These are now the foundation of your meal. The combinations are endless and provide flexible variety to every day items in your pantry and kitchen.

You customize this list to fit your flavor and food likes.

Proteins	Fruit	Fats	Grains	Legumes	Veggies	Herbs & Spices	Sea Vegetables	Fermented Foods
Halibut	Apple	Butter	Oat	Pinto	Greens	Rosemary	Dulse	Kefir Water
Salmon	Pear	Ghee	Wheat	Black	Peppers	Thyme	Kelp	Kombucha
Sardines	Peach	Lard	Barley	Navy	Chilis	Oregano	Nori	*Beer
Shrimp	Berries	Goose	Rye	Soy	Turnips	Garlic	Chlorella	*Wine
Oysters	Plums	Tallow	Spelt	Lentils	Radishes	Chive	Spirulina	Kaefer Milk
Clams	Pineapple	Coconut	Teft	Split pea	Carrots	Dill	Wakame	Yogurt
Steak	Mango	Olive	Corn	Fava	Celery	Parsley		Buttermilk
Roast	Mellon	Avocado	Buckwheat	Lima	Cabbage	Basil		*Cheese
Chops	Quince	Sesame	Millet	Mung	Yams	Black Pepper		Salami
Organ Meat	Grapes	Sunflower	Flax	Black-eyed pea	Eggplant	Chili Powder		Kimchi
Ground Meat	Kiwi	Walnut	Rice	Garbanzo	Onion	Celery Seed		Sauerkraut
Stew Meat	Tomato	Peanut	Quinoa	Peanut	Beets	Turmeric		Pickles
Eggs	Cherries	*All Nuts*	Amaranth	Snap pea	Watercress	Paprika		Sourdough
	Star Fruit	*All Seeds*			Asparagus	Cilantro		Mushrooms

** indicate foods that may contain allergens or yeasts not suitable for some individuals.*

Perspective from history

Stews have been made since ancient times. The world's oldest evidence of stew was found in Japan. Fish stew residue was found in a corded clay pot from the Jōmon period. [149]

Stews are a staple food for traditional cultures all over the world. They are affordable and allow one to combine vegetables, lentils, beans, broth, and meats; making an economical one-pot dish. The hearty stew is the first flexible, fast-cooked food in history. Stews are thick and satisfying, slow-cooked, and easier to digest for individuals with sensitive digestive systems.

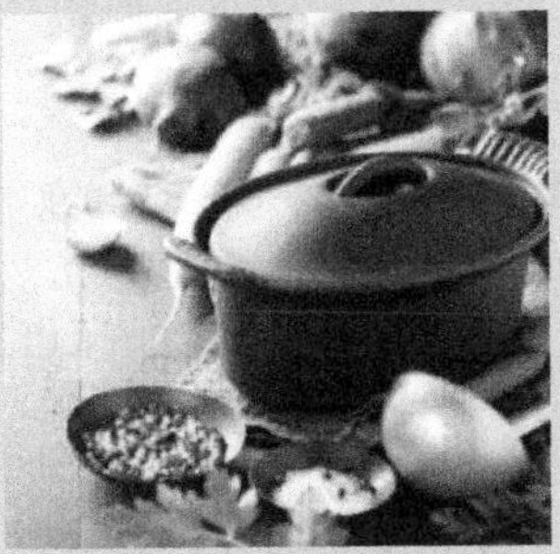

Stews are a traditional way to eat fibrous and starchy foods. The slow cooking process frees nutrients, antioxidants, minerals, amino acids, and lipids while breaking down tough protein fibers, collagen, and sugars.

The pressure cooker and Instant Pot®, cast iron or enamel Dutch-ovens, and slow cookers are all convenient ways to cook and reheat traditional stews. [150] Like bread, stews link individuals with their culture and history. The connection to personal cultures through food provides identity, comfort, and grounding.

Continued on the next page.

Amazonian tribes used the shells of turtles as vessels; boiling the turtle's entrails and various other ingredients in the shell. Other ancient coastal cultures used the shells of large mollusks to boil foods. There is archaeological evidence of these practices going back 8,000 years or more. [151] There are recipes for lamb stews and fish stews in the Roman cookery book *Apicius*, believed to date from the 4th century AD.

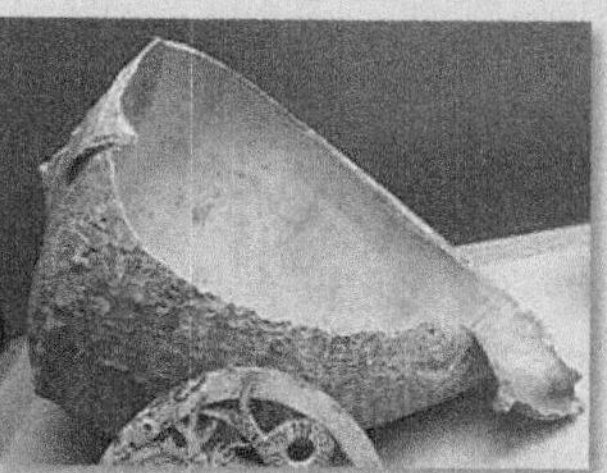

Peach State Archaeological Society. https://peachstatearchaeologicalsociety.org/index.php/26-shell-decorative/446-shell-tools-2

Modern archaeologists in Great Britain have established there was very little change in the average diet — even during conquest periods thought to be rife with famine. On the whole, a diet dominated by vegetables, cereals, beef, and mutton remained mostly unchanged.[152]

During research for this book, over 108 different names for stew from countries around the world were counted. [153, 154, 155, 156]

---

1. Catching Fire, How Cooking Made Us Human By Richard Wrangham Page 9
2. Pagel M. (2017). Q&A: What Is Human Language, When Did It Evolve And Why Should We Care?. BMC Biology, 15(1), 64. Https://Doi.Org/10.1186/S12915-017-0405-3
3. United Nations: Department Of Economic And Social Affairs Indigenous Peoples, Culture: Https://Www.Un.Org/Development/Desa/Indigenouspeoples/Mandated-Areas1/Culture.Html
4. What Is Happening To Agrobiodiversity?: Food And Agriculture Organization Of The United Nations Gender And Development Service Sustainable Development Department Fact Sheet: Http://Www.Fao.Org/3/Y5609e/Y5609e02.Htm
5. History Of Technology By Robert Angus Buchanan: Https://Www.Britannica.Com/Technology/History-Of-Technology
6. As Long Ago As 3,000 Years Ago The Egyptians Had Already Developed Advanced Methods For Building Boxes And Wooden Chests With Dovetail Joints, Including Their Ceremonial And Burial Sarcophagi With Incredible Carving, Metalwork, And Inlaid Jewels And Gilding. Even The Poorest Egyptians Would Have Used Reed Wooden Chests To Store Things: Https://Www.Scaramangashop.Co.Uk/Fashion-And-Furniture-Blog/History-Wooden-Chests-Storage-Boxes/
7. Ancestral Insight, William Schindler III, Associate Professor Of Anthropology And Archaeology At Washington College In Chestertown, Maryland. Https://Www.Drbillschindler.Com/Blog
8. Https://Www.Dictionary.Com/Browse/Homo-Sapiens-Sapiens
9. USDA Scientists Are Rethinking Calorie Counts. Good News: They're Lower Than We Thought, By Jessica Fu, 2020; Https://Thecounter.Org/Scientists-Calorie-Counts-Usda-Kind/
10. American Academy Of Neurology (AAN). (2014, September 10). Can Your Blood Type Affect Your Memory In Later Years?. Sciencedaily. Retrieved July 29, 2020 From Www.Sciencedaily.Com/Releases/2014/09/140910185913.Htm
11. Washington University School Of Medicine. (2018, May 17). Blood Type Affects Severity Of Diarrhea Caused By E. Coli: Researchers ID Protein Responsible For Blood-Group Difference. Sciencedaily. Retrieved July 29, 2020 From Www.Sciencedaily.Com/Releases/2018/05/180517123257.Htm
12. Washington University In St. Louis. (2016, August 29). Why People With Type O Blood Are More Likely To Die Of Cholera. Sciencedaily. Retrieved July 29, 2020 From Www.Sciencedaily.Com/Releases/2016/08/160829105908.Htm
13. Karolinska Institutet. (2015, March 9). How Blood Group O Protects Against Malaria. Sciencedaily. Retrieved July 29, 2020 From Www.Sciencedaily.Com/Releases/2015/03/150309124113.Htm
14. Biomed Central. (2018, May 1). Blood Type O Patients May Have Higher Risk Of Death From Severe Trauma. Sciencedaily. Retrieved July 29, 2020 From Www.Sciencedaily.Com/Releases/2018/05/180501225806.Htm

15. University Of Vermont. (2012, February 23). Blood Mystery Solved: Two New Blood Types Identified. Sciencedaily. Retrieved July 29, 2020 From Www.Sciencedaily.Com/Releases/2012/02/120223183819.Htm

16. Lund University. (2018, July 16). Researchers Crack The Code Of The Final Blood Group System. Sciencedaily. Retrieved July 29, 2020 From Www.Sciencedaily.Com/Releases/2018/07/180716103544.Htm

17. Al-Ani, H. H., Devi, A., Eyles, H., Swinburn, B., & Vandevijvere, S. (2016). Nutrition And Health Claims On Healthy And Less-Healthy Packaged Food Products In New Zealand. The British Journal Of Nutrition, 116(6), 1087–1094. Https://Doi.Org/10.1017/S0007114516002981

18. Federation Of American Societies For Experimental Biology (FASEB). (2015, March 29). Highly Processed Foods Dominate U. S. Grocery Purchases. Sciencedaily. Retrieved July 29, 2020 From Www.Sciencedaily.Com/Releases/2015/03/150329141017.Htm

19. Too much ultra-processed foods linked to lower heart .... https://newsroom.heart.org/news/too-much-ultra-processed-foods-linked-to-lower-heart-health

20. American Heart Association. (2019, November 11). Too Much Ultra-Processed Food Linked To Lower Heart Health. Sciencedaily. Retrieved July 29, 2020 From Www.Sciencedaily.Com/Releases/2019/11/191111084920.Htm

21. Ng, S. W., & Popkin, B. M. (2012). Monitoring Foods And Nutrients Sold And Consumed In The United States: Dynamics And Challenges. Journal Of The Academy Of Nutrition And Dietetics, 112(1), 41–45.E4. Https://Doi.Org/10.1016/J.Jada.2011.09.015

22. Lazzari, G., Jaquet, Y., Kebaili, D. J., Symul, L., & Salathé, M. (2018). Foodrepo: An Open Food Repository Of Barcoded Food Products. Frontiers In Nutrition, 5, 57. Https://Doi.Org/10.3389/Fnut.2018.00057

23. New evidence links ultra-processed foods with a range of https://www.sciencedaily.com/releases/2019/05/190529221040.htm

24. BMJ. (2019, May 29). New Evidence Links Ultra-Processed Foods With A Range Of Health Risks: Policies That Limit Ultra-Processed Food Intake Are Urgently Needed, Say Researchers. Sciencedaily. Retrieved July 29, 2020 From Www.Sciencedaily.Com/Releases/2019/05/190529221040.Htm

25. New evidence links ultra-processed foods with a range of https://www.sciencedaily.com/releases/2019/05/190529221040.htm

26. BMJ. (2019, May 29). New Evidence Links Ultra-Processed Foods With A Range Of Health Risks: Policies That Limit Ultra-Processed Food Intake Are Urgently Needed, Say Researchers. Sciencedaily. Retrieved July 29, 2020 From Www.Sciencedaily.Com/Releases/2019/05/190529221040.Htm

27. Processed food consumption could increase the risk of .... https://www.sanskritimagazine.com/healthy-living/processed-food-consumption-increase-risk-cancer-says-study/

28. BMJ. (2019, May 29). New Evidence Links Ultra-Processed Foods With A Range Of Health Risks: Policies That Limit Ultra-Processed Food Intake Are

Urgently Needed, Say Researchers. Sciencedaily. Retrieved July 29, 2020 From Www.Sciencedaily.Com/Releases/2019/05/190529221040.Htm

29. Critical Thinking Is The Analysis Of Facts To Form A Judgment. Critical Thinking Is Self-Directed, Self-Disciplined, Self-Monitored, And Self-Corrective Thinking. It Presupposes Assent To Rigorous Standards Of Excellence And Mindful Command Of Their Use. It Entails Effective Communication And Problem-Solving Abilities As Well As A Commitment To Overcome Native Egocentrism And Sociocentrism.

30. Food, A Culinary History From Antiquity To The Present By Jean-Lois Flandrin And Massimo Montanari, 1999 Pages 21-45

31. The Sandal And The Cave, The Indians Of Oregon By Luther S. Cressman 1981, X-Xxxiii

32. Max-Planck-Gesellschaft. (2017, July 17). Epigenetics Between The Generations: We Inherit More Than Just Genes. Sciencedaily. Retrieved July 6, 2020 From Www.Sciencedaily.Com/Releases/2017/07/170717100548.Htm

33. Mitochondrial DNA, Represents A Mainstay Of Phylogenetics And Evolutionary Biology. It Also Permits An Examination Of The Relatedness Of Populations, And So Has Become Important In Anthropology And Biogeography. *Https://En.Wikipedia.Org/Wiki/Mitochondrial_DNA*

34. University Of Southampton. (2017, April 26). Risk Of Obesity Influenced By Changes In Our Genes. Sciencedaily. Retrieved July 5, 2020 From Www.Sciencedaily.Com/Releases/2017/04/170426093316.Htm

35. Our Journey With Food By Tammera Karr, 2018 Page 18

36. Piggly Wiggly®, America's First True Self-Service Grocery Store, Was Founded In Memphis, Tennessee In 1916 By Clarence Saunders. *Http://Www.Pigglywiggly.Com/About-Us*

37. AGRICULTURAL CHEMICAL REVOLUTION, S T R A V A G A N Z A By Leopoldo Costa, Http://Www.Hort.Purdue.Edu/: *Https://Stravaganzastravaganza.Blogspot.Com/2011/03/Agricultural-Chemical-Revolution.Html*

38. In 1933 TVA Was Formed With A National Responsibility To Increase The Efficiency Of Fertilizer Manufacture And Use. More Than 75% Of The Fertilizer Produced In The United States Is Made With Processes Developed By TVA. History Of Chemical Fertilizer Development, Darrell A. Russel, Gerald G. Williams *Https://Acsess.Onlinelibrary.Wiley.Com/Doi/Abs/10.2136/Sssaj1977.03615995004100020020x*

39. The Taste Of War And The Battle For Food, 2012, By Lizzie Collingham

40. The Term First World Refers To The Developed, Capitalist, Industrial Countries, Generally Aligned With NATO And The USA. The Bloc Of Countries Aligned With The United States After World War II, Which Had More Or Less Common Political And Economic Interests, This Included The Countries Of North America And Western Europe, Japan, South Korea, And Australia. Some African Countries Were Assigned To The First World Because Of Their Links With

Western Countries.
Https://Www.Nationsonline.Org/Oneworld/Third_World_Countries.Htm

41. Source: UN Human Development Data. Http://Hdr.Undp.Org/En/Data

42. Trinkaus, Erik. "Late Pleistocene Adult Mortality Patterns And Modern Human Establishment." Proceedings Of The National Academy Of Sciences Of The United States Of America Vol. 108,4 (2011): 1267-71. Doi:10.1073/Pnas.1018700108

43. Sandle And The Cave By Luther S. Cressman, The Indians Of Oregon: Introduction By Dennis L. Jenkins, 2005 Edition Page Vi-Xxvi

44. Finding Pre-Clovis Humans In The Oregon High Desert; An Interview With Dr. Dennis Jenkins 2007: Https://Www.Archaeologychannel.Org/Video-Guide/Video-Interviews/297-Finding-Pre-Clovis-Humans-In-The-Oregon-High-Desert

45. Oregon Archaeology By Melvin C. Aikens, Thomas J. Connolly, Dennis L. Jenkins 2011

46. Nostrums And Quackery By Arthur J. Cramp, M.D. Director Of The Propaganda Department And Bureau Of Investigation Of The Journal Of The American Medical Association, Volume II, Articles On The Nostrum Evil, Quackery And Allied Matters Affecting The Public Health: Chacago 1921

47. The Tagline, Which Debuted As "Better Things For Better Living Through Chemistry" In 1935, Had Served The Company Through The Final Years Of The Great Depression, World War II, The Turbulent '60s And The Emergence Of The Global Marketplace. Dupont Replaces 1935 Tagline To Reflect Corporate Change By Sean Callahan. Published On June 01, 1999.

48. Fernandes, S. G., Rodrigues, A. M., Nunes, C., Santos, O., Gregório, M. J., de Sousa, R. D., Dias, S., & Canhão, H. (2018). Food Insecurity in Older Adults: Results From the Epidemiology of Chronic Diseases Cohort Study 3. Frontiers in medicine, 5, 203. https://doi.org/10.3389/fmed.2018.00203

49. Fernandes, S. G., Rodrigues, A. M., Nunes, C., Santos, O., Gregório, M. J., de Sousa, R. D., Dias, S., & Canhão, H. (2018). Food Insecurity in Older Adults: Results From the Epidemiology of Chronic Diseases Cohort Study 3. Frontiers in medicine, 5, 203. https://doi.org/10.3389/fmed.2018.00203

50. Frontiers | Food Insecurity in Older Adults: Results From ....
https://www.frontiersin.org/articles/10.3389/fmed.2018.00203/full

51. Causes and Consequences of Food Insecurity | Hunger and Health.
https://hungerandhealth.feedingamerica.org/understand-food-insecurity/hunger-health-101/

52. What are the Connections Between Food Insecurity and Health?
https://hungerandhealth.feedingamerica.org/understand-food-insecurity/hunger-health-101/

53. Venezuela's Food Chain Is Breaking, and Millions Go Hungry by John Otis, Wall Street Journal October 1, 2020.

54. History Of The Community Garden Movement:
Https://Www.Nycgovparks.Org/About/History/Community-Gardens/Movement

55. CDC Community Gardens: Https://Www.Cdc.Gov/Healthyplaces/Healthtopics/Healthyfood/Community.Htm

56. Beyond Food: Community Gardens As Places Of Connection And Empowerment, 2016: Https://Www.Pps.Org/Article/Beyond-Food-Community-Gardens-As-Places-Of-Connection-And-Empowerment

57. Arbuckle BS, Price MD, Hongo H, And Öksüz B. 2016. Documenting The Initial Appearance Of Domestic Cattle In The Eastern Fertile Crescent (Northern Iraq And Western Iran). Journal Of Archaeological Science 72:1-9.

58. Cai D, Sun Y, Tang Z, Hu S, Li W, Zhao X, Xiang H, And Zhou H. 2014. The Origins Of Chinese Domestic Cattle As Revealed By Ancient DNA Analysis. Journal Of Archaeological Science 41:423-434.

59. Primary Nutritional Deficiency Typically Occurs Because A Person Doesn't Get Enough Of Certain Vital Nutrients. Secondary Malnutrition Occurs When The Body's Ability To Absorb Nutrients Is Limited By A Condition Or Illness. These Conditions Can Include Celiac Disease, Cystic Fibrosis, Lactose Intolerance, Pancreatic Insufficiency And Pernicious Anemia. Https://Healthfully.Com/556049-What-Is-A-Primary-Deficiency-In-Nutrition.Html

60. Current Eating Patterns in the United States; https://health.gov/our-work/food-nutrition/2015-2020-dietary-guidelines/guidelines/chapter-2/current-eating-patterns-in-the-united-states/

61. National Center for Health Statistics: https://www.cdc.gov/nchs/nhanes/index.htm

62. Unsavory Truth Page 135-140

63. Catching Fire How Cooking Made Us Human By Richard Wrangham, 2009 Page 55-63

64. BMJ 2015;351:H4962 Doi: 10.1136/Bmj.H4962 (Published 23 September 2015)

65. Nutrition & You, 4th Edition 2016

66. Krause's Food & The Nutrition Care Process, 14th Edition, 2017

67. Fooddata Central Is An Integrated Data System That Provides Expanded Nutrient Profile Data And Links To Related Agricultural And Experimental Research. Https://Fdc.Nal.Usda.Gov/

68. Study points to consumer confusion over whole grain labeling. https://www.foodnavigator-usa.com/Article/2020/08/21/Study-points-to-consumer-confusion-over-whole-grain-labeling

69. Confused by whole grain labels on food packaging? Study .... https://www.eurekalert.org/pub_releases/2020-08/tuhs-cbw080520.php

70.Tufts University, Health Sciences Campus. (2020, August 10). Confused by whole grain labels on food packaging? Study finds you're not alone: Researchers say results provide legal evidence for proposed changes in labeling regulations. ScienceDaily. Retrieved August 12, 2020 from www.sciencedaily.com/releases/2020/08/200810103302.htm

---

71. Composition Of Foods Integrated Dataset (Cofid), Https://Www.Gov.Uk/Government/Publications/Composition-Of-Foods-Integrated-Dataset-Cofid

72. Why Board Certification is So Important to the Sustainability of Our Industry: https://www.nanp.org/board-certification

73. The Flexitarian Diet Is A Style Of Eating That Encourages Mostly Plant-Based Foods While Allowing Meat And Other Animal Products In Moderation. Https://Www.Healthline.Com/Nutrition/Flexitarian-Diet-Guide

74. Terry Wahls M.D. Blog: Https://Terrywahls.Com/Category/Blog/

75. Why I Am A Pegan – Or Paleo-Vegan – And Why You Should Be Too!: Https://Drhyman.Com/Blog/2014/11/07/Pegan-Paleo-Vegan/

76. Terry Wahls: Applying Functional Medicine to Reverse Multiple Sclerosis, 2018: https://holisticprimarycare.net/topics/functional-medicine/terry-wahls-applying-the-science-of-brain-recovery-to-reverse-multiple-sclerosis/

77. The Wahls Foundation Inc. Https://Terrywahls.Com/Research/

78. Ecowatch.Com: Why I Am A Pegan-Or Paleo-Vegan – And Why You Should Be Too, By Mark Hyman 2015

79. Why I Am A Pegan – Or Paleo-Vegan – And Why You Should Be Too! Https://Drhyman.Com/Blog/2014/11/07/Pegan-Paleo-Vegan/

80. The Wahls Protocol A Radical New Way To Treat All Chronic Autoimmune Conditions Using Paleo Principles. Avery 2020

81. The Way We Eat Now By Bee Wilson Page 238-239

82. Food-Based Dietary Guidelines In Europe: Https://Ec.Europa.Eu/Jrc/En/Health-Knowledge-Gateway/Promotion-Prevention/Nutrition/Food-Based-Dietary-Guidelines

83. Fruit And Vegetable Consumption In Europe 2012: Https://Www.Eufic.Org/En/Healthy-Living/Article/Fruit-And-Vegetable-Consumption-In-Europe-Do-Europeans-Get-Enough

84. Vadell A, Barebring L, Et Al. Anti-Inflammatory Diet In Rheumatoid Arthritis (ADIRA)- A Randomized, Controlled Crossover Trial Indicating Effects On Disease Activity. Am J Clin Nutr. 2020 Jun 1;111(6):1203-1213.

85. Trinity College Dublin. "Addressing The Safety Of High Folate Levels In The Older Population And Implications For Fortification In Ireland." Sciencedaily. Sciencedaily, 15 June 2020. Www.Sciencedaily.Com/Releases/2020/06/200615140836.Htm

86. Helmholtz Zentrum München - German Research Center For Environmental Health. "Vitamin Deficiency In Later Life." Sciencedaily. Sciencedaily, 15 December 2017. Www.Sciencedaily.Com/Releases/2017/12/171215111605.Htm

87. Chemicals and Minerals found in Drinking Water, Northwestern Health Unit: https://www.nwhu.on.ca/ourservices/EnvironmentalHealth/Pages/Chemicals-and-Minerals-found-in-Drinking-Water.aspx

88. water born pathogens | Your Whole Nutrition. https://yourwholenutrition.com/tag/water-born-pathogens/

89. Saving U.S. Water and Sewer Systems Would Be Costly - The https://www.nytimes.com/2010/03/15/us/15water.html

90. Saving U.S. Water and Sewer Systems Would Be Costly By Charles Duhigg, New York Times March 2010

91. https://www.dcwater.com/history-water-system

92. Environment Agency. Environment Agency calls for action on water efficiency - GOV.UK. https://www.gov.uk/government/news/environment-agency-calls-for-action-on-water-efficiency (2018).

93. Barton, N.A., Farewell, T.S. & Hallett, S.H. Using generalized additive models to investigate the environmental effects on pipe failure in clean water networks. npj Clean Water 3, 31 (2020). https://doi.org/10.1038/s41545-020-0077-3

94. The Mineral Content of US Drinking and Municipal Water: https://www.ars.usda.gov/ARSUserFiles/80400525/Articles/NDBC32_WaterMin.pdf

95. Azoulay, A., Garzon, P., & Eisenberg, M. J. (2001). Comparison of the mineral content of tap water and bottled waters. Journal of general internal medicine, 16(3), 168–175. https://doi.org/10.1111/j.1525-1497.2001.04189.x

96. 4. ESSENTIAL NUTRIENTS IN DRINKING WATER. https://www.who.int/water_sanitation_health/dwq/nutrientschap4.pdf

97. EPA Resources https://search.epa.gov/epasearch/?querytext=+safewater+ndwac+index&site=epa_default&result_template=2col.ftl&typeofsearch=epa&referer=https%3A%2F%2Fwww.epa.gov%2Fhome%2Fpage-not-found#/

98. Raccoons and pools, CDC: https://www.cdc.gov/healthywater/swimming/residential/animals/raccoons-and-pools.html

99. Cabral J. P. (2010). Water microbiology. Bacterial pathogens and water. International journal of environmental research and public health, 7(10), 3657–3703. https://doi.org/10.3390/ijerph7103657

100. Polyethylene Terephthalate: The Safety of Bottled Water by Jill Culora Polyethylene Terephthalate: The Safety of Bottled Water: https://www.foodsafetymagazine.com/magazine-archive1/aprilmay-2016/polyethylene-terephthalate-the-safety-of-bottled-water/

101. Yang, C. Z., Yaniger, S. I., Jordan, V. C., Klein, D. J., & Bittner, G. D. (2011). Most plastic products release estrogenic chemicals: a potential health problem that can be solved. Environmental health perspectives, 119(7), 989–996. https://doi.org/10.1289/ehp.1003220

102. BPA Exposure in the NICU by Kaitlin Mendonca, Sc.D., Russ Hauser, Sc.D., M.D. Simmons College, Harvard School of Public Health, NIEHS Grant P30ES000002: https://www.niehs.nih.gov/research/supported/sep/2013/bpa-exposure-nicu/index.cfm

103. BPA Exposure shows Transgenerational Effects on Reproductive Health by Jodi Flaws, Ph.D.; University of Illinois, Urbana-Champaign, NIEHS Grants P01ES022848, P20ES018163:

https://www.niehs.nih.gov/research/supported/sep/2015/bpa_exposure/index.cfm

104. Jobson MD, Grimm SE 3rd, Banks K, Henley G. The effects of water filtration systems on fluoride: Washington, D.C. metropolitan area. ASDC J Dent Child. 2000;67(5):350-304.

105. Health Risks from drinking demineralized water: https://www.who.int/water_sanitation_health/dwq/nutrientschap12.pdf

106. Kia Ditlevsen, Sigrid Denver, Tove Christensen, Jesper Lassen, A Taste For Locally Produced Food - Values, Opinions And Sociodemographic Differences Among 'Organic' And 'Conventional' Https://Doi.Org/10.1016/J.Appet.2019.104544

107. Local Food Directories: https://www.ams.usda.gov/local-food-directories/farmersmarkets

108. Perceptions Of Information Gaps In Farm-To-Table Studies, 2015: Https://Www.Sciencedirect.Com/Science/Article/Abs/Pii/S0956713514005544

109. Michelle R Jospe, Melyssa Roy, Rachel C Brown, Jillian J Haszard, Kim Meredith-Jones, Louise J Fangupo, Hamish Osborne, Elizabeth A Fleming, Rachael W Taylor. Intermittent Fasting, Paleolithic, Or Mediterranean Diets In The Real World: Exploratory Secondary Analyses Of A Weight-Loss Trial That Included Choice Of Diet And Exercise. The American Journal Of Clinical Nutrition, 2019; DOI: 10.1093/Ajcn/Nqz330

110. Lund University. "Original Human 'Stone Age' Diet Is Good For People With Diabetes, Study Finds." Sciencedaily. Sciencedaily, 28 June 2007. Www.Sciencedaily.Com/Releases/2007/06/070627225459.Htm

111. Umeå Universitet. "Paleolithic Diet Healthier For Overweight Women." Sciencedaily. Sciencedaily, 18 January 2018. Www.Sciencedaily.Com/Releases/2018/01/180118142911.Htm

112. Appetite Volume 147, 1 April 2020, 104544; A Taste For Locally Produced Food - Values, Opinions And Sociodemographic Differences Among 'Organic' And 'Conventional' Consumers, Kia Ditlevsen, Sigrid Denver, Tove Christensen, Jesperlassen; Http://Www.Sciencedirect.Com/Science/Article/Pii/S0195666319300273

113. Does food marketing affect children's health?: http://www.foodmarketing.org/resources/food-marketing-101/#affect_children

114. Common Thread: http://www.commonthreads.org/

115. 35 Food Education Organizations: https://foodtank.com/news/2016/09/thirty-five-food-education-organizations/

116. The Curriculum of Cuisine: http://thecurriculumofcuisine.org/

117. Jamie Oliver Launches Healthy Eating School Program: Https://Www.Educationmattersmag.Com.Au/Jamie-Oliver-Launches-Healthy-Eating-School-Program/

118. The Endocrine Society. "People Who Eat A Big Breakfast May Burn Twice As Many Calories: Study Finds Eating More At Breakfast Instead Of Dinner Could Prevent Obesity." Sciencedaily. Sciencedaily, 19 February 2020. Www.Sciencedaily.Com/Releases/2020/02/200219092539.Htm

119. Esmaeili MA, Alilou M. Naringenin attenuates CCl4 -induced hepatic inflammation by the activation of an Nrf2-mediated pathway in rats. Clin Exp Pharmacol Physiol. 2014;41(6):416-422. doi:10.1111/1440-1681.12230

120. Minato K, Miyake Y, Fukumoto S, et al. Lemon flavonoid, eriocitrin, suppresses exercise-induced oxidative damage in rat liver. Life Sci. 2003;72(14):1609-1616. doi:10.1016/s0024-3205(02)02443-8

121. Oliveira, C. P., Gayotto, L. C., Tatai, C., Della Nina, B. I., Lima, E. S., Abdalla, D. S., Lopasso, F. P., Laurindo, F. R., & Carrilho, F. J. (2003). Vitamin C and vitamin E in prevention of Nonalcoholic Fatty Liver Disease (NAFLD) in choline deficient diet fed rats. Nutrition journal, 2, 9. https://doi.org/10.1186/1475-2891-2-9

122. Does milk increase mucus production? Jim Bartleya, Susan Read mcglashanb; Division of Otolaryngology – Head and Neck Surgery, Counties-Manukau District Health Board, New Zealand; Department of Anatomy with Radiology, University of Auckland, New Zealand, Received 22 October 2009, Accepted 28 October 2009, Available online 24 November 2009. ElsevierVolume 74, Issue 4, April 2010, Pages 732-734

123. Thiara, G., & Goldman, R. D. (2012). Milk consumption and mucus production in children with asthma. Canadian family physician Medecin de famille canadien, 58(2), 165–166.

124. Effect of Hibiscus Sabdariffa on Blood Pressure in a University Population: https://clinicaltrials.gov/ct2/show/NCT03804801

125. Jalalyazdi, M., Ramezani, J., Izadi-Moud, A., Madani-Sani, F., Shahlaei, S., & Ghiasi, S. S. (2019). Effect of hibiscus sabdariffa on blood pressure in patients with stage 1 hypertension. Journal of advanced pharmaceutical technology & research, 10(3), 107–111. https://doi.org/10.4103/japtr.JAPTR_402_18

126. https://www.todaysdietitian.com/newarchives/0719p36.shtml

127. The Endocrine Society. "People Who Eat A Late Dinner May Gain Weight." Sciencedaily. Sciencedaily, 11 June 2020. Www.Sciencedaily.Com/Releases/2020/06/200611094138.Htm

128. University Of Illinois At Urbana-Champaign, News Bureau. "Control Over Work-Life Boundaries Creates Crucial Buffer To Manage After-Hours Work Stress." Sciencedaily. Sciencedaily, 25 June 2020. Www.Sciencedaily.Com/Releases/2020/06/200625122734.Htm

129. Staffordshire University. "Why Do So Many Of Us Feel Guilty About Taking A Lunch Break?." Sciencedaily. Sciencedaily, 17 June 2020. Www.Sciencedaily.Com/Releases/2020/06/200617121453.Htm

130. European Society of Cardiology. (2020, August 28). Nurses burned out and want to quit. ScienceDaily. Retrieved October 7, 2020 from www.sciencedaily.com/releases/2020/08/200828081037.htm

131. Vanderbilt University Medical Center. (2019, October 23). Consensus report shows burnout prevalent in health care community. ScienceDaily. Retrieved October 7, 2020 from www.sciencedaily.com/releases/2019/10/191023172121.htm

132. The Way We Eat By Bee Wilson Page 127

133.European Society of Cardiology. (2020, August 28). Nurses burned out and want to quit. ScienceDaily. Retrieved October 7, 2020 from www.sciencedaily.com/releases/2020/08/200828081037.htm

134. Comprehensive Guidelines For Food Recovery Programs, Developed By The Food Recovery Committee 2000 Conference For Food Protection / Council I, Updated March 2007: Www.Foodprotect.Org/Media/Guide/Food-Recovery-Final2007.Pdf

135. Gleaning is the act of collecting leftover crops from farmers' fields after they have been commercially harvested or on fields where it is not economically profitable to harvest.

136. Why We Eat What We Eat By Bee Wilson Page 36, 38

137. Lopez And Jacobs 2018: Hawkes 2006: Eckhardt Et Al. 2006

138. Obesity Growing Among Adults With Diabetes. https://www.webmd.com/diabetes/news/20041118/obesity-growing-among-adults-with-diabetes

139. Hawkes 2006

140. Improving Livelihood Opportunities For Rural Women In Pakistan 2018: Https://Www.Nestle.Pk/Media/Newsandfeatures/Improving-Livelihood-Opportunities-For-Rural-Women-In-Pakistan

141. Door To Door Sales Of Fortified Products Nestle: Https://Www.Nestle.Com/Ask-Nestle/Health-Nutrition/Answers/Addressing-New-York-Times-Obesity-Junk-Food-Brazil

142. Top 10 Best Meal Delivery Services Cook Fresh Meals At Home: Https://Www.Top10bestmealdelivery.Com/?Bkw=Home%20meal%20kits&Bcampid=267541954&Bcamp=MD%20Search&Bagid=1177577510137141&Bag=Meal%20Kit&Btarid=Kwd-73598650469777:Loc-4129&Bidm=Be&Bnet=S&Bd=C&Bmobval=0&Bt=Search&Utm_Source=Bing&Utm_Medium=Cpc&Utm_Term=Home%20meal%20kits&Utm_Campaign=Bing+CPC+Campaign&C=73598797705415&M=E&K=73598650469777&Binterest=&Bphysical=87047&Bfeedid=&A=B9504&Ts=Delivery&Topic=&Test=DT_Bing_Search_General&Msclkid=39d98d449d5912cd9660d3a26e350d2f

143. The Rise Of Food Delivery In The United States Was Caused By Economic Necessity, As During The 1950s, The Growing American Middle-Class Were Content To Stay At Home Watching Their New Television, And To Make Their Food In Their Own Kitchens. Https://Www.Thevintagenews.Com/2019/01/08/Food-Delivery/

144. Traditional Food Products And Consumer Choices: A Review: Https://Www.Researchgate.Net/Publication/320979697_Traditional_Food_Products_And_Consumer_Choices_A_Review

145. A Low-Carb Strategy For Fighting The Pandemic's Toll, Federal Dietary Guidelines Don't Reflect The Evidence That Eating Fewer Carbohydrates Can Help To Reduce Obesity, Diabetes And Heart Disease. By Nina Teicholz May 30, 2020: Https://Www.Wsj.Com/Articles/A-Low-Carb-Strategy-For-Fighting-The-Pandemics-Toll-11590811260?Mod=Searchresults&Page=1&Pos=1

146. Male Athletes And Eating Disorders By Sansone, Randy A MD; Sawyer, Robert MD, Clinical Journal Of Sport Medicine: March 2005 - Volume 15 - Issue 2 - P 45-46 Doi: 10.1097/01.Jsm.0000157794.85381.C5

147. 2016 Update On Eating Disorders In Athletes: A Comprehensive Narrative Review With A Focus On Clinical Assessment And Management, By Elizabeth Joy, Andrea Kussman, Aurelia Nattiv: Https://Bjsm.Bmj.Com/Content/50/3/154

148. Underdiagnosed Male Eating Disorders Are Becoming Increasingly Identified, NPR March 2019: Https://Www.Npr.Org/2019/03/02/699733879/Underdiagnosed-Male-Eating-Disorders-Are-Becoming-Increasingly-Identified

149. World's Oldest Pottery Used To Cook Fish In Japan | JOMON FOOD | Facts And Details: Http://Factsanddetails.Com/Japan/Cat16/Sub105/Entry-5279.Html#Chapter-5

150. Presto with its vast experience in manufacturing pressure canners and to more adequately meet the needs of the consumer, the company created the first saucepan-style pressure cooker in 1939 and gave it the brand name "presto." This revolutionary pressure cooker eliminated cumbersome lug nuts and clamps and, instead, featured a rotating cover with a simple gasket sealing design that is still being used in modern day pressure cookers. Https://Www.Gopresto.Com/Content/Corporate-Information/Company-History

151. Bowls like this one from the etowah mound complex were the result of trade, perhaps in exchange for steatite items or copper. Bowls made from horse conch were recovered from the late archaic sections of the tick island site in volutia county, florida had burned bottoms, indicating an attempt at cooking in shell vessels. This did not prove to be a successful approach as all of the bottoms of the shell vessels had burned out.

152. Cardiff University. (2020, July 6). Norman Conquest Of 1066 Did Little To Change People's Eating Habits. Sciencedaily. Retrieved July 10, 2020 From Www.Sciencedaily.Com/Releases/2020/07/200706140915.Htm

153. Stew: Https://En.Wikipedia.Org/Wiki/Stew

154. The British Museum- A History Of The World, Episode 10: Http://Www.Bbc.Co.Uk/Ahistoryoftheworld/About/Transcripts/Episode10/

155. "Taillevent, Viandier (Manuscrit Du Vatican)". Www.Staff.Uni-Giessen.De. Retrieved 2017-01-27.

156. Food.Com, Stew: Https://Www.Food.Com/Topic/Stews

Chapter Two
Sustainability From the Ground Up

Loaves and Fishes

This is not the age of information.

This is <u>not</u>
the age of information.

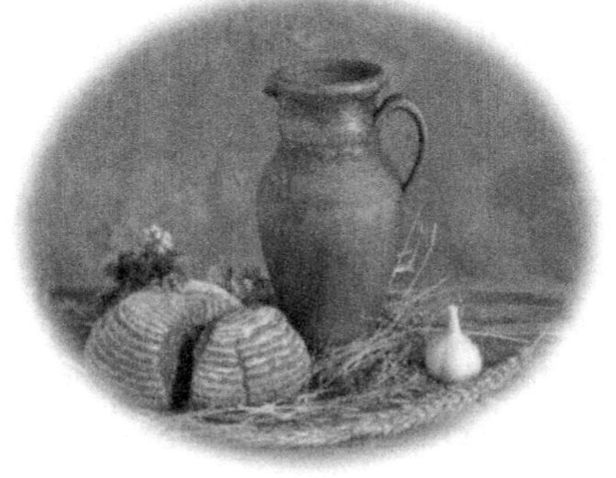

Forget the news,
and the radio,
and the blurred screen.

This is the time
of loaves
and fishes.

People are hungry,
and one good word is bread
for a thousand. [1, 2, 3]

~ David Whyte

What is a sustainable life? When looking at history and archaeology, certain areas line up with humanity's ability to cultivate a sustainable population. Paleo societies first required a nutrient-dense food supply, followed by drinkable water and, of course, breathable air. It would be incorrect to believe the environment of ancient peoples was devoid of heavy metals and pollution. Modern research is finding evidence of high levels of heavy metal contamination at ancient villages and settlements was found in the soil and sediment of lake beds. The planet is continuously off-gassing heavy metals through the soil, water, and air; it is a natural process. Radon gas is the natural result of uranium in the ground degrading. [4]

Additionally, volcanic eruptions along with regular occurrences of forest and range fires added toxins to the air and increased sediment run-off; in the case of fires, early paleo-populations and the indigenous populations that followed; routinely used fire to regenerate feed for wildlife and increase available plant foods. This practice continues even today with wild and forest land management. History provides perspective and understanding of the lifestyle of Paleo-people. Ancient peoples of the western United States lived in a changing climate 10,000 years ago and became increasingly nomadic as food became scarce. [5] These inland food scarcities moved the population from the Great Basin in the western U.S. to Pacific coastal areas. Archaeologists estimate this migration took place over 2,000 years after the Great Basin was populated. Most of the Great Basin populations of Paiute bands continued living a sparse and primitive lifestyle in the Great Basin well into the 1900s. The select populations that developed permanent villages and a permanent population base were located near sites with a rich and varied abundance of foods. [6, 7, 8]

When it comes to health in the modern age, what is the one area in which almost everyone has control? Just a clue here; *it is not* which doctor you select or which annual tests you have done, nor the area of the country/world in which one resides, nor choices a person may make about which church to attend or not.

Like populations of the past, the bottom line for a sustainable life today is food availability, and it is far easier to acquire calorie-dense foods today. Just as ancient societies were at the whim of a changing environment and migratory patterns, modern populations are being challenged by industrial food sources and by discerning nutrients' quality within available quantity. Unlike hunter-gathers of old, most people today have a measure of control over their income and lifestyle.

> *"I believe food is the single most important factor in health. Few are born requiring medication, but all require food.*
>
> *The number one leading cause of chronic illness in America is the modern diet."*
>
> ~Tammera J. Karr

Examining our empty plate pattern expands the common understanding of diet to incorporate lifestyle; this greatly expands our knowledge of what is otherwise a limited concept solely relating to food. In this expanded way of thinking, the diet of *lifestyle* is not singularly composed of food but also contains water, chemicals, drugs, sights, sounds, experiences, and external influences ingested into our beings. To understand why all of these multiple factors

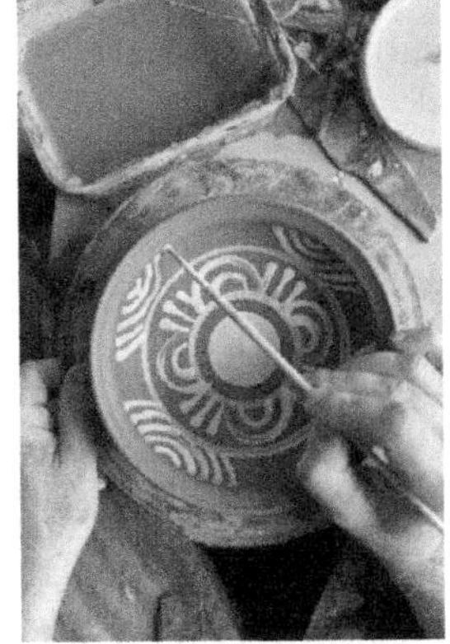

matter and why they should be considered forms of nourishment, understanding one word is necessary.

sustainable

1: capable of being sustained

2 a: of, relating to, or being a method of harvesting or using a resource so that the resource is not depleted or permanently damaged

b: of or relating to a lifestyle involving the use of sustainable methods.

Merriam-Webster Dictionary third edition

Over the last twenty years, small communities have begun returning to more sustainable practices; reclaiming local food with the resurgence of farmers' markets, local bakeries, old school general stores, and mercantile and community-supported agriculture (CSA). The visible results of these efforts are rebuilding communities, increasing food security, and improving connections between generations and individuals once more.

The return to sustainable agriculture practices also comes with changes in lifestyle choices: Do individuals use glass or plastic for food storage? What is the impact of sustainable practices on local and regional environments? How do agricultural changes and other aspects of sustainable living impact drinking water? We will look further at the question concerning water and agriculture shortly. Are agricultural chemicals affecting health? What are chemicals doing to children? Are microplastics going to affect sustainability for seven generations?

To consider these questions can be overwhelming and could almost drive a person crazy if they were not careful. Once again, we can employ the lens of mindfulness to focus on one, two, or three potential changes each person can embrace.

> *Principle 1:* Lasting lifestyle and health changes require allowing one to be empowered; small changes can take up to eight weeks to become sustainable.

One person may be able to incorporate more whole foods sustainably. Another may be able to limit their plastic consumption. In contrast, others may throw the net wide and take on water filtration, gardening, and/or many other aspects of a mindful and sustainably balanced lifestyle. It is important to acknowledge that each person will integrate reasonable, achievable, and sustainable changes to find their own balance. When historians look at the food movements like fusion (combining different cultural foods into one dish) and diet trends such as the plant-based movement; perspective comes into play and is important. [9]

Of course, some trends can be good and others not so much. Take for example, the current plant-based diet movement, which can have pros and cons depending on the person and the food sources they utilize.

Benefit: Plant-based diets, in general, help individuals lose weight and lower cholesterol while increasing the volume of healthy vegetables consumed. [10]

Findings do not always provide expected results: Food manufacturer, Beyond Meat®, funded a small study in 2020 comparing meat's health effects with plant-based alternatives. Most meat alternatives have high levels of saturated fat, sodium and are highly processed; made with food isolates and extracts as opposed to whole beans or chopped mushrooms. [11] These factors contribute to cardiovascular disease. A bacterium in the digestive tract — Trimethylamine N-oxide, or TMAO — is thought to be a risk factor for cardiovascular disease. Researchers expected vegetarian subjects to have lower levels of TMAO. However, results were mixed, and the findings were not conclusive. [12]

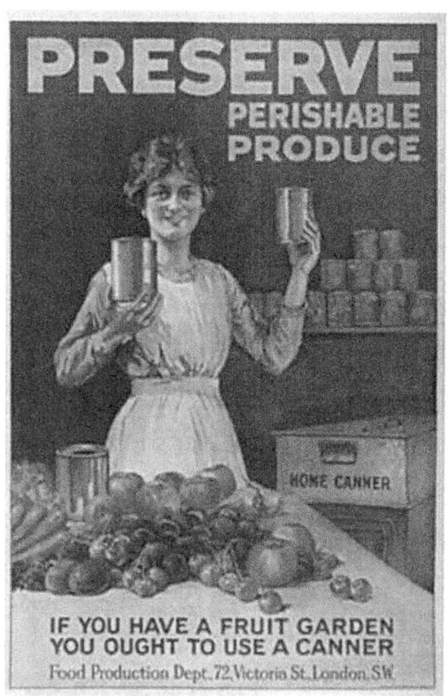

So, what is it that makes the difference? It is pretty simple; Grandma was right when she told you to eat your vegetables. The diet should be made up of roughly 45% plant-based foods, of which 15% should be from starches. When individuals consume more vegetables, all risk factors go down. Raw vegetables require far more energy to break down and metabolize, so individuals lose weight when consuming more raw vegetables. Cooked plant-based foods, on average, provide more calories and are easier to digest than raw, so a vegetarian may find they are challenged by the battle of the bulge and type 2 diabetes if they eat only cooked plant-based foods.

Negative effect: Going vegetarian is not always a sustainable approach for everyone due to differences in genetics, lifestyle, food sourcing, and accessibility. [13]

Next: If an individual has elevated risk factors for type 2 diabetes, Alzheimer's, Parkinson's, and nerve disorders; a strict plant-based diet can increase the likelihood of developing these conditions. [14, 15, 16, 17]

However, a flexible plant-based approach can increase the consumption of vegetables and quality fats and protein; decreasing risk factors for certain diseases. How well individuals respond to whole foods, plant-based, omnivore, or keto diet approaches translates into the quality of the foods consumed and each individual's unique biology. These effects have to do with the type of fats, inflammation-causing compounds, and upregulation of single nucleotide polymorphism (SNPs). [18, 19] As unique individuals, each person has their own balance point regarding nutrient utilization from food.

> *Principle 2*: *A* strict *one-diet* approach may not work for everyone, even if they are in the same *family*.

It follows that for many, good health will not be sustainable when consuming industrial produced vegetarian foods, like Beyond Meat®, soy noodles, soy milk, BOCA Burgers®, or

Soylent® meal replacement. While these are plant-based, they are also highly processed industrial foods. More than the fact they are industrially fabricated foods — even if labeled organic, vegan, or GMO-free — their primary nutrient makeup will still lack vital cofactors lost during processing. Once again, we direct you to whole locally produced foods when it comes to quality plant-based foods. In fact, industrial vegan foods are poor substitutes for whole plants prepared and cooked in traditional ways. This is also a key point when looking at the longevity information on the *Blue Zones* like Loma Linda, California, and Okinawa, Japan. When reviewing the research information, the original statements said; community, connection, activity, and a sense of purpose (in essence, lifestyle) were stronger contributing factors to longevity than any single dietary approach. [20, 21, 22]

> *Principle 3*: Connection with community and culture combined with a sense of value and purpose contribute to health as much or more than foods consumed.

No matter how hard the tech-industry tries, these synthetic foods do not contain the same nutrients, co-factors, amino acids, lipids, and natural compounds found in whole foods from nature. Another point to consider: it requires a huge amount of natural resources to manufacture food from refined extracts, and the process creates an additional burden of waste byproducts that are potential pollutants to groundwater, fisheries, and air.

Humans have historically sought out animal-based foods such as fish, poultry, beef, lamb, pork, and wild game to fill nutrient requirements when it comes to amino acids and lipids. [23] Poultry's popularity has surpassed beef in the last five years; however, it is incorrect to believe that eating poultry is a superior protein or that it is better for the environment than cattle, sheep, or pigs. [24, 25, 26] Those who have raised poultry can attest to the challenges of dealing with ventilation and litter from chicken coops and yards. [27]

It was once believed the biological function of various dietary proteins depended entirely upon the percentage of the individual amino acids contained in each protein type. Current research, however, shows each form of protein, in addition to the benefits of its amino acid composition, also provides a unique set of functional properties that are separate and distinct from the amino acid profile that it contains. [28]

	Fresh Peas	Wheat flour	Chicken breast	Beef steak	Whole egg	Cow's milk	Human milk	Cod fillet
				g/100 g total protein				
Lysine	8.0	1.9	9.3	8.7	6.3	7.4	7.1	9.6
Cysteine	1.2	2.6	1.3	1.2	1.8	0.8	2.0	1.1
Tyrosine	3.0	2.6	3.6	3.7	4.0	4.1	3.0	3.4
Tryptophan	1.0	1.1	1.1	1.2	1.8	1.3	2.3	1.1

Each form of animal protein contains its own unique amino acid profile. Poultry contains higher levels of tryptophan and tyrosine. Lamb contains one of the best all-around amino acid profiles in combination with vital minerals. The balance of amino acids present in red meats such as lamb reduces amino acid sensitivity in some individuals. [29,30] The amino acids tryptophan (via 5-HTP), tyrosine, glutamic acid, and aspartic acid seem to have an increasingly negative impact on individuals with family histories of migraine headaches. They may experience increased occurrence or likelihood from foods such as poultry higher in these amino acids. [31,32]

In many coastal areas, food tradition dictates that wild oysters should only be eaten in months whose name ends with the letter *r* to avoid watery shellfish or food poisoning. Research published in 2019 suggests people have been following this practice for over 4,000 years. [33] Seasonal bivalves contain high levels of specific lipids, rare amino acids, and zinc in the spring. [34] These nutrients are vital for reproduction. Additionally, these nutrients bring balance to hormones in older individuals; aiding in a smooth transition to the last decades of life.

All of this also explains why ancient peoples sought out these nutrient-rich foods from coastal waters. [35] The concept of sustainability involves thinking about seasonal foods. Consider young greens, tender herbs, berries, fruits, poultry, and eggs that have been traditionally harvested in spring and summer. Red meats such as bison, deer, moose, salmon (historically fish was seen as meat or flesh equal to land animals — distinctions occur in culinary terminology and religious dietary laws.), beef, goat, and sheep contain heme-iron and vitamin B_{12}. [36] These proteins were traditionally prepared with savory herbs, starchy roots, nuts, and seeds in the fall and winter. Pork also has a long history of being harvested in the late fall after the first freeze, which helped reduce the risk of trichinosis and spoilage. Pork and apples are classical images. In TCM the combining of the two lends to digestion. In traditional Asian culture venison, beef, and pork are considered *hot* foods and prepared during winter months when human bodies need more energy to stay warm. Mushrooms have more than one season and are traditionally harvested in both spring and fall; not only do they provide valuable minerals, but more importantly, is their value in supporting the immune system against viruses and parasites.

Traditional food choices, such as those of Alaska's native population, reflect long-standing generational values of sustainable practices. The kinds of seafood and land foods harvested by this heavy meat-eating culture are prepared and consumed with reverence and respect during its appropriate season. [37]

When individuals recognize the importance of growing and harvesting traditional whole foods; it is easier to understand why one should be eating a varied diet — that includes animal and plant foods during the season when they are at their best. [38] Eating plant-based foods in season and naturally sustainably harvested animal protein sources, ensures a broader spectrum of quality nutrition, reduced food sensitivities, and encourages a diverse microbiome that supports sustainable health. [39, 40, 41]

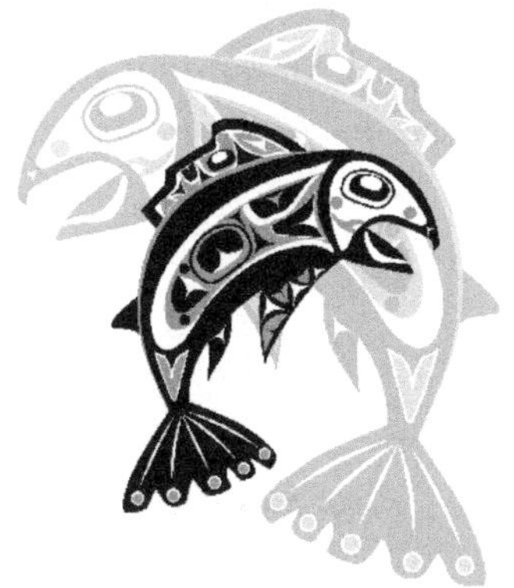

What we have learned

Through archaeology and anthropology studies modern humans have learned which foods made up ancient peoples' cultural diets from the first ice age to 1950. Until World War II, regional and local foods were the norm, even within cities. Produce, milk, butter, fish, and fruits came primarily from regional sources.

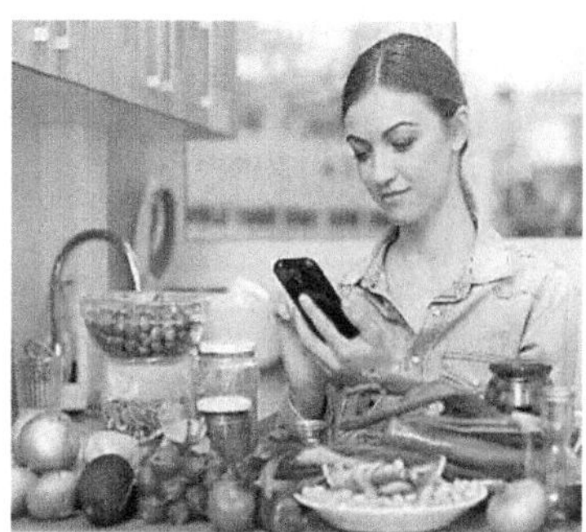

Locally produced foods contain the minerals and microbiota of the area they are grown in. [42] They are adapted to local environmental cycles, and the overall nutrient content of local foods is higher and safer than those shipped in from neighboring states or countries. Almost every food recalled in the last ten years for *listeria*, *salmonella*, or *E. coli,* plastic and/or glass contamination has been produced at industrial-farms, factories, or processed and shipped in from another country. [43, 44, 45, 46]

Sustainability from the soil up

Soil and dirt are not the same — in the case of dirt, it is listed as unable to sustain or grow vegetation. [47] By contrast, soil is rich in microbes and organic material that foster vegetation growth. Soil composition varies in the mineral and microbial content in relation to location. Some areas have high levels of selenium, others almost none. The plants and animals of each particular region contribute to and farm the microbes in that region's water and soil. Soil scientists have learned trees send signals to microbes in the soil when it is time to harvest or plant-specific fungi that the tree is dependent on for nourishment. Each domain in nature has its own unique micro-ecosystem comprised of diverse colonies of fungi and bacteria. [48] These colonies of microbiota form the grocery store for humans, animals, plants, and insects.

> *"The golden sweet pools of maple syrup on the plate is stored summer sunshine."*
>
> ~Robin Wall Kimmerer, PhD
> author of *Braiding Sweetgrass*

Traditional fishing, ranching, and farming practices are dependent on sustainable ecosystems to thrive. The healthier the rangeland, the healthier the livestock and wild animals. The same is true of farming; those who practice sustainable agriculture employ fewer chemicals and have greater diversity in soil microbiota supporting disease-resistant crops. In permaculture, ground cover crops replace nutrients in the soil and promote healthier microbes while retaining moisture content and reducing the damaging loss of topsoil and runoff. [49, 50, 51]

Beneficial bacteria building sustainable health

"It isn't the Cows; it is the How." This statement from Diana Rodgers at the Sustainable Dish and *Sacred Cow* author says it all in a nutshell. [52]

When pioneers followed the call of *manifest destiny* across the North America continent, advancement of the United States boundaries resulted. They encountered massive herds of herbivores who groomed and tended the soil. Birds followed the herds gleaning nourishment from the droppings and spreading them for easier decomposition into the soil. Researchers have found the diversity of soil microbiota and mycorrhiza is dependent on transportation by migratory herbivores. [53, 54] Modern cattle on rangelands add to the naturally occurring bacteria and fungi diversity of countless migratory grazing and foraging animals. This is achieved through soil disturbance, vegetation cropping, urination, defecation, and decay following birth and death. [55, 56]

Herbivores have been part of the environment and are responsible for the health of grasslands, prairies, and forest fringes since the Cenozoic era. Humans have eaten herbivores from the dawn of time. In nature, each life form adds to or takes from an ecosystem. [57]

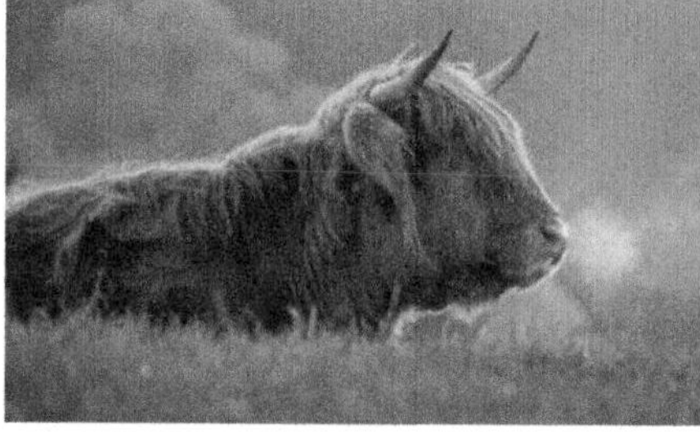

Large industrial farms apply tons of chemicals and fertilizers to crops every year, putting groundwater at risk. A study released in 2020

from the University of Colorado at Boulder highlighted sulfur as a growing environmental challenge.

Researchers examined sulfur applications across multiple crops in the United States: corn in the Midwest, sugarcane in Florida, and wine grapes in California. Models of sulfur in surface waters in areas recovering from acid rain are increasing again. The scientists predict that increasing sulfur levels will continue in croplands worldwide; including China and India, that are still working to regulate fossil fuel emissions.

The report emphasized that simply documenting the impacts of increased sulfur on the environment and human health isn't enough. Increased monitoring and research should include farmers, regulatory agencies, and land managers to increase collaboration and collective action. "We have an imperative to understand the impact that we're having on the environment," said lead author Eve-Lyn Hinckley. "And then we need to work together towards solutions to mitigate those effects." [58]

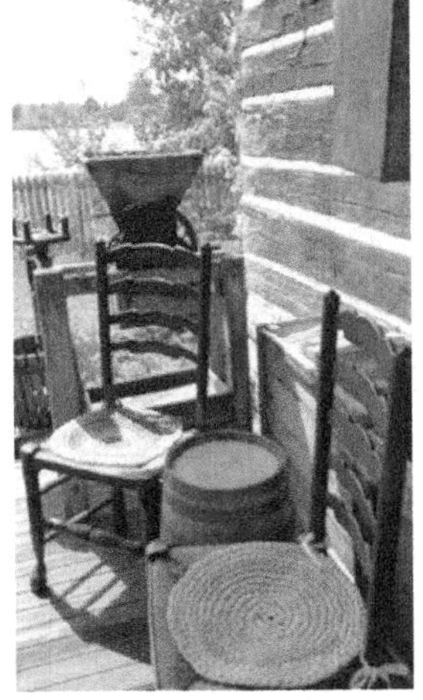

When individuals buy foods from factory farms (a large industrialized farm, especially a farm on which large numbers of livestock are raised indoors in conditions intended to maximize production at minimal cost) they have no control over the food quality. [59] Nor where it comes from, or the impact on soil and groundwater; and their money ends up in the hands of large multi-national businesses outside of the country of residence.

There was a 24% increase in American farm bankruptcies in 2019. The good news is, at the same time, more young Americans started up small permaculture farms. [60, 61, 62]

Agriculture, water, and climate

For sustainable health, folks cannot overlook the role of clean and safe drinking water. Just like one must have clean holistic nutrition to maintain health, safe drinkable water and breathable air are necessary for life. [63, 64, 65, 66] When looking back at history, the lessons of the great Dust Bowl illustrate what happens when topsoil is lost, choking the air and blocking out the sunlight. [67, 68, 69, 70] The loss of nutrient-rich topsoil is not a thing of the past; today, the average soil loss rate is 5.8 tons per acre per year. Over ten years, 0.37-inch topsoil loss totals about $12,225 in lost yield and nutrients on 40 acres. [71]

Just as humans have a microbiome system, so do animals and environments. This is especially important when discussing agriculture and its effects on water stores and the climate. We may be under the impression one area or another is suffering from drought due to climate change. The more important question is how much water holding capacity does the soil in a given area have?

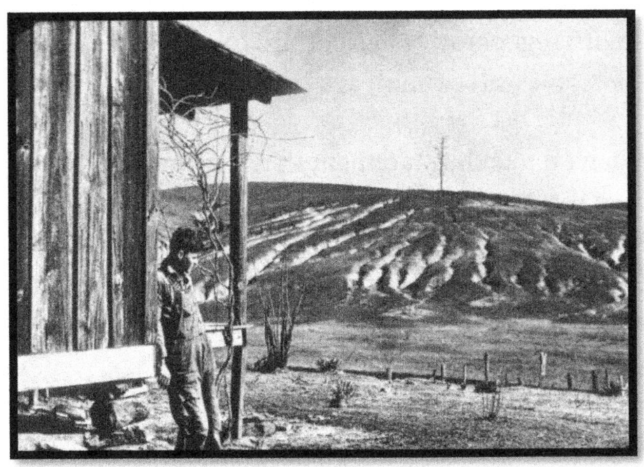

Eroded topsoil during the Dust Bowl 1930s
Image Credit USDA NRCS Georgia

Gabe Brown writes in his book, *Dirt to Soil,* that by changing farming practices to sustainable no-tillage methods and utilizing diverse crop blends, farmers not only increase production they also improve the health of the soil, the infiltration of water, and the water-holding capacity of the soil also significantly increases.

"For every 1% increase in organic matter, we can store between 17,000 and 25,000 gallons of water per acre," Brown goes on to explain. [72] This approach means one farm using industrial farming methods of tillage and chemical fertilizers can apply hundreds of gallons of water per acre per day that largely evaporates or runs off because it cannot penetrate the soil. These monoculture crops have shallow root systems that increase susceptibility to disease and heat. Brown says, "This is a perfect example of how we "create" our own drought."

More — with regenerative agriculture topsoil stays in place, and erosion and water runoff are mitigated.

> When I make the statement that the amount of rainfall an area receives is not relevant, I get a lot of disgusted looks — especially from farmers in drier climates. It is true though. How much rainfall you get is not important; what is important is how much rainfall can infiltrate the soil, says Brown.

By rebuilding *soils* from compacted, lifeless *dirt*, robust microbiome systems take hold, feeding and supporting the plants with nutrients. In turn, the animals that feed on the plants are healthier, and eventually, we as humans are healthier from eating quality foods.

Beneficial bacteria to the rescue

Beneficial bacteria in our digestive systems metabolize indigestible compounds, supply essential nutrients like vitamin K, enhancing mineral absorption, and balances immune function. Additionally, commensal bacteria increase utilization of *omega*-3 fatty acids. A diverse and resilient microbiome defends against colonization by opportunistic pathogens, aids in hormone clearance, supports healthy cell replication, and reductions in inflammation. All of which contributes to the prevention of chronic illness. [73, 74]

Researchers believe the human body contains at least 1,000 different known bacteria species, all of which amounts to 150 times more microbial genes than are found in the entire human genome. [75, 76] Furthermore, human microbial composition and function differ according to different locations, ages, sexes, races, and diets. [77, 78] From 1960 to the present, the population's use of chemical disinfectants in their homes has significantly altered the population's microbial diversity. [79, 80]

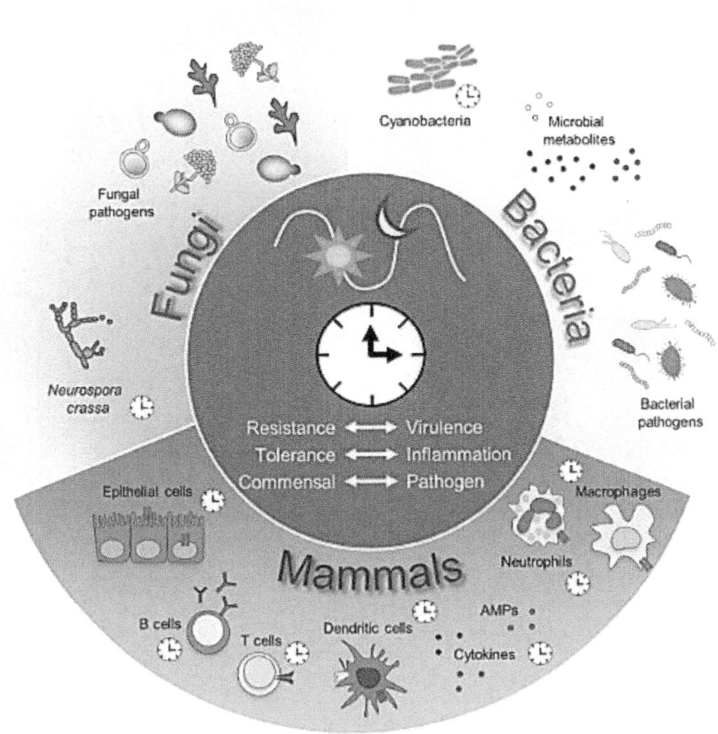

Graphic Credit: Costantini C, Renga G, Sellitto F, et al. Microbes in the Era of Circadian Medicine. Front Cell Infect Microbiol. 2020;10:30. Published 2020 Feb 5. doi:10.3389/fcimb.2020.00030

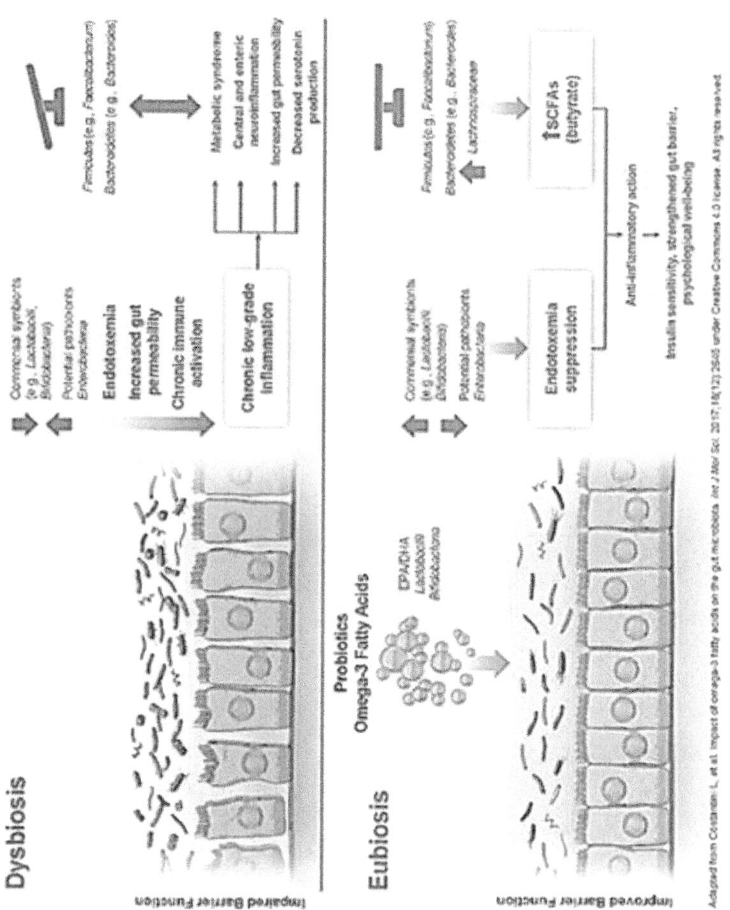

Image credit/Reference: Hutchinson, A.N.; Tingö, L.; Brummer, R.J. The Potential Effects of Probiotics and ω-3 Fatty Acids on Chronic Low-Grade Inflammation. Nutrients 2020, 12, 2402.

Dangers of disinfecting

The modern human diet has lost much of its diversity in content, nutrients, and micro-nutrients from pre-World War II. [81, 82, 83] In a nursing textbook from 1934; under disinfection methods, the first recommended option reads as follows: *Fresh air, Sunlight, and Cleanliness.* [84] The use of steam sterilizing and principles was not set in healthcare until 1956 by J.J. Perkins. [85] Modern industrial foods have little, if any, of the microbes necessary for digestion, and they are essentially *dead*, providing no sustainable nutrition. These foods are sterile and incapable of supporting healthy immune function and protecting gut permeability. Centuries of traditional foods and their preparation came about through an understanding of the balance of nature.

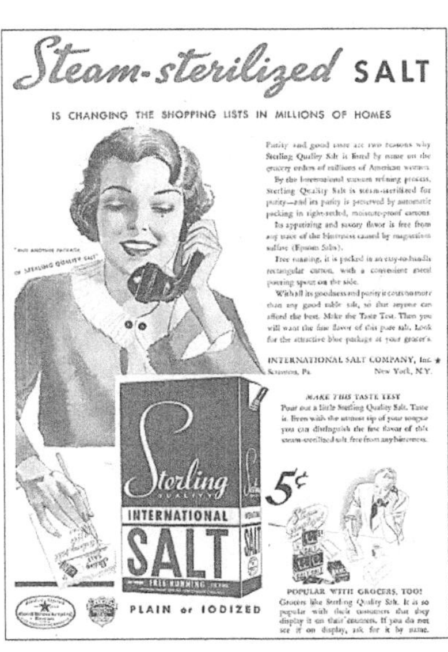

Sterling Salt, 1935
Good Housekeeping Magazine

When we combine disinfectants, hormone-disrupting agents, and industrial food chemicals, the result is all-out *germ warfare*; wiping out the good with the bad, leading to a perfect storm for poor health. [86, 87, 88] While the use of these substances and methods has been touted by the modern food industry as necessary for food safety, in theory the reality is turning out to be very different.

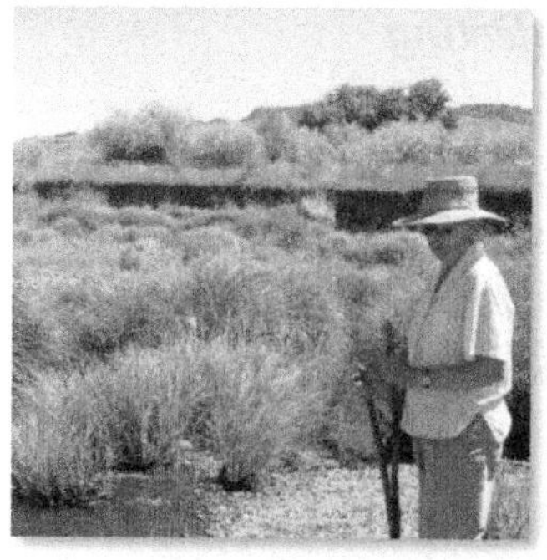

Betty Sitz 1920-2018
Sitz Ranch Drewsey Oregon 2017

To have sustainable health, just like the herbivores, humans need a balanced relationship with traditional whole foods; along with mindful choices regarding chemically altered and industrial foods ingested, and connection to nature and family. Otherwise, the modern standard American diet (SAD) will continue to bulldoze traditional foods, plant diversity, safe water, and microbiota sources out of existence. By making one small change in their food and lifestyle habits, individuals can stop the proverbial stampede of degeneration and move forward to a mindful and sustainable lifestyle.

Mindful shopping: the new hunting and gathering

Today's grocery stores have changed a lot over the past twenty years. Gone in many areas are the local specialty grocers seen in films from the 1950s; replaced by mega-sized Walmart or warehouse stores. The hardest part about this change for individual buyers is the overwhelming volume of food products; over 40,000 are vying for consumers' attention. When folks are tired and stressed from work or family needs, trips to the market are even more problematic. This is prime time to be tempted by those cleverly colored and displayed industrial foods. Market researchers fully understand what is happening inside consumers' overwhelmed brains; they know what colors, flavors, and even sounds will attract individuals to buy. [89, 90] Just like a skilled hunter knows how to find and lure the food sources in the wild — so do modern food marketers and retailers in the wilds of the grocery store aisles.

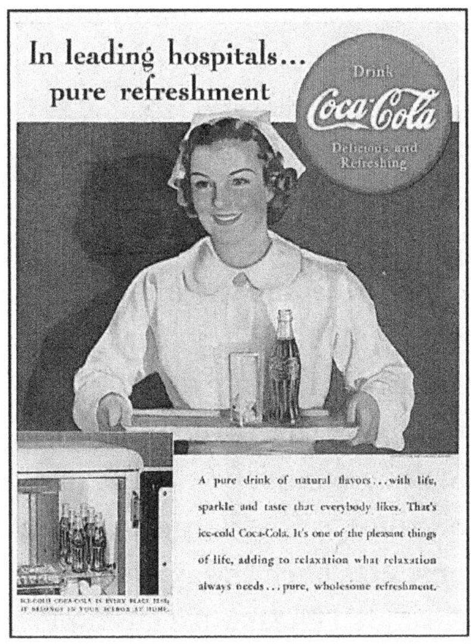

Life Magazine 1938

Meaning of "safe"

"Safe" for food additives is defined to mean a reasonable certainty in the minds of competent scientists that the substance is not harmful under the intended conditions of use. [91]

Congress set standards in 1958 to encourage innovation while ensuring public confidence that chemicals added to food would not have harmful effects years later. The benefits of an additive are not a factor in determining whether it is safe. [92]

Shopping the outer fringe

For decades, clinicians have told clients to limit their shopping to the grocery store's outer edge — the problem is marketing experts know healthcare providers are telling clients to avoid the inner aisles. The center and endcaps are where many highly processed, refined, and denatured industrial foods are located. However, with increasing frequency, ultra-refined industrial food items are now making their way into the produce area. Additionally, produce is now being paired with companion industrial products such as salad dressings and dips. Croutons and shredded cheese are interspersed with vegetables. Colored sugar glazes, caramel dips, and chocolate sit alongside fruits.

The mindful and sustainable alternative? Local farmers' markets and butcher shops have always been a sustainable way to purchase food. This way of shopping supports businesses in communities, and it also increases the nutritional value of the foods consumed. This is a win-win choice when looking at cost; communities are a big part of who we are as a people, so keeping the local economy healthy involves more sustainable choices than supporting franchise chains. The closer to us that food is grown, the higher the immune-boosting nutrients because of the microbiota of species within the same area.

When we take that moment of pause and calm our minds, we begin to see possibilities and solutions lost when highly stressed or working from a place of fear. During these times of clarity, we can mindfully evaluate what can be done to manage stressful situations.

With food prices ever increasing, having the pantry shelves full before winter reduces stress and frees-up limited resources during the winter. Some individuals, especially in rural areas, practice home food fermenting, drying, and canning. All of these mindful measures can ease stress or food insecurity fears. When utilizing drying, fermenting, and canning techniques people are more flexible over food spoilage if the power goes out for extended periods.

Each time you take a moment of pause and think clearly about the *what ifs* within your control; stress goes down, and feelings of helplessness diminish. Research has confirmed when individuals are under heightened pressure, the enormity of the uncertainties become overwhelming, increasing the stress hormone cortisol and suppressing dopamine production. The more uncertainties in an individual's life, the more likely they are to make potentially dangerous decisions.

A historical example would be the multitude of events that led up to the Donner Party tragedy. The Donner Party was a group of American pioneers who migrated to California from 1846–47. Delayed by a series of mishaps, being unprepared and inexperienced, resulted in them getting trapped and snowbound in the Sierra Nevada mountain range. Some survived through cannibalism of deceased party members. [93] The stigma of events never left those who survived.

It is easier to plan and prepare for events than recover from devastation; whether it is unexpected company, road closures, forest fires, power outages, increasing food prices or goods shortages. This became all too clear for the authors during the late summer firestorm of 2020, which devastated areas of western Oregon. By mindfully thinking through the *what ifs*, the authors dealt with inconveniences versus trauma and retained resilience during these traumatic events.

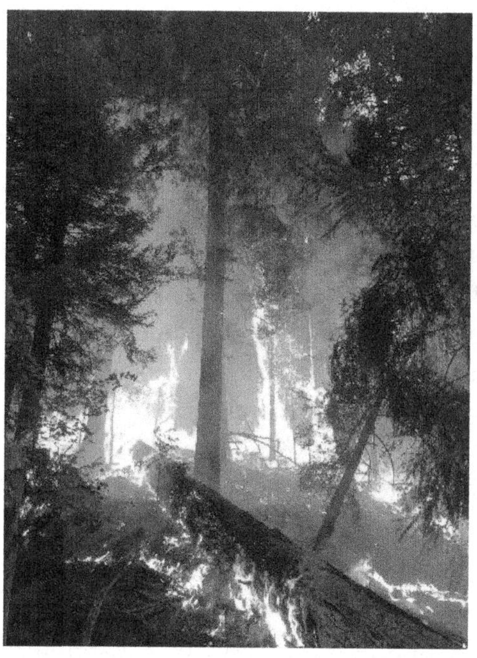

(*Firestorm 2020 Umpqua National Forest — home of author Tammera Karr and others working on Empty Plate* – the Archie Creek fire (one of seven massive fires in western Oregon) destroyed over 109 residences along with campgrounds, millions of dollars of private timber, state and federal structures, and power grid infrastructure in forty-eight hours. Over six-weeks, the authors and those working with them on *Empty Plate* were challenged by evacuations, dense smoke, closed highways, utilities outages, and restricted access to food sources.)

Where to begin?

- Plan your excursions into the grocery stores just as you would a family camping trip or vacation. Consider those items you need, have room for and want. Placing the importance on *need* and *room* before *want.* A flashlight without batteries cannot provide light in the dark, for example. Writing a list versus typing one on your phone places information into the brain's memory regions more efficiently; a written list does not depend on battery life for accessibility. Planning ahead, plus, buying dry goods and staples (paper products, pet food, laundry soap...) in bulk (bulk foods may come from store bins or larger packaging), saves money and frustration.

  - Buy in bulk: flour, rice, beans, lentils, seeds, nuts, dried fruit, pasta, oatmeal, sugar, tea, and coffee. Buy in bulk **only** those foods that will be used over two to three months. Rotate older dry goods forward in cupboards each time you restock.

- On average, frozen foods have a four to six month shelf life; canned goods twenty-four months, and dry goods like beans, grains, and flour average eighteen months in sealed packaging. It is best if these are stored in a cool, dry area, not in a freezer.

- Take advantage of sales on favorite canned goods and condiments. Depending on the *best by dates*, these items may last six to twelve months, saving you trips to the store and allowing for creative flexibility in the kitchen.

  - Limit the foodstuffs that are a specialty items; it is better to have tomato sauce than spaghetti sauce, for example. A simple base food such as tomato sauce can be used in meatloaf, soups, sauces, and made into tomato soup.

- Change the frequency of trips to the market. Individuals are more prone to spontaneous, unhealthy purchases when they shop for food daily or even weekly. Limit weekly shopping to fresh produce; better yet, make an event out of frequenting local farmers' markets or farm stands, avoiding mega-stores altogether.
    - Take advantage of u-pick farms if you have children, so they learn about where food comes from and the pure pleasure of a berry bursting in their mouth fresh off the vine.
    - Don't be afraid of blemishes on fresh produce at farm stands or markets. Save money by buying seconds. Seconds are produce that is deemed to have *defects*; fruit that may be too large or small, have bruises or scars on the skins, or be older. Seconds can be found in farm markets, local farm stands, or conversing with a local produce manager at your favorite store. Many merchants will place custom orders for customers. Seconds work great for smoothies, hot cereal, compotes, desserts, and salads.
- Buy large cuts of meat: by buying a whole chicken, turkey, fish or roast, you can downsize your purchase later at home into a multitude of meal options and save money.
    - One turkey thigh in an InstantPot with vegetables and water makes several meals for one or two people.

- A pork loin or beef roast can be cut into cubes (stew meat), chops, roast, stir-fry, and ground meat. One pork loin or round roast of 3-pound; can produce up to ten servings.

- A whole chicken can be boned and sectioned; the bones and trimmings make broth, breast meat shredded for tacos, thighs for pot pie, and so forth.

- Utilize leftovers for breakfasts, lunches, and snacks.

➢ Buy organic quality cooking oils and butter — the healthy fats people consume are worth the extra money. This single food group is where the most significant chemical exposure may be. Animal fats are designed to trap substances in an animal's body for safety. Fats and oils hold toxins and environmental chemicals. Individuals should strive to use organic products, not wrapped in plastic, to reduce exposure to hormone-disrupting chemicals.

➢ Invest in a whole-home or multi-stage water filtration system. *We will cover this more momentarily.* If you are sure your water is safe and clean, there is no need to buy bottled water, which reduces plastic bottle waste and saves money. **see additional recommendations at the back.*

All of these suggestions save money, time, and frustration, especially when local stores are having difficulty due to seasonal weather or travel restrictions. When you keep a well-stocked pantry and freezer it is a positive step for sustainability.

> *"Avoiding or running away from challenges doesn't give meaning to our lives, but discovering our values and virtues as we struggle through them does. When we're forced to dig deep, we tap into reserves of power we never dreamed we had. Our inner warrior rises to meet us, and we're able to face hardship with strength and grace."*
>
> ~ Tieraona Low Dog, MD

Modern innovation and unintended consequences

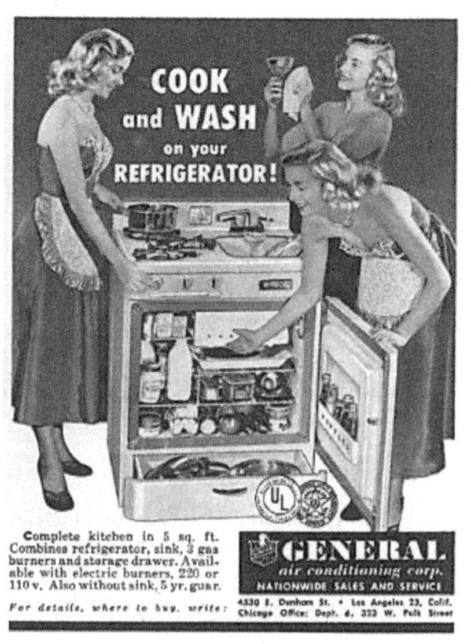

General Air Conditioning 1952
Collier's Magazine

The 21st century has presented more than one challenge to healthy living. How can it be that a seemingly innocent or benign factor could be the cause of so many health problems? Modern innovation has provided us with countless tools and conveniences that make our jobs and lives easier. The *unintended* consequences of innovation have resulted in more plastic trash, an increasingly fractured sense of time, escalating health challenges, and the prevalence of industrial denatured foods.

How do folks take out the trash both figuratively and physically without driving themselves and others around the bend? By looking back at what was the norm in the days before the advent of drinking water packaged in plastic bottles or artificial flavorings. Two of the most proactive and sustainable suggestions for achieving health are adding more vegetables to your daily intake and removing 300 calories per day of refined/processed foods.

> *Principle 4*: The most proactive thing we can do for our health is cut 300 calories daily from industrially processed foods and add 300 calories of locally produced vegetables.

Here is one scenario: Client "A" works as a long-haul truck driver. He tries to eat healthy on the road five days a week, but there is not much of a fresh food selection in truck stops. Even if he tries to make some food that he can take on the road, only a tiny refrigerator is available, and there is no real way to cook.

Solutions: Incorporate a shake once a day with freeze-dried fruit and vegetable powders. The use of a 12-volt blender makes smoothie mixes palatable. The freeze-dried blends add in greater nutrient variety; freeze-dried vegetable and fruit mixtures can be used as seasoning, provided.

On a day off, client "A" could plan two hours for food preparation; making up small airtight containers with raw vegetables, nuts, and fruit. It is much easier to eat a handful of sugar snap peas, kohlrabi, turnip, broccoli stems, or yam slices than to stop and peel them or try to eat them whole. *Recommendation:* The glass canning jars or Snapware brand containers seal tight and do not leak. These glass containers fit easily in a small soft-sided cooler and work in a *HotLogic* heated lunchbox. Experience has shown foods hold up in these containers in the fridge or cooler for three to four days.

Hard-boiled eggs in the shell, canned chicken, pork, beef, or fish like sardines and salmon are easy proteins. The eggs last in a small refrigerator or cooler with ice for three to four days. The low sodium canned meats do not require refrigeration and can be used with convenience store salads, rye crackers, or a loaf of hearty bread. Pre-cook brown rice, baked sweet or red potatoes, can add more variety.

Next, purchase a small HotLogic personal oven. Before heading down the road, combine the prepped vegetables in their glass dish, a small sliced parboiled potato, one can of meat with liquid, and plug into a 12-volt outlet on the dash. In two to three hours, a meal is hot and ready to eat during fuel up or at the end of shift.

For many individuals, spending a little time prepping for the coming week and investing in a couple of small appliances can result in dropping 400 calories without having to think about it or go hungry. Increasing raw vegetable consumption provides crunchy foods that help replace chips and other processed snack foods, which are often eaten to combat boredom, stress, and/or sleep. By making this one dietary change to save calories, individuals who work on the road can relax and enjoy eating with family or friends guilt-free on their weekends off.

The additional increase in vegetables in a daily routine does more than act as fuel; vegetables provide dietary fiber that feeds the gut microbiota responsible for removing toxins and chemicals. Fresh whole foods nourish the brain for improved cognition, support healthy blood sugar levels, support commensal bacteria, build immune function and remove excess cholesterol and sodium while providing potassium and magnesium for heart health. [94]

To answer the questions about many of our present food dilemmas, all one has to do is think back to times before we had prepackaged, processed foods and fried convenience foods from gas station quick-marts.

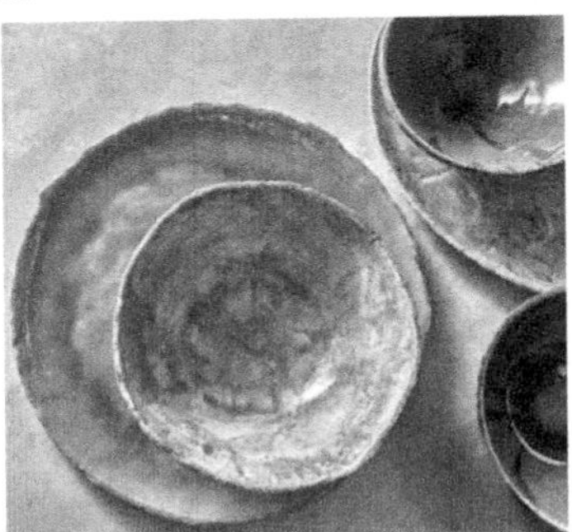

Principle 5: Planning ahead for the manageable *what ifs*, adds a level of freedom from fear and worry — allowing for more enjoyable adventures in life.

Plastics come of age and bring unintended consequences

Plastics are almost exclusively made from fossil fuels and led to a market ripe for development. In 1935 the development of *plastic fibers* rayon and nylon, came into use as synthetic silk and, were used during World War II. The use of synthetic silk materials filled a need for parachutes, ropes, body armor, helmet liners, and more. World War II necessitated a significant expansion of the plastics industry. Plexiglass provided an alternative to glass for aircraft windows. During World War II, plastic production increased by 300% in the United States. [95]

It wasn't long until plastic was everywhere, and thousands of products were being made. By the mid-1960s American perceptions changed, and plastics were no longer seen as entirely positive. [96] Plastic debris in the oceans was first observed in the 1960s when Americans became increasingly aware of environmental problems.

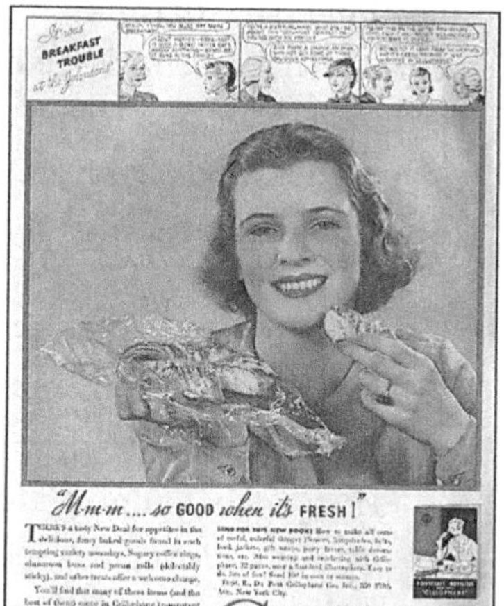

1935 DuPont Chemical Comp.
Good Housekeeping Magazine

Unlike natural fibers, such as fur, paper, and metal — which break down organically over time, plastics last in the environment forever. They break down into microplastic beads that are ingested by birds, fish, humans, and animals. [97,98] In addition to the ease with which natural fibers break down into the soil, they are also traditional materials that connect people with their culture and nature. When cared for properly, an Irish wool sweater will last for one's lifetime and into the next person's with little impact on the environment.

The reality is our lives are inextricably linked with all forms of plastics; cars to computers, medications to diapers, and bottled water — nearly everything we need or do has plastic involved. As such, the mindful serving on our empty plate urges us to think twice before buying or replacing items made from plastic and seek out those made traditionally from natural materials.

Unintended consequences to health

Phthalates are the most common form of plastics that are found in animals and humans. When viewing government and industry websites, it is easy to see reports slanted to protect industry versus human health. Again and again, statements like *more research needs to be done, effects are unknown at this time*, and *small studies whose results cannot be generalized* will appear at the end of research studies on phthalates' effects on living creatures.

Phthalate studies released in 2020 linked long-lasting adverse effects on motor function in children whose mothers were exposed to phthalates during late pregnancy. [99] And in a 2019 study from the Department of Genetic Medicine and Development at UNIGE Faculty of Medicine affect gene expression. The study revealed, "Phthalates, one of the most common endocrine disruptors, are commonly used by industry in many plastic products; toys, clothing, baby bottles, or even medical equipment; as well as in cosmetics. Guidelines are beginning to be imposed to limit their use; their toxic effect on the endocrine system is worrying." [100, 101]

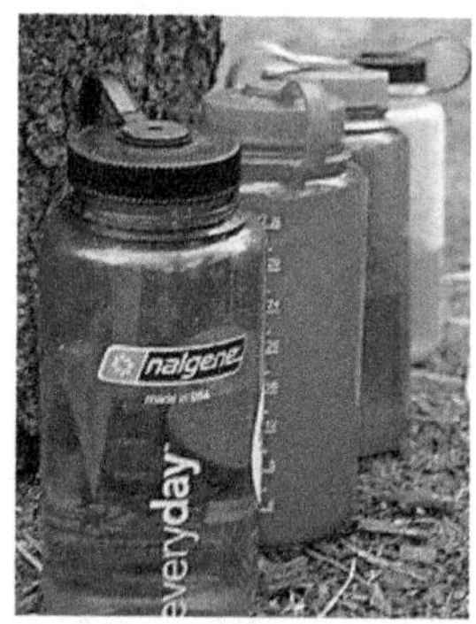

The *PLOS One* magazine raises the question of individual vulnerability to phthalates and the possible transmission to future generations of epigenetic changes that should normally be erased during fetal development.

> Indeed, the exposure of male fetuses to phthalates can have devastating consequences for the fertility of future individuals by modifying the regulatory elements of the expression of genes responsible for spermatogenesis — phthalate susceptibility depends mainly on the genetic heritage of each individual. [102, 103]

Studies from 2015 and 2017 reveal exposures to specific phthalates used in consumer products from plastic toys, household building materials, and personal care products including toothpaste and shampoos, were associated with depressed thyroid function in girls at age 3, and early exposure in the womb to phthalates disrupts the masculinization of male genitals. [104, 105]

Phthalates are just one of the hundreds of human-made chemicals being found in humans. The research reported on through the Environmental Working Group (EWG) revealed the average male has over fifty chemicals present in blood tests and women over 168. [106, 107]

> *"Once you were a child. Once you knew what inquiry was for.*
> *There was a time when you asked questions because you wanted answers and were glad when you had found them.*
> *Become that child again: even now."*
> ~ C.S. Lewis [108]

Putting toxins in perspective

With the growing exposure to hormone-disrupting phthalates and heavy metals in food supplies, one may ask themself questions on future generations' sustainability and health. One area of concern is baby food, especially when looking at heavy metals and fluoride. [109, 110, 111]

Many health professionals, nutritionists, and biologists misuse the word *mineral*. When they say *mineral* in the context of human nutrition, they really mean *dietary element*. An *element* is a pure substance that cannot be broken down into anything simpler by chemical means. The one exception in a healthy human is bone mineral hydroxyapatite, found in bones and teeth. Bone mineral is an inorganic, crystalline, solid with a single chemical formula and qualifies as a genuine mineral.

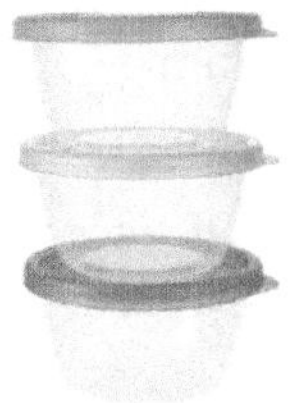

Organic dietary elements — these were living and can bring life to cells. Organic dietary elements contain carbon, and their electrons spin clockwise, like those of the human body. Additionally, these cells can form an ionic bond and easily break down to help with bodily function, such as tissue repair. [112]

Inorganic elements — these were never living without carbon and cannot bring life to cells. The body treats these elements as toxins. These materials are tightly held together; they cannot easily be broken down. And, their electrons spin counterclockwise, out of sync with animal and human cell function. [113]

In 2016, the European Union (EU) set new allowable inorganic arsenic standards for food manufacturers. Research out of Queen's University Belfast found in 2017 that almost half of all rice baby food products contained dangerous levels of inorganic arsenic despite new regulations. [114]

What to know about arsenic

Next to baby cereals made from rice, which absorbs more arsenic than any other food crop; juice is the next leading source of arsenic in the diet, followed by tap water. For parents concerned about arsenic exposure from fruit juices, the American Academy of Pediatrics (AAP) recommends that: [115, 116]

- Infants under 1 year of age should not drink juice.
- Toddlers ages 1–3 should not drink more than 4 ounces of juice per day.
- Children ages 4–6 should not drink more than 4 to 6 ounces of juice per day.
- Children ages 7–18 should not drink more than 8 ounces of juice per day.

The good news: Research has once again confirmed what past generations already knew about traditional food preparation. When baby food is made fresh each day at home; phthalate, heavy metal, and chemical exposure significantly decrease. Research published in 2019 in the journal *Environmental Science & Technology* found inorganic arsenic in rice is reduced when traditional parboiling methods are used. Also, the calcium content in rice is increased. [117]

According to the World Health Organization (WHO), mercury is one of the most harmful substances for human health. Mercury can influence the nervous system and the development of the brain. Mercury exposure is particularly detrimental to children and can also be transmitted from a mother to a fetus during pregnancy. [118]

The good news: Traditional water filtration methods involving wood, bacteria impregnated tiles, and the sun through the forms of carbon and steam are affordable for most. [119] Municipalities and industry may soon be employing filtration systems developed in Sweden; where researchers developed a method of removing mercury from large-scale water sources in 2018. The process works via extracting the heavy metal ions from water by encouraging them to form an alloy with another metal. [120]

> Today, cleaning away the low, yet harmful, levels of mercury from large amounts of water is a major challenge. Industries need better methods to reduce the risk of mercury being released in nature, says Björn Wickman at the Department of Chemistry and Chemical Engineering at Chalmer. [121]

Vintage dishes and lead

Plastic and disposable paper plates are loaded with chemicals; these chemicals are called xenoestrogens, and they displace endogenously produced hormones on cell receptor sites. [122] But these chemicals are not the only thing that alters hormone function. Heavy metals, mercury, and lead also alter hormone pathways, uptake and the commensal bacteria in the large intestine that facilitate excess estrogens (there are four estrogens) clearance. [123]

With the resurgence of repurposing, many are seeking out vintage dishware in thrift stores. The problem with vintage dishware; it can be a dangerous source of heavy metals (HM); lead, arsenic, and cadmium, especially for children. [124] As many as 800 million children have dangerously high lead values in their blood. [125] No

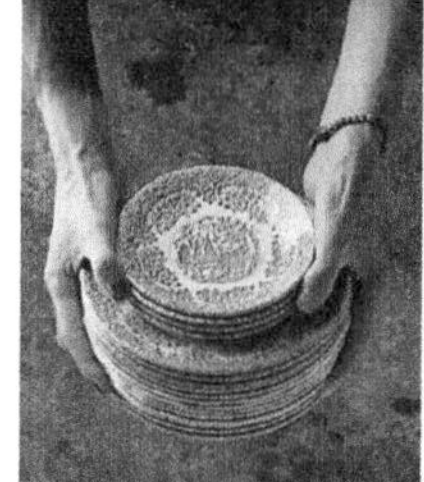

value limit has been established that is considered safe, and, therefore, the number of children affected could be much higher both in Norway and in other countries. The report from Pure Earth and UNICEF, published in late 2020, "shines the spotlight on lead as an important global environmental and health problem that is especially tied to children's health and development," says Heidi Aase, who heads the NeuroTox study at the Norwegian Institute of Public Health.

The NeuroTox study examines relationships between environmental toxins in the mother's womb, including lead, and various brain development measures. ADHD, autism and cognitive functions are considered in a large sample of Norwegian children. Environmental toxins found in the mother's body during pregnancy can affect the baby's development.

"A child's earliest years of life are characterized by rapid growth and brain development. This makes children particularly vulnerable to harmful substances in the environment," says Kam Sripada, a postdoc at the Norwegian University of Science and Technology (NTNU). [126]

When looking at lead safety levels, consider the following: Greater than 45 micrograms per deciliter of lead in blood is unsafe for children. [127]

What is vintage dishware? It may be surprising to learn dishes in the cupboards from as recent as 1998 are listed right alongside grandma's vintage dishware. According to the Corning website and customer service, *lead* and *cadmium* are present in their dishware manufactured up until 2005.

Vintage dishes to replace due to lead and cadmium on the eating surface [128]

Manufacturer's Style	Lead ppm	Cadmium ppm	Arsenic ppm
Vintage Cream	28,000	150	
Vintage Blue and Yellow Floral with Butterflies	41,500		
Spice and Leaf pattern	42,900	557	
Old Franciscan Desert Rose China made in England	47,800		
Desert Rose earthenware China c. 1941 made in the USA	122,000		
Johnson Bros. Willow pattern China post-1912	43,100		
Glass Measuring cup c. 1994 Red lettering on the outside	6,253		
Red vintage Pyrex Refrigerator Food storage container With glass lid	310,000	33,200	14,200

Tupperware, a better pick?

Yellow Tupperware: 2677 ppm cadmium, 15 ppm mercury
Green Tupperware: 2,780 ppm lead, 234 ppm arsenic [129]

It is noteworthy that the lead is in the outer colored surface of vintage Pyrex dishes and containers. Other listings refer to the surface area where food touches the glazed area.

In a statement answering a customer question on safety and use of their vintage Corelle dinnerware circa 2000 (note:

vintage is older than twenty years), a Corelle customer service representative replied with: "Prior to the 1990s, virtually all glass and ceramic ware made *anywhere* in the world contained *lead*." Happily, as of 2018, Corelle is a market leader in creating lead-free dishware. That is great as long as an individual buys only plain white dinnerware. Even though their new products do tend to be completely *lead-free*, these products have been testing positive for cadmium (in specific colors) — at levels considered potentially concerning, given cadmium is a known carcinogen. [130, 131, 132]

Ways to reduce plastic through clothing: Use natural fibers like linen, cotton, bamboo, hemp, fur, leather, wool, and silk over polyester, rayon, fleece, or nylon; and reduce clothing and shoe purchases. Buy quality classic styles that fit well, feels good, and lasts.

> *Principle 6:* Select glass, low toxin/HM ceramic, metal, wood, bamboo, and high-grade gloss paper over plastic or vintage dishware.

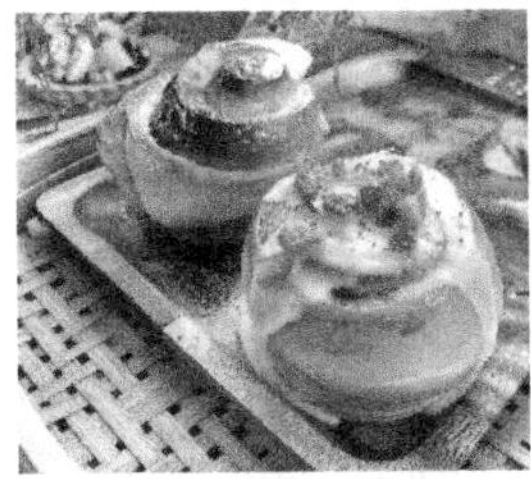

While we can't all be the *Don Quixote* of the 21st century, tilting at every windmill of concern; we can still make mindful choices. After reading all of this information on toxins in dishware, the simple banana leaf plate and the bread trencher sound pretty safe!

How is it that so many generations have passed without toxic levels of lead?

Well, they haven't is the answer. Childhood mortality was enormous before the 1960s, so there is no clear way of knowing how many newborns to three-year-old children before the 1960s died because of heavy metal toxicity. The next part of the answer lies in relationship to vegetable consumption by earlier populations; especially those foods capable of trapping and removing heavy metals and chemical toxins such as garlic, cilantro, and flat-leaf parsley, as well as blueberries, lemon water, sea vegetables like dulse, cabbage, cauliflower, Brussels sprouts, greens of all kinds, black and green tea, tomatoes, and naturally fermented foods. [133, 134] All of these foods were eaten at much higher levels from 1900 to 1960. [135]

Recommendations

- Replace old dinnerware with certified lead and cadmium free dinnerware. There are quite a few American-made dishes now available. HF Coors dinnerware, established in 1925, is a disabled veteran-owned company and certified lead-free.

- Eat plenty of vegetables and fermented foods that are vital to health in every aspect.

- Clean house; save those vintage pieces that have emotional significance to family members, but reconsider their daily use, especially when children are eating.

Three questions to ask

Intolerances to chemicals, foods, and drugs impact 8%–33% of individuals, yet few people are screened for it at their doctors' offices. To address this and increase awareness of chemical intolerance, researchers at The University of Texas Health Science Center at San Antonio (UT Health San Antonio) developed and validated a three-question, yes-or-no survey. This easy to use test for primary care providers, allergists, dermatologists, and other specialists can be incorporated into client visits. The survey is called the *Brief Environmental Exposure and Sensitivity Inventory,* or *BREESI.*

The *BREESI* focuses on three different exposure categories: chemical inhalants, drugs/medications, and foods/food additives. The research team enrolled 293 volunteers from a university-based primary care clinic and online to complete the BREESI and QEESI.

- Of respondents who said *yes* to all three BREESI questions, 90% had scored *very suggestive* of chemical intolerance.

- Of those who said *no* to all three BREESI questions, 95% had scored *not suggestive* of chemical intolerance.

Currently, Claudia S. Miller, MD, MS, professor emeritus in the Joe R. and Teresa Lozano Long School of Medicine at UT Health San Antonio, is concerned that misuse of disinfectants to combat COVID-19 may be endangering susceptible individuals. Combustion products from the 2020 California and Oregon wildfires are another concern.

Outgassing volatile organic chemicals (VOCs) from new construction, remodeling, and *sick* buildings frequently triggers chemically intolerant individuals' symptoms.

> Quick screening questionnaires are used routinely in clinics today, e.g., for quality of life or substance abuse, or reactions to antibiotics or latex, and we believe chemical intolerance also needs to be assessed routinely, given its high prevalence, [136]

The Brief Environmental Exposure and Sensitivity Inventory [137]

1. Do you feel sick when you are exposed to tobacco smoke, certain fragrances, nail polish/remover, engine exhaust, gasoline, air fresheners, pesticides, paint/thinner, fresh tar/asphalt, cleaning supplies, new carpet, or furnishings? *By sick, we mean: headache, difficulty thinking, difficulty breathing, weakness, dizziness, upset stomach, etc.*

Yes No

2. Are you unable to tolerate or do you have adverse or allergic reactions to any drugs or medications (such as antibiotics, anesthetics, pain relievers, X-ray contrast dye, vaccines, or birth control pills) or to an implant, prosthesis, contraceptive chemical, or device, or other medical/surgical/dental material or procedure?

Yes No

3. Are you unable to tolerate, or do you have adverse reactions to any foods such as dairy products, wheat, corn,

eggs, caffeine, alcoholic beverages, or food additives (e.g., MSG, food dye)?

Yes No

- The research revealed that 97% of persons answering **Yes** to all three items on the BREESI had high CI scores as assessed by the QEESI.
- If two items were endorsed, approximately 84% of the sample had high CI scores.
- If one item was endorsed, 48% had high CI scores. 100% of those who answered **No** to all of the BREESI items showed no evidence of CI on the QEESI.

Any individual answering **Yes** to one or more of the three BREESI screening items should take the full QEESI at www.TILTresearch.org.

Sustainability is a multifaceted process

Americans do not need more food — it is quite the reverse; what is desperately needed is more nutrition. There is no nutrition in a calorie; it is a measure of heat energy output. Nutrition provides the building blocks for health, growth, repair, cognitive elasticity, and longevity. Without the incorporation into the food of vitamins, minerals, co-factors, sugars, enzymes, and amino acids, there would be no life as we know it. One cannot live a sustainable life on calories alone.

Just as the use of calories as a measure of food quality is flawed, so is the popular rhetoric on *Farmers Feeding the World*. Humans do not need more food produced; worldwide, there are tons of food wasted every day. The answer is far simpler; a return to diverse and sustainable practices that do not feed off the empty calories of subsidies and farm policies driven by the multinational food and drug industries.

The original intention of farm subsidies was to reduce the risk farmers endure from the weather, commodities brokers, and demand disruptions. Due to the complexity of subsidies, only large producers can take advantage and qualify. [138] There are only five crops subsidized by the federal government: corn, soybeans, wheat, cotton, and rice; raised in Texas, Nebraska, Kansas, Arkansas, and Illinois. In 2017, these five states received 38.5% of the $7.2 billion distributed. Producers of foods such as meat, fruits, and vegetables can only benefit from crop insurance and disaster relief. Between 1995 and 2017, $369.7 billion was paid out to a handful of industrial farms. [139]

According to the United States Department of Agriculture (USDA), the total U.S. corn crop for 2018–19 was projected at 14 billion bushels. Food, seed, and industrial use were expected to increase 75 million bushels, reaching 7.1 billion, an increase associated with ethanol production. [140, 141] By comparison, California produces the most food by value: almonds, wine, dairy, walnuts, and pistachios; these crops, however, are not subsidized. [142]

Subsidies act like a regressive tax that helps high-income businesses, not rural farmers. Between 1995 and 2017, the top 10% of recipients received 77% of the $205.4 billion in federal subsidies. The top 1% of industrial farms received 26% of the subsidy payments. [143] That averages out to $1.7 million per corporate industrial farm company. Fifty people on the Forbes 400 list of the wealthiest Americans own industrial farm companies that received farm subsidies. By comparison, 62% of U.S. farms did not receive any subsidies. This 62% is made up of many rural farmers who augment their income through local-direct-to-consumer sales at local businesses and markets.

Since 2013, America's farmers and ranchers have weathered a 45% drop in net farm income; the largest three-year drop since the start of the Great Depression. This wrongdoing is the result of policies designed to enrich corporations at the expense of farmers and ranchers. [144] Those who have lived around agriculture know that the modern food system's problems are not with the farm or the volume being produced. The problems of waste, cruelty, and denaturing of food happens after food leaves the farm when it enters the industrial machine of *Big Food.*

In 1996, Via Campesina coined the expression *food sovereignty*. *Food sovereignty* is defined as "the right of peoples to healthy and culturally appropriate food produced through ecologically sound and sustainable methods, and their right to define their own food and agriculture systems." [145, 146]

Sustainability is a multifaceted process that begins with turning the soil and planting of seed and ends with consumers' daily choices. Unfortunately, we are at a time in history when large multi-national corporations own 80% of our manufactured foods and meats. In the present scenario, our food is far from local.

Permit yourself to enjoy simple food

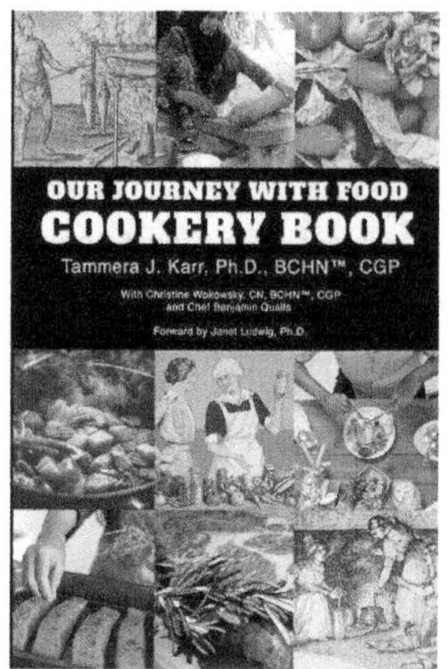

Older print versions of cookbooks like *Joy of Cooking* and *Better Homes and Garden Cookbook* or modern "homesteader" cookbooks like *Our Journey with Food Cookery Book* by Tammera Karr *or The Prairie Homestead Cookbook* by Jill Winger (2019) are filled with basic recipes. These recipes provide freedom and flexibility and do not require boxed or canned mixes. Older cookbooks additionally provide information on fermenting and even simple canning.

Suggestion: Use *Post-it Notes* (stiff page markers), in cookbooks to write recipe modifications on so they do not fall out. There are thousands of cookbooks available electronically, but recipe accuracy does not always occur in many newer versions. There is also a loss of valuable information on altitude adjustments and substitutions found in older cookbooks.

These reliable cookbooks are just as valuable today as they were to the pioneers or families of the 1940s. They represent simpler times and comfort for us, knowing we can make almost anything from scratch if we have a well-stocked pantry. The value of printed cookbook copies is they do not depend on electricity or technology to function. Print cookbooks can be used while camping without fear of draining the battery or a network failure.

> *"By matter we are nourished, lifted up, linked to everything else, invaded by life."*
>
> ~ Pierre Teilhard de Chardin

How do food traditions help?

Food equals memories: Traditional foods based on heritage, culture, and location vary widely. Foods also carry strong memories of events and people. Fragrances from spices, herbs, and foods can comfort people when they are lonely, overwhelmed, or anxious. Food is a simple way to honor one's connection to culture, family, friends, and the environment.

Because the motions associated with cooking are familiar, there is a type of muscle memory— it is almost automatic; the chopping or slicing, the heating of the oil, the stirring and seasoning — these are practiced and deeply ingrained actions that do not require intense thought. Their repeated performance acts as a tonic to calm stress hormones and the central nervous system. The benevolent and reverent motions of hands combined with the smells of cooking and eating food can be a form of meditation.

A peek at genetics: past, present, and future

Our physical environment, stress, lifestyle, and food nutrients determine our health from before conception to death. What we eat is related to how and when our genes are activated, decreasing or increasing genetic predispositions. Research supports the fact that lifestyle has a more significant effect on our health than our DNA. [147, 148] In 2011, researchers began publishing findings on lifestyle effects on gene expression, and the science of epigenetics was born. Epigenetics has changed the predominant scientific view from DNA ruling our course to **us** ruling our DNA. [149, 150, 151, 152]

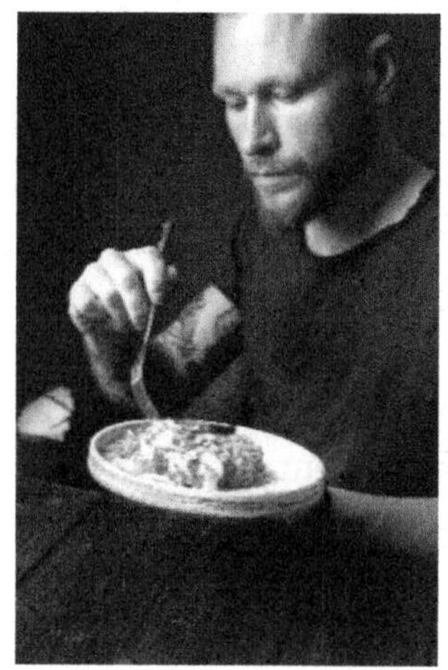

Individuals are more than their DNA. The foods we take in, the various chemicals and substances we are exposed to in our environment, and life events; all work to activate and deactivate genetic regulation.

For health to be sustainable, one has to look beyond the surface of events. The sustainability of humanity's health incorporates the past, present, and future. Let's look for a moment at one virus: Smallpox *(variola virus)* holds a unique position in medical history. It was the first disease for which a vaccine was developed and remains the only human disease eradicated by vaccination.

After years of fishing for viral DNA in ancient human remains, genetic evidence is revealing more of the evolutionary and necessary role of viruses. The information on the human virome is just beginning to emerge. Scientists have identified 33,242 unique viral populations that are present in the human gut. This is not cause for alarm; most viruses don't cause disease. According to researchers out of Ohio State University, each person's gut virus composition is as unique as a fingerprint. [153]

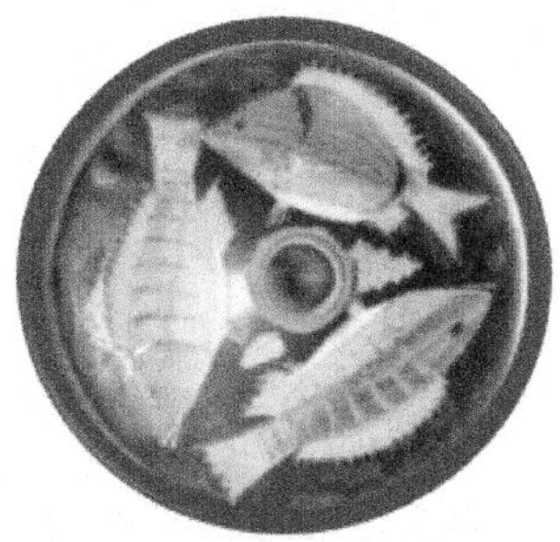

Humans as far back as 600 A.D. carried the *variola virus.* [154, 155] Smallpox is only one example of a severe infectious disease whose history has been suddenly and substantially rewritten by ancient DNA analysis. [156] Equally, researchers are showing the history of viruses jumping from one species to humans is not new. DNA research is in the earliest days of looking at the human virome and how viruses make up human DNA. [157]

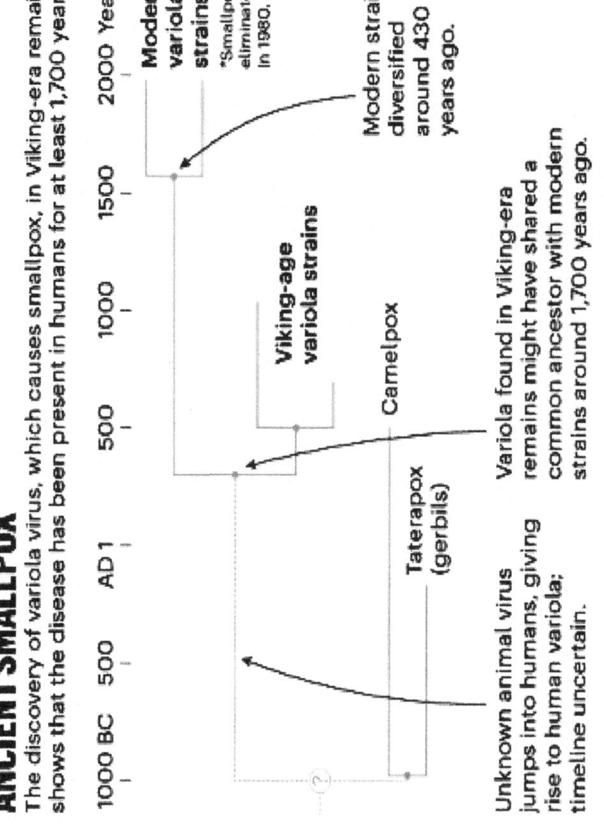

Nature Research Journal - Smallpox and other viruses plagued humans much earlier than suspected. https://www.nature.com/articles/d41586-020-02083-0

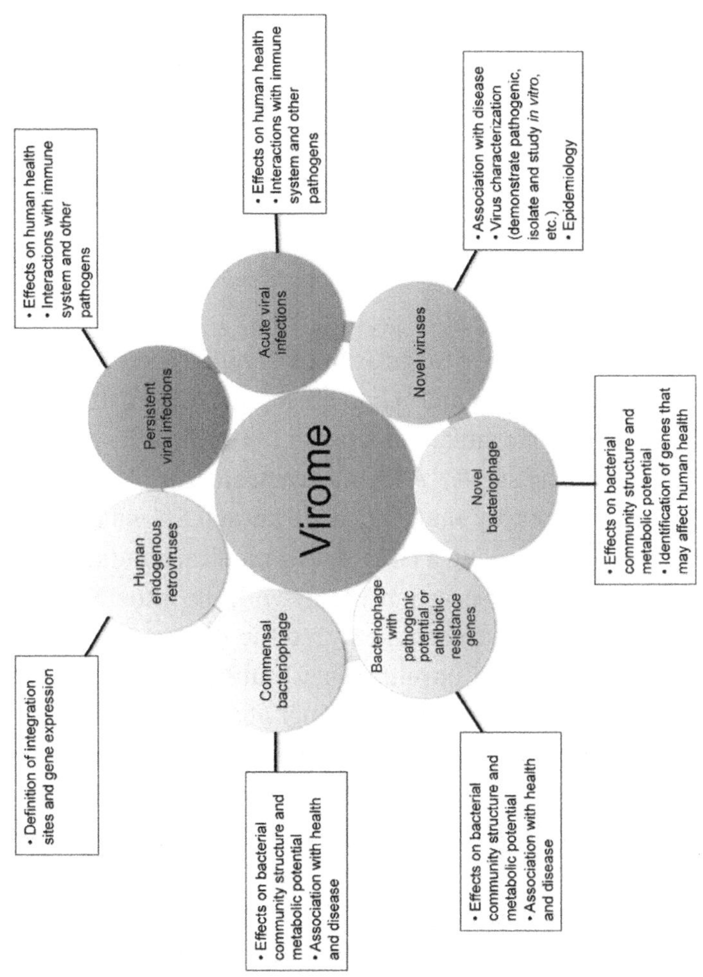

From page 128. Components of the human virome. Circles represent components of the virome that can be characterized by metagenomic sequencing.
Wylie, K. M., Weinstock, G. M., & Storch, G. A. (2012). Emerging view of the human virome. Translational research: the journal of laboratory and clinical medicine, 160(4), 283–290. https://doi.org/10.1016/j.trsl.2012.03.006

Principle 7: Eat those foods from your personal genetics that make your DNA sing.

The next generation

Children inherit four times as many new gene mutations from their fathers than their mothers. According to research, this fact suggests faults in the male DNA are a driver for rare childhood diseases. [158] Allan Pacey, professor of andrology at Sheffield University said: "We have known for many years that the risk of having a child with a medical condition of genetic origin increases noticeably with the father's age at conception." Researchers analyzed the DNA of 1,500 Icelanders and their parents. They found new mutations from mothers increased by 0.37 per year of age; one-quarter of the rate found in men. While most new mutations are harmless, they can occasionally disrupt the workings of important genes for health.

In one section of chromosome *8*, scientists found new mutations were passed on from mothers. The researchers found fifty-times more mutations from the mother in chromosome *8* than in any other genome part.

> It seems that when a chromosome breaks in an egg, it can sometimes be repaired, avoiding a chromosomal catastrophe but leaving a scar of small mutations, said Martin Taylor, a geneticist at the University of Edinburgh. [159]

Men passed on one new mutation for every eight months of age, compared with women who passed on a new mutation for every three years of age. The figures mean that a child born to 30-year-old parents would, on average, inherit eleven new mutations from the mother but 45 from the father. [160]

> *Principle 8*: Diets should be based on individual needs, not agendas, politics, philosophy, or dogma. One size does **not** fit All.

The 1998 ACE Study revealed adverse childhood experiences (ACEs) could contribute significantly to negative adult physical and mental health outcomes and affect more than 60% of adults. This continues to be reaffirmed with more recent studies. [161] The effect of toxic stress resulting from trauma may not appear right away or as expected. Traumatic sources of toxic stress may not be apparent to a clinician. Psychological maltreatment can be traumatic and stressful. [162]

In 2010, researchers asked the question, *Does the Impact of Psychological Trauma Cross Generations?* An individual's age, gender, and culture play a role in how *lonely they feel*, for example. Mitochondrial DNA may be responsible for transmitting generational information; memories of past generations.

Their findings?

> "It is fascinating that clinical observations in humans have suggested the possibility that specific traits acquired during life and influenced by environmental factors may be transmitted across generations," said lead researcher Dr. Mansuy. [163]

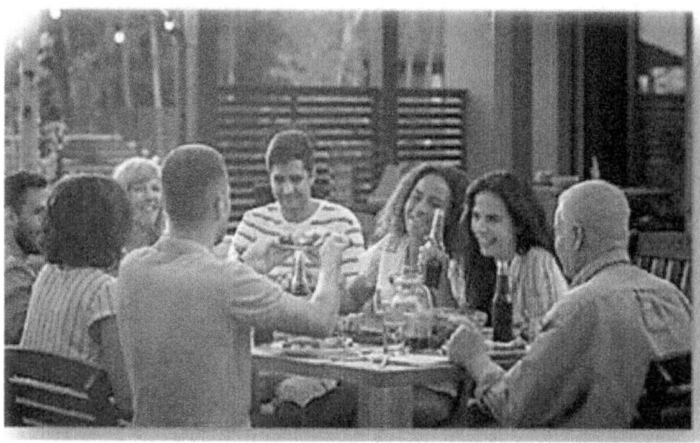

The human body and the DNA within are intimately connected to the environment and Nature's natural cycles. In recent years, several genome-wide association studies (GWAS) of sleep-related traits have identified a number of single nucleotides polymorphism (SNPs), but their relationships with insomnia symptoms were not known. [164] Sleep is an essential state of decreased activity and alertness. Through genome-wide association analysis in 446,118 adults of European ancestry, researchers found that 5% of participants carrying the most sleep duration-increasing alleles reported 22.2 minutes longer sleep duration compared to the 5% carrying the fewest.

The disruption of healthy sleep patterns from artificial and natural light activates or deactivates aspects of SNPs' genetic variants.[165, 166]

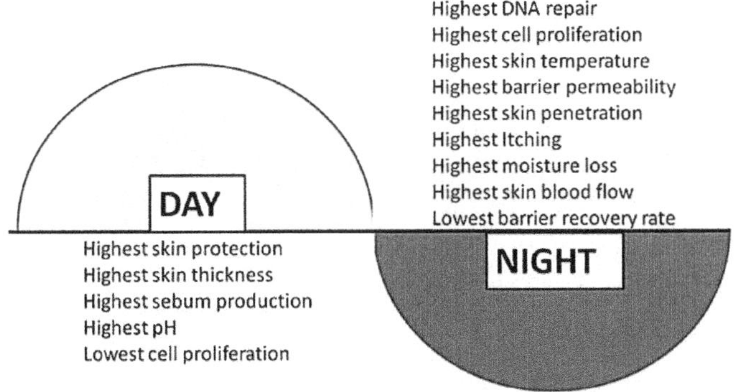

Image Credit: Matsui MS, Pelle E, Dong K, Pernodet N. Biological Rhythms in the Skin. Int J Mol Sci. 2016;17(6):801. Published 2016 May 24. doi:10.3390/ijms17060801

The pattern is emerging on the empty plate: it connects people to the past, forms connections with one another here and now, and offers a peek into the future.

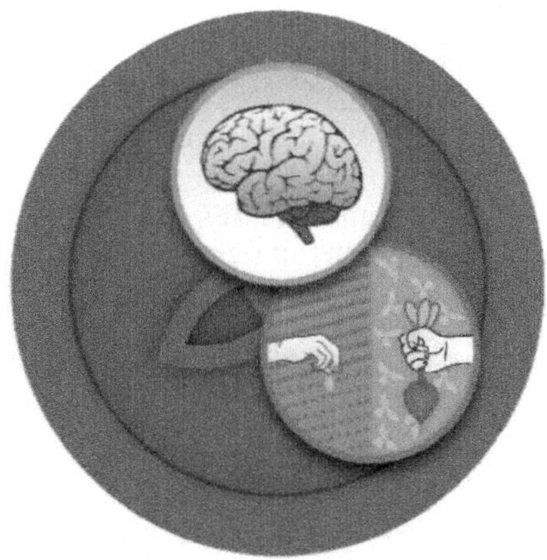

---

1. David Whyte, Poet, Author, Speaker: Https://Www.Davidwhyte.Com/#Home
2. Natural Capitalism 2000, Opening Page
3. Https://Livingonthefaultlines.Com/David-Whyte-Poems-Loaves-And-Fishes/
4. Radon - National Institute of Environmental Health Sciences https://www.niehs.nih.gov/health/topics/agents/radon/index.cfm
5. 10,000 BC: Paleo-Indian Era (Stone Age Culture) The Earliest Human Inhabitants Of America Who Lived In Caves And Were Nomadic Hunters Of Large Game Including The Great Mammoth And Giant Bison. Https://Www.Warpaths2peacepipes.Com/History-Of-Native-Americans/History-Of-Oregon-Indians.Htm
6. The Oregon Encyclopedia, Paisley Caves; Https://Oregonencyclopedia.Org/Articles/Paisley_Caves/#.Xwnonod7nb0
7. Cressman, Luther S. The Sandal And The Cave: The Indians Of Oregon. Corvallis: Oregon State University Press, 2005.
8. Jenkins, Dennis, Et Al. "Clovis Age Western Stemmed Projectile Points And Human Coprolites At The Paisley Caves." Science 337.6091 (July 13, 2012): 223-228.
9. The History Of Fusion Cuisine By Exquisite – 2015; Https://Exquisite-Taste-Magazine.Com/The-History-Of-Fusion-Cuisine/
10. Diabetologia. (2017, November 9). Consumption Of Antioxidant-Rich Foods Is Associated With A Lower Risk Of Type 2 Diabetes, Study Shows. Sciencedaily. Retrieved July 10, 2020 From Www.Sciencedaily.Com/Releases/2017/11/171109224048.Htm
11. Plant-based 'meats' improve some cardiovascular risk https://www.sciencedaily.com/releases/2020/08/200811125045.htm
12. Stanford Medicine. (2020, August 11). Plant-based 'meats' improve some cardiovascular risk factors compared with red meat. ScienceDaily. Retrieved August 12, 2020 from www.sciencedaily.com/releases/2020/08/200811125045.htm
13. University Of Southampton. (2017, April 26). Risk Of Obesity Influenced By Changes In Our Genes. Sciencedaily. Retrieved July 5, 2020 From Www.Sciencedaily.Com/Releases/2017/04/170426093316.Htm
14. Research Milestones For MS And Autoimmune Patients: By Wahls Team *Https://Terrywahls.Com/Research-Milestones-For-Ms-And-Autoimmune-Patients/*

15. Fast Food Makes The Immune System More Aggressive In The Long Term, 2018: *Https://Www.Uni-Bonn.De/News/010-2018*

16. Processed Sugars Vs. Natural Sugars: What's The Difference?, 2017: *Http://Blogs.Oregonstate.Edu/Moore/Processed-Vs-Natural-Sugar/*

17. University Of South Florida (USF Innovation). (2020, July 6). People With High Cholesterol Should Eliminate Carbs, Not Saturated Fat, Study Suggests. Sciencedaily. Retrieved July 7, 2020 From Www.Sciencedaily.Com/Releases/2020/07/200706113955.Htm

18. Processed Sugars Vs. Natural Sugars: What's The Difference?, 2017: Http://Blogs.Oregonstate.Edu/Moore/Processed-Vs-Natural-Sugar/

19. NIH Study Finds Heavily Processed Foods Cause Overeating And Weight Gain, 2019: Https://Www.Nih.Gov/News-Events/News-Releases/Nih-Study-Finds-Heavily-Processed-Foods-Cause-Overeating-Weight-Gain

20. Takata H, Suzuki M, Ishii T, Sekiguchi S, Iri H. Influence of major histocompatibility complex region genes on human longevity among Okinawan-Japanese centenarians and nonagenarians. Lancet. 1987;2(8563):824-826. doi:10.1016/s0140-6736(87)91015-4

21. Passarino, G., De Rango, F., & Montesanto, A. (2016). Human longevity: Genetics or Lifestyle? It takes two to tango. Immunity & ageing : I & A, 13, 12. https://doi.org/10.1186/s12979-016-0066-z

22. vB Hjelmborg J, Iachine I, Skytthe A, et al. Genetic influence on human lifespan and longevity. Hum Genet. 2006;119(3):312-321. doi:10.1007/s00439-006-0144-y

23. Laskowski W, Górska-Warsewicz H, Kulykovets O. Meat, Meat Products And Seafood As Sources Of Energy And Nutrients In The Average Polish Diet. Nutrients. 2018;10(10):1412. Published 2018 Oct 2. Doi:10.3390/Nu10101412

24. Wójcik, Oktawia P Et Al. "The Potential Protective Effects Of Taurine On Coronary Heart Disease." Atherosclerosis Vol. 208,1 (2010): 19-25. Doi:10.1016/J.Atherosclerosis.2009.06.002

25. Poultry Production And The Environment – A Review, P. Gerber, C. Opio And H. Steinfeld; Animal Production And Health Division, Food And Agriculture Organization Of The United Nations, Viale Delle Terme Di Caracalla, 00153 Rome, Italy: Https://Sciencing.Com/Ecological-Impact-Chicken-Farming-5005.Html

26. Poultry Farms In Virginia - Eastern Shore Environmental Impact Of Chicken Farming, 2020; Https://Www.Waterfrontpropertylaw.Com/Blog/Posts/Poultry-Farming-Affect-Eastern-Shore/

---

27. Ecological Impact Of Chicken Farming: Https://Sciencing.Com/Ecological-Impact-Chicken-Farming-5005.Html

28. Hall, B., R.D. Protein Powder Passion: A Closer Look At One Of The Hottest Topics In Sports Nutrition. Muscle Media. 63:56-64, 1997.

29. Górska-Warsewicz, Hanna Et Al. "Food Products As Sources Of Protein And Amino Acids-The Case Of Poland." Nutrients Vol. 10,12 1977. 13 Dec. 2018, Doi:10.3390/Nu10121977

30. University Of Sydney. (2019, April 30). Put Down The Protein Shake: Variety Of Protein Better For Health: Popular Protein Great For Increasing Muscle Mass, But Could Reduce Your Life-Span -- Researchers Say To Vary Protein Intake. Sciencedaily. Retrieved July 3, 2020 From Www.Sciencedaily.Com/Releases/2019/04/190430091826.Htm

31. Liang, X., Wang, S., Qin, G., Xie, J., Tan, G., Zhou, J., Mcbride, D. W., & Chen, L. (2017). Tyrosine Phosphorylation Of NR2B Contributes To Chronic Migraines Via Increased Expression Of CGRP In Rats. Biomed Research International, 2017, 7203458. Https://Doi.Org/10.1155/2017/7203458

32. Low levels of serum serotonin and amino acids identified in migraine patients: Biochemical and Biophysical Research Communications, Volume 496, Issue 2, 5 February 2018, Pages 267-273, https://www.sciencedirect.com/science/article/abs/pii/S0006291X1732380X

33. Nicole R. Cannarozzi Et Al, Seasonal Oyster Harvesting Recorded In A Late Archaic Period Shell Ring, PLOS ONE (2019). DOI: 10.1371/Journal.Pone.0224666: Https://Phys.Org/News/2019-11-Oysters-Months-Thumb-Years.Html

34. Mirzal, R. "Do Marine Mollusks Possess Aphrodisiacal Properties?" Presented At The American Chemical Society Meeting, March 13-17, 2005, San Diego.

35. Pacific Oysters, Contain 1,550 Milligrams Of Omega-3 Fatty Acids (Eastern Oysters Contain About 500-550 Milligrams). Omega-3 Fatty Acids In Oysters Occur In Two Forms: Eicosapentaenoic Acid (EPA) And Docohexaenoic Acid (DHA). These Long-Chain Forms Of Omega-3 Are Considered Particularly Potent Because They Don't Have To Be Converted Into Other Compounds Before The Body Can Make Use Of Them. Source: Https://Www.Healwithfood.Org/Best-Dietary-Sources/Oysters-Omega-3-Content.Php#Ixzz6rb0udqfu

36. Mirriam-Websters second edition- Meat: animal tissue considered especially as food. Distinctions occure in culinary and religious dietary presets.

37. Food The Chemistry Of Its Components, 5th Edition By Tom Coultate 2009: Page 160-173

38. Believe It Or Not: Some Shellfish Contains Carbohydrate By Loren Cordain, Ph.D., 2014: Https://Thepaleodiet.Com/Believe-Shellfish-Contains-Carbohydrate

39. Wilson RP. Protein And Amino Acid Requirements Of Fishes. Annu Rev Nutr. 1986;6:225-244. Doi:10.1146/Annurev.Nu.06.070186.001301

40. Wójcik, Oktawia P Et Al. "The Potential Protective Effects Of Taurine On Coronary Heart Disease." Atherosclerosis Vol. 208,1 (2010): 19-25. Doi:10.1016/J.Atherosclerosis.2009.06.002

41. Not All Animal Foods (Meat, Poultry, Pork, Lamb, Beef, Eggs, Fish, Shellfish, Organ Meat, Etc.) Are Completely Composed Of Only Protein And Fat. Supermarket Meats Contained Almost No Carbohydrate For A Basic Physiologic Reason – Rigor Mortis – A Condition In Which The Muscles Go Into Rigid Contraction For The Few Minutes And Hours After Death. The Fuel That Supplies Rigor Mortis Is Stored Muscle Glycogen, And Once This Fuel Is Expended, Rigor Mortis Resides And Muscle Meats Contain Virtually Zero Glycogen And Hence Zero Carbohydrate.

42. Microbiota (N.)(Used With A Sing. Or Pl. Verb) The Microorganisms That Typically Inhabit A Particular Environment, Such As The Soil, A Body Of Water, Or A Site On Or In An Organism, Considered As A Group. Also Called Microbiome. Https://Medical-Dictionary.Thefreedictionary.Com/Microbiota

43. Industrial agriculture refers to a process of mechanizing the growing, harvesting, and processing of food. Rather than having a multitude of small family farms producing a variety of healthful, wholesome foods, we have huge, multinational, multibillion-dollar corporations that have maximized their ability to provide food by making every natural step in the life cycle of a crop or animal

44. United States Department Of Agriculture Food Safety And Inspection Service: Https://Www.Fsis.Usda.Gov/Wps/Portal/Fsis/Topics/Recalls-And-Public-Health-Alerts/Current-Recalls-And-Alerts

45. The Debate Over The Health Effects Of Food Processing By Colby Vorland, 2017: Https://Nutrition.Org/The-Debate-Over-The-Health-Effects-Of-Food-Processing/

46. The Local Food Movement As A Catalyst For Community By Tobias Roberts, 2017: Https://Permaculturenews.Org/2017/08/22/Local-Food-Movement-Catalyst-Community/

47. The Difference Between Soil And Dirt; Https://Www.Naturespath.Com/En-Us/Blog/Difference-Soil-Dirt/

---

48. A Mycorrhiza Is A Symbiotic Association Between A Green Plant And A Fungus. The Plant Makes Organic Molecules Such As Sugars By Photosynthesis And Supplies Them To The Fungus, And The Fungus Supplies To The Plant Water And Mineral Nutrients, Such As Phosphorus, Taken From The Soil.

49. Joel Salatin's Pattern For Carbon Farming At Polyface Farm, 2013: Https://Www.Permaculture.Co.Uk/Articles/Joel-Salatins-Pattern-Carbon-Farming-Polyface-Farm

50. Articles By Joel Salatin; Http://Www.Polyfacefarms.Com/Articles/

51. The Ecology Center; Https://Www.Theecologycenter.Org/

52. Sustainable Dish By Diana Rodgers, RD: Https://Sustainabledish.Com/

53. Biocodex Microbiota Institute: Https://Www.Biocodexmicrobiotainstitute.Com/En Human Microbiome

54. The mycorrhizal mutualistic association provides the fungus with relatively constant and direct access to carbohydrates, such as glucose and sucrose. The carbohydrates are translocated from their source (usually leaves) to root tissue and on to the plant's fungal partners. In return, the plant gains the benefits of the mycelium's higher absorptive capacity for water and mineral nutrients.

In some more complex relationships, mycorrhizal fungi do not just collect immobilized soil nutrients, but connect individual plants together by mycorrhizal networks that transport water, carbon, and other nutrients directly from plant to plant through underground hyphal networks; Https://En.Wikipedia.Org/Wiki/Mycorrhiza

55. Gut Microbiomes Of Herbivores And Carnivores October 29, 2015 By Oliver: Http://Cohanlab.Research.Wesleyan.Edu/2015/10/29/Gut-Microbiomes-Of-Herbivores-And-Carnivores/

56. Gut Microbiomes Lose Diversity With Immigration: Study As People Move To The United States From Southeast Asia, The Microbes In Their Digestive Tracts Begin To Westernize, Possibly Explaining High Rates Of Obesity And Other Metabolic Issues In These Immigrant Populations. Https://Www.The-Scientist.Com/News-Opinion/Gut-Microbiomes-Lose-Diversity-With-Immigration--Study-65029

57. Soil From A Northern Ireland Graveyard May Lead Scientists To A Powerful New Antibiotic, By Franz Lidz, 2020; Https://Www.Smithsonianmag.Com/Science-Nature/Astonishing-Medical-Potential-Soil-Northern-Ireland-Graveyard-180973741/

58. University of Colorado at Boulder. (2020, August 10). Agriculture replaces fossil fuels as largest human source of sulfur in

the environment. ScienceDaily. Retrieved August 12, 2020 from www.sciencedaily.com/releases/2020/08/200810113214.htm

59. Factory Farming | Definition of Factory Farming by Merriam https://www.merriam-webster.com/dictionary/factory%20farming

60. The Economic Impact Of Locally Produced Food, 2017: Https://Www.Stlouisfed.Org/On-The-Economy/2017/December/Economic-Impact-Locally-Produced-Food

61. Permaculture (the word, coined by bill mollison, is a portmanteau of permanent agriculture and permanent culture) is the conscious design and maintenance of agriculturally productive ecosystems which have the diversity, stability, and resilience of natural ecosystems. It is the harmonious integration of landscape and people — providing their food, energy, shelter, and other material and non-material needs in a sustainable way. Without permanent agriculture there is no possibility of a stable social order.

62. Permaculture integrates land, resources, people and the environment through mutually beneficial synergies – imitating the no waste, closed loop systems seen in diverse natural systems. Permaculture studies and applies holistic solutions that are applicable in rural and urban contexts at any scale. Https://Www.Permaculturenews.Org/What-Is-Permaculture/

63. Swansea University. "Removing Toxic Chemicals From Water: New Environmentally-Friendly Method." Sciencedaily. Sciencedaily, 30 June 2020. Www.Sciencedaily.Com/Releases/2020/06/200630155750.Htm

64. Something In The Water: Pollutant May Be More Hazardous Than Previously Thought Https://Www.Sciencedaily.Com/Releases/2020/06/200605121514.Htm

65. Rural Water Wells In High Plains Aquifer Show Large Increase In Nitrate Levels Https://Www.Sciencedaily.Com/Releases/2020/01/200107122259.Htm

66. How US Sewage Plants Can Remove Medicines From Wastewater, New Research Shows That Technologies Are Available, But The Upgrades Can Be Expensive Https://Www.Sciencedaily.Com/Releases/2020/01/200108160330.Htm

67. Mcleman, Robert A Et Al. "What We Learned From The Dust Bowl: Lessons In Science, Policy, And Adaptation." Population And Environment Vol. 35,4 (2014): 417-440. Doi:10.1007/S11111-013-0190-Z

68. Cook BI, Miller RL, Seager R. Amplification Of The North American "Dust Bowl" Drought Through Human-Induced Land Degradation. Proc Natl Acad Sci U S A. 2009;106(13):4997-5001. Doi:10.1073/Pnas.0810200106

69. Lynch KM, Lyles RH, Waller LA, Abadi AM, Bell JE, Gribble MO. Drought Severity And All-Cause Mortality Rates Among Adults In The United States: 1968-2014. Environ Health. 2020;19(1):52. Published 2020 May 18. Doi:10.1186/S12940-020-00597-8

70. The Need For Conservation Of Natural Springs In Drying Climate Https://Www.Sciencedaily.Com/Releases/2020/06/200603132548.Htm

71. Economics of Soil Loss by Kurt Lawton, 2017: https://www.farmprogress.com/soil-health/economics-soil-loss

72. Soil to Dirt, one families journey into regenerative agriculture by Gabe Brown, 2018 pg 129-130

73. J.L. Round, S.K. Mazmanian The Gut Microbiota Shapes Intestinal Immune Responses During Health And Disease Nat Rev Immunol, 9 (5) (2009), Pp. 313-323

74. University of Illinois at Chicago. (2020, September 2). Links among poor sleep, high blood pressure, gut microbiome discovered: Study shows potential negative effects of disrupted sleep. ScienceDaily. Retrieved September 4, 2020 from www.sciencedaily.com/releases/2020/09/200902182439.htm

75. L.K. Ursell, H.J. Haiser, W. Van Treuren, N. Garg, L. Reddivari, J. Vanamala, Et Al. The Intestinal Metabolome: An Intersection Between Microbiota And Host Gastroenterology, 146 (6) (2014), Pp. 1470-1476

76. Wang, B., Yao, M., Lv, L., Ling, Z., & Li, L. (2017). The Human Microbiota In Health And Disease. Engineering, 3(1), 71-82.

77. E.B. Hollister, C. Gao, J. Versalovic Compositional And Functional Features Of The Gastrointestinal Microbiome And Their Effects On Human Health Gastroenterology, 146 (6) (2014), Pp. 1449-1458

78. National Academies Of Sciences, Engineering, And Medicine. (2018). Environmental Chemicals, The Human Microbiome, And Health Risk: A Research Strategy. National Academies Press.

79. Wiley. (2020, July 8). Links Between Parents' And Children's Asthma And Allergies. Sciencedaily. Retrieved July 10, 2020 From Www.Sciencedaily.Com/Releases/2020/07/200708105941.Htm

80. Insider Money: 15 Household Products That Contain Cadmium, Methanol, Or Benzene By Amber Hewitt, 2017: Https://Www.Insidermonkey.Com/Blog/15-Household-Products-That-Contain-Cadmium-Methanol-Or-Benzene-529244/?Singlepage=1

81. Baylor College Of Medicine, Department Of Molecular Virology And Microbiology, The Human Microbiome Project; Https://Www.Bcm.Edu/Departments/Molecular-Virology-And-Microbiology/Research/The-Human-Microbiome-Project

82. Ohio State University. (2020, July 8). How Good Gut Bacteria Help Reduce The Risk For Heart Disease: Researchers Identify A Protein Responsible For Bacteria's Beneficial Behavior. Sciencedaily. Retrieved July 10, 2020 From Www.Sciencedaily.Com/Releases/2020/07/200708150606.Htm

83. University Of Würzburg. (2020, July 6). Location, Location, Location: Even Gut Immune Response Is Site-Specific. Sciencedaily. Retrieved July 7, 2020 From Www.Sciencedaily.Com/Releases/2020/07/200706100820.Htm

84. Text-Book Of The Principles And Practice Of Nursing, 1934 Page 584

85. In 1956, Principles And Methods Of Sterilization In Health Care Sciences By J.J. Perkins Was Published. This Textbook Set The Standard And Methodology For Processing And Sterilization Of Reusable Medical Devices. Https://Books.Google.Com/Books/About/Principles_And_Methods_Of_Sterilization.Html?Id=-Lyppqaacaaj&Redir_Esc=Y

86. The Human Microbiota In Health And Disease, Engineering Volume 3, Issue 1, February 2017, Pages 71-82: Https://Www.Sciencedirect.Com/Science/Article/Pii/S2095809917301492

87. United States Environmental Protection Agency, Safer Choice: Https://Www.Epa.Gov/Saferchoice

88. Institute Of Medicine, Division Of Health Promotion, Indoor Air And Disease Prevention. Clearing The Air: Asthma And Indoor Air Exposures. Washington, DC: National Academies Press, 2000. Kanchongkittiphon W, Et Al. Indoor Environmental Exposures Of Asthma: An Update To The 2000 Review By The Institute Of Medicine. Environmental Health Perspectives. 2015; 123: 6-20.

89. An Introduction To Sensory Marketing; How Our Senses Sell Us, By Robert Longley 2019: Https://Www.Thoughtco.Com/Sensory-Marketing-4153908

90. How Food Packaging Color Influences Consumer Behavior By Nikki Clark 2016; Https://Hartdesign.Com/Industry-News/Food-Packaging-Color-Influences-Consumer-Behavior/

91. Fixing the Oversight of Chemicals Added to Our Food. https://www.pewtrusts.org/~/media/legacy/uploadedfiles/phg/content_level_pages/reports/foodadditivescapstonereportpdf.pdf

92. Determining The Regulatory Status Of A Food Ingredient: Https://Www.Fda.Gov/Food/Food-Ingredients-Packaging/Determining-Regulatory-Status-Food-Ingredient

93. Snowbound:Two Accounts of Donner Party Tragedy by Various https://www.barnesandnoble.com/w/snowbound-various/1027081068

94. BMJ. (2020, July 8). Higher Fruit, Vegetable And Whole Grain Intake Linked To Lower Risk Of Diabetes: Findings Further Support Advice To Eat More Of These Foods To Prevent Disease. Sciencedaily. Retrieved July 10, 2020 From Www.Sciencedaily.Com/Releases/2020/07/200708213317.Htm

95. Joseph L. Nicholson And George R. Leighton, "Plastics Come Of Age," Harper's Magazine, August 1942, P. 306.

96. Science Matters: The Case Of Plastics: Https://Www.Sciencehistory.Org/The-History-And-Future-Of-Plastics

97. Microplastics In Seafood And The Implications For Human Health, 2018: Https://Www.Ncbi.Nlm.Nih.Gov/Pmc/Articles/PMC6132564/

98. University of California - Santa Barbara. (2020, September 16). The persistence of plastic: New report reveals for the first time the level of terrestrial synthetic microfiber emission on a global scale. ScienceDaily. Retrieved September 29, 2020 from www.sciencedaily.com/releases/2020/09/200916154851.htm

99. Arin A. Balalian, Robin M. Whyatt, Xinhua Liu, Beverly J. Insel, Virginia A. Rauh, Julie Herbstman, Pam Factor-Litvak. Prenatal And Childhood Exposure To Phthalates And Motor Skills At Age 11 Years. Environmental Research, 2019; 171: 416 DOI: 10.1016/J.Envres.2019.01.046

100. Ludwig Stenz, Rita Rahban, Julien Prados, Serge Nef, Ariane Paoloni-Giacobino. Genetic Resistance To DEHP-Induced Transgenerational Endocrine Disruption. PLOS ONE, 2019; 14 (6): E0208371 DOI: 10.1371/Journal.Pone.0208371

101. Genetic inequity towards endocrine disruptors -- ScienceDaily. https://www.sciencedaily.com/releases/2019/06/190613121100.htm

102. Rachelle Morgenstern, Robin M. Whyatt, Beverly J. Insel, Antonia M. Calafat, Xinhua Liu, Virginia A. Rauh, Julie Herbstman, Gary Bradwin, Pam Factor-Litvak. Phthalates And Thyroid Function In Preschool-Age Children: Sex-Specific Associations. Environment International, 2017; 106: 11 DOI: 10.1016/J.Envint.2017.05.007

103. Genetic inequity towards endocrine disruptors. https://medicalxpress.com/news/2019-06-genetic-inequity-endocrine-disruptors.html

104. Endocrine Society. (2015, March 5). Prenatal Exposure To Common Chemical, Phthalates, Found In Some Plastics Disrupts Masculinization Of Male Genitals. Sciencedaily. Retrieved June 18,

2020 From
Www.Sciencedaily.Com/Releases/2015/03/150305125150.Htm

105. Columbia University's Mailman School Of Public Health. (2017, May 30). Household Chemicals May Impair Thyroid In Young Girls. Sciencedaily. Retrieved July 12, 2020 From
Www.Sciencedaily.Com/Releases/2017/05/170530140719.Htm

106. Nicole W. (2014). A question for women's health: chemicals in feminine hygiene products and personal lubricants. Environmental health perspectives, 122(3), A70–A75.
https://doi.org/10.1289/ehp.122-A70

107. Women and Chemicals – WECF, 2018;
https://www.wecf.org/wp-content/uploads/2018/12/WomenAndChemicals_PublicationIWD2016

108. C.S. Lewis Quotes, Thirst Was Made for Water.
https://cslewisquotes.tumblr.com/post/28563319480/thirst-was-made-for-water

109. BMJ. (2015, February 24). Water Fluoridation In England Linked To Higher Rates Of Underactive Thyroid. Sciencedaily. Retrieved July 11, 2020 From
Www.Sciencedaily.Com/Releases/2015/02/150224083811.Htm

110. University Of Bath. (2017, November 13). Simple Water Test Could Prevent Crippling Bone Disease. Sciencedaily. Retrieved July 10, 2020 From
Www.Sciencedaily.Com/Releases/2017/11/171113195013.Htm

111. University Of East Anglia. (2017, June 21). Common Water Treatments Could Damage DNA. Sciencedaily. Retrieved July 7, 2020 From
Www.Sciencedaily.Com/Releases/2017/06/170621113954.Htm

112. Difference between Organic and Inorganic Minerals | APEC Water. https://www.freedrinkingwater.com/water-education3/25-water-organic-inorganic-minerals.htm

113. Difference between Organic and Inorganic Minerals | APEC Water. https://www.freedrinkingwater.com/water-education3/25-water-organic-inorganic-minerals.htm

114. Queen's University Belfast. (2017, May 4). New Research Shows Illegal Levels Of Arsenic Found In Baby Foods. Sciencedaily. Retrieved July 6, 2020 From
Www.Sciencedaily.Com/Releases/2017/05/170504161538.Htm

115. Parent Plus: Limit infants' exposure to arsenic by feeding a variety of grains Trisha Korioth, Staff Writer, 2016:
https://www.aappublications.org/news/2016/05/19/Arsenic051916

---

116. USDA, Arsenic in Food and Dietary Supplements: https://www.fda.gov/food/metals-and-your-food/arsenic-food-and-dietary-supplements

117. American Chemical Society. (2019, April 17). Parboiling Method Reduces Inorganic Arsenic In Rice. Sciencedaily. Retrieved July 10, 2020 From Www.Sciencedaily.Com/Releases/2019/04/190417084610.Htm

118. Mercury And Health, World Health Organization 2017: Https://Www.Who.Int/News-Room/Fact-Sheets/Detail/Mercury-And-Health

119. American Chemical Society. (2020, July 8). Purifying Water With The Help Of Wood, Bacteria And The Sun. Sciencedaily. Retrieved July 11, 2020 From Www.Sciencedaily.Com/Releases/2020/07/200708105959.Htm

120. Removing toxic mercury from contaminated water -- ScienceDaily. https://www.sciencedaily.com/releases/2018/11/181121073214.htm

121. Chalmers University Of Technology. (2018, November 21). Removing Toxic Mercury From Contaminated Water. Sciencedaily. Retrieved July 11, 2020 From Www.Sciencedaily.Com/Releases/2018/11/181121073214.Htm

122. Lead Paint Trial: Did Industry Promote Product Knowing Of Its Toxic Dangers?: Https://Www.Huffpost.Com/Entry/Lead-Paint-Trial_N_3612546

123. The four major naturally occurring estrogens in women are estrone (E1), estradiol (E2), estriol (E3), and estetrol (E4). Estradiol is the predominant estrogen during reproductive years both in terms of absolute serum levels as well as in terms of estrogenic activity.

124. European Lung Foundation. (2020, September 2). Exposure to cadmium in the womb linked to childhood asthma and allergies. ScienceDaily. Retrieved September 4, 2020 from www.sciencedaily.com/releases/2020/09/200902182433.htm

125. Norwegian University of Science and Technology. (2020, October 1). 800 million children still exposed to lead: Study documents a persistent, dangerous problem. ScienceDaily. Retrieved October 7, 2020 from www.sciencedaily.com/releases/2020/10/201001113555.htm

126. Norwegian University of Science and Technology. Original written by Steinar Brandslet.

127. Centers for disease control and prevention: what has not changed is the recommendation for when to use medical treatment for children. Experts recommend chelation therapy when a child is found with a test result of greater than or equal to 45 micrograms

per deciliter of lead in blood.
Https://Www.Cdc.Gov/Nceh/Lead/Prevention/Blood-Lead-Levels.Htm

128. Lead Safe Mama:
Https://Tamararubin.Com/Category/Vintage-Dishes/

129. Hazardous Metals In Vintage Plastic Toys Measured By A Handheld X-Ray Fluorescence Spectrometer By Gillian Zaharias Miller, Phdecology Centerzoe E. Harrisst. Ambrose University:
File:///C:/Users/Holistic%20Nutrition/Appdata/Local/Temp/JEH-Janfeb2015-Vintage-Toys.Pdf

130. De Burbure, C., Buchet, J. P., Leroyer, A., Nisse, C., Haguenoer, J. M., Mutti, A., Smerhovsky, Z., Cikrt, M., Trzcinka-Ochocka, M., Razniewska, G., Jakubowski, M., & Bernard, A. (2006). Renal And Neurologic Effects Of Cadmium, Lead, Mercury, And Arsenic In Children: Evidence Of Early Effects And Multiple Interactions At Environmental Exposure Levels. Environmental Health Perspectives, 114(4), 584–590.
Https://Doi.Org/10.1289/Ehp.8202

131. Pan S, Lin L, Zeng F, Et Al. Effects Of Lead, Cadmium, Arsenic, And Mercury Co-Exposure On Children's Intelligence Quotient In An Industrialized Area Of Southern China. Environ Pollut. 2018;235:47-54. Doi:10.1016/J.Envpol.2017.12.044

132. Koike S. Nihon Eiseigaku Zasshi. 1997;52(3):552-561. Doi:10.1265/Jjh.52.552

133. Heavy Metal Detox Diet:
Https://Www.Healthline.Com/Health/Heavy-Metal-Detox

134. 8 Foods To Help You Detox Naturally:
Https://Www.Amymyersmd.Com/2018/05/8-Foods-To-Help-You-Detox-Naturally/

135. What Is A Heavy Metal Detox?:
Https://Www.Medicalnewstoday.Com/Articles/327317.Php

136. University of Texas Health Science Center at San Antonio. (2020, September 21). Think you have chemical intolerance? Answer three questions: COVID-19 disinfectants, wildfire smoke and mold endanger chemically susceptible individuals; new brief inventory can help identify those at risk. ScienceDaily. Retrieved September 29, 2020 from
www.sciencedaily.com/releases/2020/09/200921170345.htm

137. https://chemical-free-life.org/2020/09/23/do-you-have-chemical-sensitivity-answering-just-three-questions-can-tell-you/

138. Farm Subsidies With Pros, Cons, And Impact;
Https://Www.Thebalance.Com/Farm-Subsidies-4173885

139. Commodity Subsidies In The United States Totaled $7.2 Billion In 2017;

Https://Farm.Ewg.Org/Progdetail.Php?Fips=00000&Progcode=Totalfarm&Yr=2017&Page=States&Regionname=Theunitedstates

140. WASDE: Corn Use For Ethanol Up In 2018-'19; Http://Ethanolproducer.Com/Articles/15282/Wasde-Corn-Use-For-Ethanol-Up-In-2018-Undefined19

141. Land Usage Attributed To Corn Ethanol Production In The United States: Sensitivity To Technological Advances In Corn Grain Yield, Ethanol Conversion, And Co-Product Utilization; Https://Www.Ncbi.Nlm.Nih.Gov/Pmc/Articles/PMC4022103/

142. Five Facts You Need To Know About The US Farming Industry; Https://Www.Realclearpolicy.Com/Articles/2018/08/01/Five_Facts_You_Need_To_Know_About_The_Us_Farming_Industry_110740.Html

143. Five Facts You Need To Know About The US Farming Industry; Https://Www.Realclearpolicy.Com/Articles/2018/08/01/Five_Facts_You_Need_To_Know_About_The_Us_Farming_Industry_110740.Html

144. A Looming Crisis On American Farms By Alicia Harvie; Https://Www.Farmaid.Org/Issues/Farm-Economy-In-Crisis/Looming-Crisis-American-Farms/

145. Feeding The World Intelligently By John Ikerd: Prepared For Presentation At The Tennessee Local Food Summit, Organized By The Barefoot Farmer, Hosted By Tennessee State University, Nashville, TN, December, 1-3, 2017. Https://Faculty.Missouri.Edu/Ikerdj/Papers/Tennesseelfsfeedingtheworldintelligently.Pdf

146. American Farmers Say They Feed The World, But Do They? By Dan Charles Https://Www.Npr.Org/Sections/Thesalt/2013/09/17/221376803/American-Farmers-Say-They-Feed-The-World-But-Do-They S3

147. Tiffon, Céline. "The Impact Of Nutrition And Environmental Epigenetics On Human Health And Disease." International Journal Of Molecular Sciences Vol. 19,11 3425. 1 Nov. 2018, Doi:10.3390/Ijms19113425

148. Olden, Kenneth Et Al. "Discovering How Environmental Exposures Alter Genes Could Lead To New Treatments For Chronic Illnesses." Health Affairs (Project Hope) Vol. 30,5 (2011): 833-41. Doi:10.1377/Hlthaff.2011.0078

149. Lund University. "How Lifestyle Affects Our Genes." Sciencedaily. Sciencedaily, 23 April 2019. Www.Sciencedaily.Com/Releases/2019/04/190423133451.Htm

150. Max-Planck-Gesellschaft. "A Healthy Lifestyle Increases Life Expectancy By Up To Seven Years: Maintaining A Normal

Weight, Not Smoking, And Drinking Alcohol At Moderate Levels Are Factors That Add Healthy Years To Life." Sciencedaily. Sciencedaily, 20 July 2017.
Www.Sciencedaily.Com/Releases/2017/07/170720113710.Htm

151. Harvard T.H. Chan School Of Public Health. "Following Five Healthy Lifestyle Habits May Increase Life Expectancy By Decade Or More." Sciencedaily. Sciencedaily, 30 April 2018.
Www.Sciencedaily.Com/Releases/2018/04/180430075619.Htm

152. Uppsala University. "Genetic Effects Are Influenced By Lifestyle." Sciencedaily. Sciencedaily, 6 September 2017.
Www.Sciencedaily.Com/Releases/2017/09/170906103749.Htm

153. Ohio State University. (2020, August 24). Each human gut has a viral 'fingerprint': New database consists of over 33,000 unique viral populations in the gut. ScienceDaily. Retrieved August 25, 2020 from
www.sciencedaily.com/releases/2020/08/200824131803.htm

154. Duggan AT, Perdomo MF, Piombino-Mascali D, Et Al. 17th Century Variola Virus Reveals The Recent History Of Smallpox. Curr Biol. 2016;26(24):3407-3412. Doi:10.1016/J.Cub.2016.10.061

155. A History Timeline of Epidemics & Plagues - The History https://www.futuretimeline.net/forum/topic/22820-a-history-timeline-of-epidemics-plagues/

156. Düx A, Lequime S, Patrono LV, Et Al. Measles Virus And Rinderpest Virus Divergence Dated To The Sixth Century BCE. Science. 2020;368(6497):1367-1370. Doi:10.1126/Science.Aba9411

157. University of Otago. (2020, September 21). Archaeology uncovers infectious disease spread 4000 years ago. ScienceDaily. Retrieved September 29, 2020 from
www.sciencedaily.com/releases/2020/09/200921091535.htm

158. Jónsson, H., Sulem, P., Kehr, B. et al. Parental influence on human germline de novo mutations in 1,548 trios from Iceland. Nature 549, 519–522 (2017). https://doi.org/10.1038/nature24018

159. Fathers pass on four times as many new genetic mutations as mothers – study by Ion Sample, 2017 The Guardian:
https://www.theguardian.com/science/2017/sep/20/fathers-pass-on-four-times-as-many-new-genetic-mutations-as-mothers-study

160. Jónsson, H., Sulem, P., Kehr, B. et al. Parental influence on human germline de novo mutations in 1,548 trios from Iceland. Nature 549, 519–522 (2017). https://doi.org/10.1038/nature24018

161. Adverse Childhood Experiences and the Lifelong ....
https://www.aap.org/en-us/Documents/ttb_aces_consequences.pdf

162. Adverse Childhood Experiences ACEs:
https://www.aap.org/en-us/Documents/ttb_aces_consequences.pdf

163. Elsevier. "Does The Impact Of Psychological Trauma Cross Generations?." Sciencedaily. Sciencedaily, 8 September 2010. Www.Sciencedaily.Com/Releases/2010/09/100908102058.Htm

164. Bragantini, D., Sivertsen, B., Gehrman, P. et al. Genetic polymorphisms associated with sleep-related phenotypes; relationships with individual nocturnal symptoms of insomnia in the HUNT study. BMC Med Genet 20, 179 (2019). https://doi.org/10.1186/s12881-019-0916-6

165. Kripke, D. F., Kline, L. E., Nievergelt, C. M., Murray, S. S., Shadan, F. F., Dawson, A., Poceta, J. S., Cronin, J., Jamil, S. M., Tranah, G. J., Loving, R. T., Grizas, A. P., & Hahn, E. K. (2015). Genetic variants associated with sleep disorders. Sleep medicine, 16(2), 217–224. https://doi.org/10.1016/j.sleep.2014.11.003

166. Dashti, H.S., Jones, S.E., Wood, A.R. et al. Genome-wide association study identifies genetic loci for self-reported habitual sleep duration supported by accelerometer-derived estimates. Nat Commun 10, 1100 (2019). https://doi.org/10.1038/s41467-019-08917-4

Chapter Three
Mindfulness

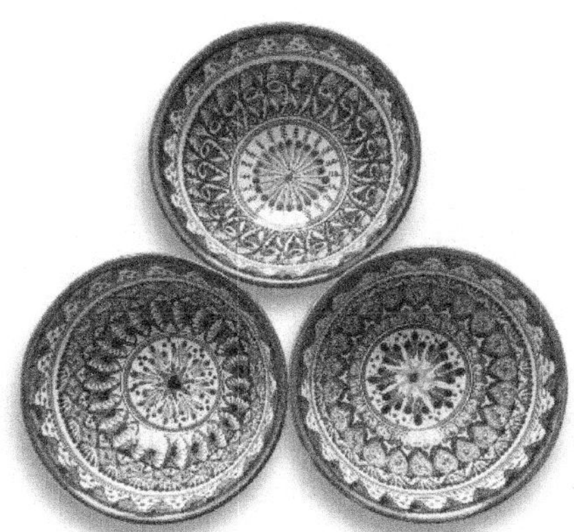

Remain quiet.
Discover the harmony in your own being.
Embrace it.
If you can do this, you will gain everything,
and the world will become healthy again.

~Lao Tzu [1]

Nutrition and mindfulness have been interwoven in Kathleen's experience since the beginning of her formal meditation training in 2006. Kathleen's first meditation teacher grew up in an ashram, steeped in Ayurvedic tradition and yogic science, and later studied nutritional biochemistry. At one of her training sessions, while viewing photographs of research done in Japan by Masaru Emoto (New York Times bestselling author of *Hidden Messages in Water*) on the energetic effects that emotions, words, music, and prayer have on water; Kathleen was deeply affected by what she saw. [2]

Emoto had taken droplets from each of the water samples and had frozen them on glass slides, then examined and photographed them under a powerful microscope (the work done by Masaru Emoto 1943–2014 is controversial). Some of the droplets were prayed over by Buddhist monks or were exposed to *grace* said by a family before a meal. Some of them were exposed to words of love and gratitude. Some had been collected from horribly polluted lakes and streams in Japan, and some had been cursed in anger by a person saying, "I hate you." Other droplets were exposed to different kinds of music — Beethoven's exquisitely beautiful *Ode to Joy*, a Mozart symphony, loud and angry *heavy metal* music, and a death march.

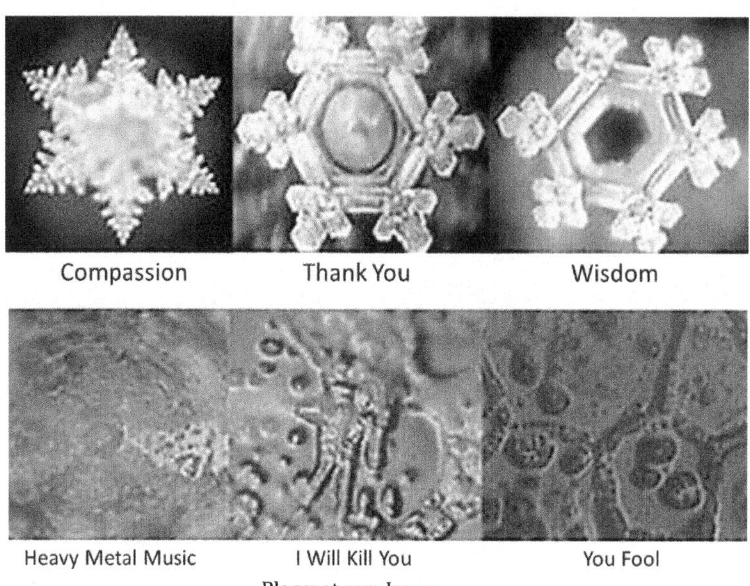

Blogspot.com Image

After the presentation, Kathleen wrote in her journal: "As I looked at the images of the frozen water crystals, each labeled with the energetic element it had been exposed to in the experiment, **I was astonished**. Water that had been infused with gratitude by saying grace before meals or blessed by a prayer recited by a Buddhist priest formed the most amazingly beautiful snowflake shapes and intricate fractal patterns. Each was unique and perfect. Water that had been cursed or that came from a polluted source assumed chaotically foul and evil-looking patterns. To my medically trained eyes, the resemblance to cancer cells was uncanny. I vividly remember the visceral reaction I experienced when the thought crossed my mind, "That is what cancer cells look like!!" The next equally stunning thought was a question, "How much of our bodies are made of water??" Immediately followed by, "And how much of our food?"

In Kathleen's eyes, the visible change in the water's substance crystalized on those slides was nothing less than what could be described as a *miracle* — the alteration of physical form and substance by the energy created from a human mind. This training served as an awakening for Kathleen; solidly grounding her in the value of meditation for patients and students and introducing the role of mindfulness for health.

> *"Mindfulness is paying attention on purpose, in the present moment, non-judgmentally."*
>
> ~Jon Kabat-Zinn, MD [3]

In 1979, while he was on the faculty at the University of Massachusetts School of Medicine, Dr. Jon Kabat-Zinn took a group of (stressed-out) medical students into the library's basement to practice techniques that eventually became the Mindfulness-Based Stress Reduction (MBSR) program. The first Western program to apply mindfulness practices to wellbeing and health. [4]

In 2020, the word mindfulness seems to pop up everywhere, from product advertising to business planning to school curricula. The media is saturated with articles and opinions about this ancient and simple (though not always easy) practice. Once associated with Eastern spiritual and mystical beliefs, mindfulness continues to be promulgated, secularized, and popularized via many *programs* throughout the Western world.

One working definition of mindfulness is a process of openly attending, with awareness, to one's present moment experience. This process of conscious awareness of present moment experience contrasts sharply with much of our usual daily life experience. How often do we find ourselves unintentionally letting our minds wander? Or run on automatic pilot? The mind is much more inclined toward suppressing unwanted thoughts about experiences in the past or future than paying undivided attention to what one is presently experiencing. [5, 6, 7, 8]

> *Principle 1*: Mindfulness is not about paying more attention but involves paying attention differently.

Mindfulness is about intentionally paying attention to one thing at a time — not dividing our attention. In the words of Dr. Deepak Chopra, Dr. Rudolph Tanzi, Dr. Jon Kabat-Zinn, and many other scientists: "Multitasking doesn't work." Neuroscientists who study the human brain's workings are concerned that the modern myth that supports the value of multi-tasking — actually just encouraging the tendency to divide our attention — hampers the ability to perform even simple tasks. [9]

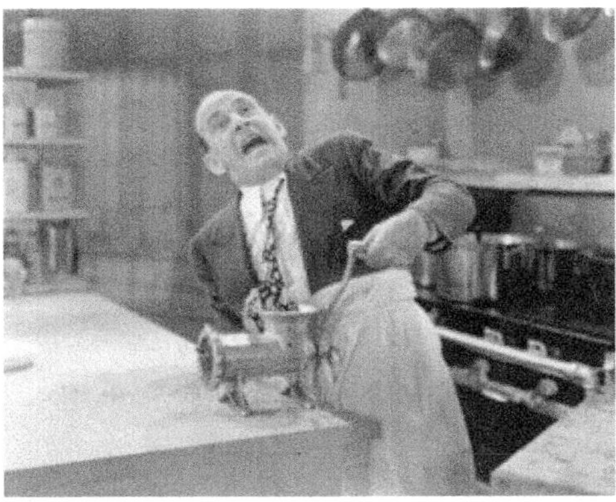

Many individuals spend their waking hours in a distracted state, aided by multiple technologic devices and resources that support the multi-tasking myth; rarely paying full attention to what they are doing/thinking/feeling in the here and now. At the end of the day, a person can feel like the victim of a constantly busy and chattering mind (what Buddhists call the *monkey mind*), which does not allow one to be present and enjoy daily life. [10]

Studies show that the hypothalamus, thymus glands, and brain function of individuals who practice mindfulness display more elasticity and resiliency to the impact of stress, due in part to the physiologic changes that accompany relaxation in the body. Relaxation's effects on balancing the hypothalamic-pituitary-adrenal-thyroid (HPAT) axis have been well documented in decades of research. [11, 12, 13]

Contemplation and introspection have been part of human existence for so long they may even be coded into our DNA. Regardless of one's belief system, a person who practices prayer, intention-setting, meditation, gratitude, and chants/mantra stimulates slow, deep-breathing, and elicits a relaxation response in the body. These proven methods down-regulate the central nervous system, calming brain chemistry, and stress hormones, and facilitating increased resilience needed to weather periods of disaster, strife, and upheaval with greater ease and flexibility.

Harvard professor Dr. Ellen Langer has westernized mindfulness with the following definition: *"Mindfulness is the process of actively noticing new things, relinquishing preconceived mindsets, and then acting on the new observations."* [14] Mindfulness is a basic human ability, awakening the skill of moment by moment awareness is possible for all. We just need to develop our *mindfulness muscle*, which gets stronger and more proficient with practice, just like any other muscle.

Mindfulness is not about paying more attention but paying attention differently, using the whole mind and heart, using the body's full resources and all its senses. One *practices* being aware of what is happening in the moment through undivided attention to the present moment. Foundational present moment experiences involve focusing on oneself with an awareness of body sensations, emotions, and thoughts. Mindfulness practice offers a way to step — if just for a short time — out of the chaotic world, with all of its' seductions and addictions. It can introduce a person to their own real power by creating some distance and internal detachment from ever-present thoughts, reactions/feelings and allowing their awareness to move to a place of calm stillness and focus.

Through her initial meditation training, Kathleen learned to practice bringing calm, non-judgmental attention to a point of focus in the present moment — her own breathing, physical sensations, or sounds. Later she adopted the mantra, which means silently repeating and concentrating on a word or phrase. Meditation is an exercise in letting go of distractions and returning one's attention again and again to the chosen object of focus. Over time, Kathleen began to understand that her meditation practice allowed her to experience mindfulness, and her definition evolved: mindfulness is the capacity for awareness and increase in self-awareness that results from a regular meditation practice.

Importantly, mindfulness can introduce a person to their own real power by creating some distance and internal detachment from ever-present thoughts, reactions/feelings and allowing their awareness to move to a place of calm stillness and focus.

> *Principle 2*: Mindfulness practice encourages an individual to become a compassionate and non-judgmental observer of oneself.

As one begins to develop the ability to simply observe behaviors, thoughts, and feelings; undoubtedly, patterns will begin to emerge. After all, we humans are creatures of habit! When observing these patterns, an instrumental question to ask oneself, in order to stay neutrally curious and not revert to judgment, is this: " Hmm, just look at that! Isn't that interesting?"

When an individual becomes aware of repetitive personal reactions or behaviors and is able to examine them from a non-judgmental perspective, they are practicing mindfulness. It is useful to remember that the word practice is both a noun and a verb; that is, practice does not become a practice unless it is practiced regularly. Importantly, it does not really matter how long the attitude of mindful presence is maintained because almost immediately, the practice decreases stress, anxiety, and fear and can create a mood of calm and peace. [15]

> *There are few people I know on the planet who couldn't benefit more from a greater dose of awareness.*
>
> ~Jon Kabat-Zinn [16]

Ama and Agni: using Ayurveda (the oldest healing system in the world) to explain healthy digestion

Ayurveda is a 6,000-year-old health system that combines science, philosophy, and spirituality as necessary aspects for healthful living. In contrast with most Western philosophies regarding diet — which mostly focus on serving sizes and caloric intake — Ayurveda acknowledges that a healthy diet can contain both plant and animal-based nutrients and that portion sizes should be individualized. It also considers the energetic qualities of foods. In the spirit of developing new awareness — in other words, becoming mindful of — about how our conscious choices influencing diet and health. More than what one eats — let's examine how Ayurveda explains the workings of the body, as it processes nourishment. It may lead to a greater understanding of what really powers health, happiness, wellness, and longevity.

Advice on how to achieve a balanced state of (digestive) health from Simon Chokoisky, a Medical Astrologist and Sanskrit scholar at the Ayurvedic Institute in Albuquerque, New Mexico, is contained in two words: *eliminate Ama.* [17] No equivalent for the Sanskrit word *Ama* exists in English. Still, the concept is related to inefficient digestive processes that lead to a sort of *toxic sludge* or *morbid mucoid plaque* in the body. *Ama* can be grossly visible; the best example of it is the yellowish, sticky mucous found on your tongue when you wake from sleep. And it is certain that if *Ama* is visible on your tongue, it is also present in your body in many subtle ways that are invisibly damaging: circulating systemically via the bloodstream and lymphatic system and causing chronic inflammation, cell toxicity, and energetic *congestion*.

Ayurveda and Traditional Chinese Medicine (TCM) share the concept stating that disease results from vital energy, or life force, blockages along channels/Nadi/meridians that circulate this energy throughout the body. In yogic science (Ayurveda), this life force is called *Prana*; in TCM, it is called chi or qi. [18] According to Ayurveda, which means the *science of life* in Sanskrit, Ama is the root cause of all disease. One Ayurvedic practice is to scrape it from the tongue every morning.

Modern medical research is beginning to prove the wisdom of this ancient concept. Today, research studies on the insidious damage of chronic inflammation abound, pointing to it as the probable underlying cause of diabetes, kidney and cardiovascular diseases, autoimmune disorders, and relating it to amyloid plaque formation in the brain that is found in Alzheimer's disease. [19, 20]

If an individual wakes up with fresh-smelling breath, no ama on their tongue, and the (not smelly) morning bowel movement floats in the toilet bowl. They know their body is relatively *Ama*-free, with good gut flora from eating enough fiber. Research now tells us that our prehistoric ancestors ate up to 100 grams of fiber per day. [21] The Standard American Diet (SAD) usually contains fewer than twenty!

If a person is not quite ready for a bowel movement first thing in the morning, Simon recommends drinking a tall glass of room-temperature water (16 ounces) after scraping the tongue. [22] The body and brain have been without fluids for the hours spent sleeping and will welcome hydration. Drinking water also encourages peristalsis and flushing of any toxins in the digestive system. This could be the most important drink of the day!

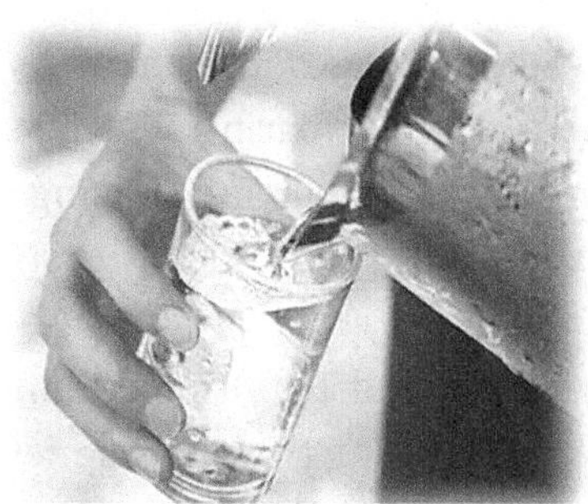

Kindling the metabolic *fire* of the body, called *Agni* in Sanskrit, is the way to eliminate *Ama*. Agni's concept is more comprehensive than just the biologic and enzymatic processes involved in physically digesting food. Metabolism is the process that must happen within the holistic body/mind/spirit in order for an individual to absorb all that is ingested via our five senses. What is seen, heard, smelled, tasted, and felt.

All that we experience can either support our health or work against it. Ayurveda teaches that literally everything encountered in our lives becomes assimilated as part of each individual person's body/mind/spirit. The energetic qualities of everything we are exposed to must be *digested* efficiently and thoroughly via *Agni*, including the transformation of food

into consciousness. Ayurveda maintains that if this vital metabolic process is deficient, disease results.
Agni is the balanced opposite of *Ama* in the body: when one is high, the other is low and vice versa. According to Ayurveda, impaired *Agni* is the root cause behind many modern addictions: tobacco, coffee, drugs, even sex. When the body's metabolic fire turns sluggish, stimulating activities and/or substances are sought. But chemical or emotional *crutches* are no substitute for the wealth of our own inner pharmacy. Ayurvedic wisdom states that building strong *Agni* to burn *Ama* will curb cravings for substances that we seek to either calm or stimulate our bodies and minds. Eating with awareness will kindle *Agni* and facilitate healthy digestion. [23]

The energetic qualities of foods

What provides the proper nourishment for the mind to remain calm yet alert — in other words, the best state for mindfulness practice? Ayurveda breaks the energetics of foods themselves into three categories: *physical, mental, and causal.* [24, 25] Vedic science teaches that human bodies are made of the same five elements that comprise everything in the Universe: *Earth, Water, Air, Fire, and Ether* (Space). We ingest serve as building blocks for the nervous system and fuels processes within individual cells' (all 50 trillion of them, remember?) needed to sustain their cellular intelligence. [26]

Indeed, it is the combination of all this intrinsic information, which creates our own personal *awareness*, that is, our bodymind's inner wisdom and unique capacity to make choices about what is needed for the organism to sustain itself. For example, the neuronal cells which make up the central nervous system have the amazing ability to choose the amino acids and B vitamins (from all of the nutrients dissolved in the blood) that are required to make up the fats that supply them with materials to create neurotransmitters. [27, 28]

The cellular intelligence required to power the billions of life processes encompassed by a living human being is governed by the universal life force itself. In yogic science (Ayurveda), this life force is called *Prana;* in TCM, it is called *chi or qi.* [29] When the cells lose their GPS connection to this governing force, they lose this innate intelligence — just like someone traveling loses their way — and disease sets in.

Foods have their own *physical* quality of energy, related to each of the five elements that are projected in our minds and bodies when we eat them. [30, 31, 32, 33]

Earth energy is needed for stability and creates the physical structure of the body: teeth, bones, cells, tissues, organs. The more stable our physical structure is, the more stable mental processes, such as mindfulness, can be.

Water energy relates to the fluid component, which is also the most substantial portion of the human body: blood, cerebrospinal fluid, secretory fluids, and digestive juices. It is the largest component of cells themselves.

Fire is the element that transforms. This version of fire, however, is not damaging like inflammation. Fire governs our will, transforming ideas, desires, and power into action. It is needed for the bodymind to be alert and focused. Digestion transforms food into necessary physical substances that the body absorbs.

Air supports the life force; *Prana* or *Chi* is carried by air. It is not the breath itself, but the breath moves it dynamically throughout every single respiration of our lives. It is the primary force for mental balance. It is important to keep this element nourished well because it tends to an imbalance with age; many body fluids dry up.

Lastly, *Ether or Space.* The micro spaces that exist in the body are critical: the crucial spaces maintained between the synapses in the brain, each small alveoli in the lungs that needs to remain open for optimal breathing, the exact time between each phase of the heartbeat (as seen in the QRS complexes on an EKG reading). Dr. Deepak Chopra calls all of these infinitesimal spaces in the body, taken together, "the ground of infinite possibility." [34]

Importantly, when we feed our bodies with genetically modified substances and not real whole foods, we *create chaos* among these elements and their inherent information systems. The body literally does not know what to do with them!

The *mental* category of food energies comes from the sensory input the brain receives about the colors, shapes, smells, and sounds of food. Perception of these sensory stimuli affects the *outer mind, - Mana* in Sanskrit, which is the conscious or thinking mind, as well as our *inner mind* or deep subconscious known as *Chitta.*

How sensory input is perceived creates personal feelings and thoughts, which give rise to emotions. Have you heard the term *emotional eating*? Are there foods you eat just because you can guarantee they make you feel good? Freeing oneself from 'knee-jerk' responses to foods, behavior patterns that are long ingrained as conditioned reactions, is possible by employing mindfulness in the present moment. Learning to regulate what we actually need versus what we want to take in, or eat, significantly affects well-being. Being calm and deliberately mindful of choices relies on one's ability to create a *PAUSE.*

A useful mindful behavior sequence to memorize is:

PAUSE, BREATHE, OBSERVE, RESPOND

"Be aware of your breathing.

Notice how this takes attention away from your thinking and creates space."

~ Eckhart Tolle

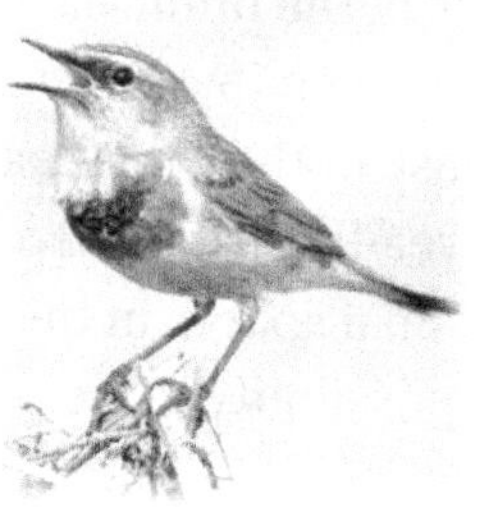

In the consciously created space of a pause, with room to breathe, one can detach from the event at hand and observe it without judgment. An individual is then free to choose a response and does not just react out of habit or (sometimes unconscious) conditioning. As an added benefit to adopting this practice, one might begin to be cognizant of patterns or behaviors that seem to occupy precious mental space without express consent. How much in the way of *old habits* do we carry around with us? Do you find yourself donating mental space to these encroachers who are not paying any rent?

> *Principle 3*: Being aware of the breath takes attention and creates mental space.

Food is essential for the health of the body, but it also provides nourishment for the mind. The Upanishads (ancient Ayurvedic text) state that food consumed is divided by a person's being into parts: the gross part is converted into flesh, and the subtle (causal) energy feeds the mind. Since what a person eats is transformed energetically into that individual's consciousness, examining the causal energy in foods is important.

Nutritional qualities that impress the holistic mind/body/spirit are called *Gunas* in Sanskrit. [35, 36, 37] The first quality is *Satwa*, which brings a state of harmony, balance, joy, and intelligence. Foods with this quality encourage serenity and peaceful awareness. They are fresh, juicy, light, and naturally sweet: fruits and vegetables, whole grains, legumes, and fresh organic dairy foods from well-cared-for cows. A sattvic diet leads to true health: a peaceful mind in control of a fit body, with a balanced flow of energy between them.

The second quality is *rajas*, which brings a state of action and change in movement. It is an uplifting and vibrant energy that feeds attraction, longing, and attachment. Foods that are bitter, sour, salty, pungent, hot (spicy) have a lot of this energetic quality. They include fish, eggs, sweets, desserts, raw onions and garlic, fried bread, tea, coffee, and tobacco. Ayurveda teaches that an overabundance of *Rajas* feeds jealousy and anger, ego, delusions, and fantasies. An overabundance can also create over-stimulation, hyperactivity, and insomnia.

Ayurveda teaches that an overabundance of *Rajas* feeds jealousy and anger, ego, delusions, and fantasies. An overabundance can create over-stimulation, hyperactivity, and insomnia.

The third quality is *Tamas*, which is associated with solidarity. Processed or frozen foods, carbohydrates, red meats, and chemically treated foods often cause heaviness, lethargy, and stupor after eating, leading to fatigue and even confusion. According to Ayurvedic wisdom, too much *Tamas* can be related to abusive or addictive behaviors. [38]

Being aware of these energetic qualities of food can help the mind be in the best possible state for mindfulness practice. If there is a need to increase peaceful awareness and serenity, one can eat more *satwa* foods to achieve the desired state. When there is a need for more stimulation, energy, or action to eliminate dullness or boredom, eating more *raja* foods can fuel a change in the state of mind.

It is essential to realize that these three energetic qualities are *found within all things* that people ingest and are exposed to, not just in foods. We need to be mindful of keeping in balance all that we allow ourselves to *take in* through our senses in order to sustain the mind's ability to remain resilient, focused, and clear; maintain the body in good health, and allow the spirit to be light and bright.

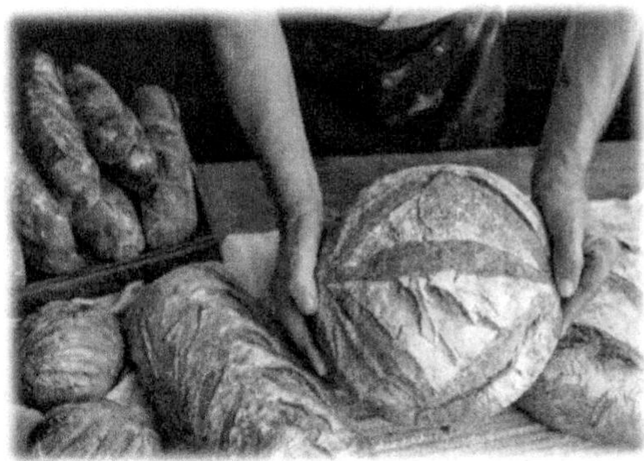

"Love doesn't sit there like a stone; it has to be made, like bread; re-made every day, made new." [39]

~Ursula LeGuin

Mindful food preparation

To prepare food and cook it, a place must be dedicated to these tasks — a kitchen. People shop, barter for, or grow the necessary ingredients and store them until they are ready to take them out of cupboards, cabinets, and refrigerators. Then ingredients are assembled so they can be seen and used. To do this mindfully, we must honestly know and understand all that is there.

> *"Bread, like love, must be made every day."*
>
> ~Ancient proverb

And what is there? "The earth under our feet. The water in our glasses. The simple tastes of sweet and salt. The seasons. The very rhythm of life. The list can go on." [40] We can pause, breathe, and observe — taking time to see and appreciate these ordinary gifts — things we see every day and mostly ignore. How often do we really appreciate the gift of food as a continual ingredient in our lives?

For many of us, the answer is not often enough — unless we deliberately make time to recognize it as such and to recognize it repeatedly. When we do so, we honor the goodness around us, allowing our awareness to expand beyond a more accustomed, narrow, self-absorbed viewpoint.

Not only do we need a kitchen to cook in, but we must also be willing to engage in the process. Tension can enter the picture here, for the will can just as easily lean towards willfulness as willingness. Mindfulness is the direct opposite of trying (using force) to make happen what we want to happen. Force is often met with resistance. There is an old saying, "*What you resist, persists.*" Have you found this to be true?

The power of mindfulness is related to willing participation. "Willingness, on the other hand," according to Gunilla Norris, "allows life to show us the way." [41, 42] When we are willing to feel hunger, willing to prepare and cook food, and then willing to receive its sustenance, we "open the door in the heart's kitchen" and can joyfully participate in the moments that occupy these daily activities.

Kitchen Yogi meditation

Any activity can be transformed into meditation, even washing, and chopping vegetables. Remember, the key to mindfulness is paying attention to what is happening in the present moment. It is not the activity itself that elevates the quality of mental awareness, but the energy of mindful attentiveness that an individual brings to it. Inspired by Joel and Michelle Levy in their book, *Luminous Mind,* [43] here is an exercise to transform a routine kitchen chore, chopping vegetables, into an experience of mindfulness:

- Begin by grounding yourself. Feel the contact points between the soles of your feet and the floor, feeling your feet touching the ground. Sense how the floor beneath you connects you to the earth.

- With your knees slightly bent, imagine that you can feel your feet and legs growing down into the earth — like the roots of a plant. Using your attention, move this rooted feeling upward from your feet through your lower legs to your knees, then your thighs, into your hips and your entire legs.

- Next, move your awareness upwards to your navel in the center of your body. Feel the Earth's energy that is rising through your feet and legs, moving now through the middle of your body, and feel the balance that is centered there. At your navel, the energy that is rooted in your lower body equals the energy that is rising in your upper body. Remember, the energy center located around the navel is where *Agni* resides.

- Now allow that same energy to continue moving upwards into the upper part of your body. Breathe it in, and as you exhale, feel your upper body open up and become more alive, with your arms energized like the branches of a tree move gently with the wind. On an exhale, allow your shoulders to drop. With another exhale, allow your jaw to relax, loose and soft. Inhale and let your eyes soften to a wide gaze.

- Inhaling and exhaling slowly, sense your whole body's upright posture as being connected to the Earth.

- Be receptive. **Allow the sensations** of *sight* (color/shape/form/symmetry), *sound* (snap/squish/pop), *taste* (bitter, sweet, sour), *smell* (spicey/pungent/sharp), and *touch/feel* (hard/soft/slippery/juicy) **of each vegetable to come to you, and receive them,** as you hold them in your hands and chop with the knife.

- Feel the sensation of the knife in your hand, its hardness, its cold, sharp edge. Become aware of the contact points between your hand and the knife. Are you squeezing more than necessary or using too much force to chop? Soften your grip a bit; you can safely lighten up!

- As you chop, go back to the beginning step and feel your feet on the floor, soften the knees.

- Moving from a grounded center, stay aware of your body and your breathing.

- Keep eyes/gaze soft.
- Continue to focus on being open and receptive, staying in touch with the flow of sensations.
- Attend to every moment of this task as if this was your first time doing this — or your last.
- Remain alert, relaxed, and precise; mindfully moving from moment to moment for as long as you are working.
- When you have finished, release the focus on sensations.
- Thank your body/mind/spirit for the experience, and the Universe for your good fortune to have food to prepare and eat today.

Vastu: Keeping the center clear

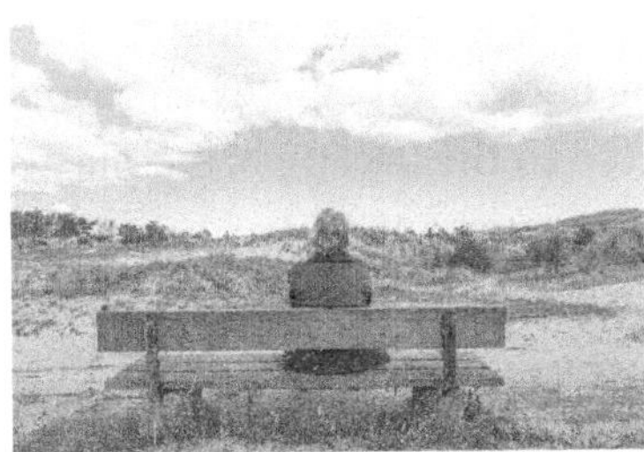

One final principle of Ayurveda deserves mention, *Vastu Shastra.* This ancient Vedic science of placement is similar to the Chinese science of *Feng Shui*, and both hold that the centers of home/work/living spaces need to be kept clear for greatest health and prosperity. [44, 45] The corollary of this principle for the body is keeping the

GI tract clear. The intestines include millions of villi and microvilli; small finger-like projections into the lumen of the GI tract that move in wavelike pulses to push food through the system. These work best if given ample time to rest and replenish between meals. And they welcome periods of complete rest for rejuvenation — the fast that accompanies eight hours of sleep, for instance. Most large mammals, including humans, have bodies that were built too fast. The fasting period of *emptiness* in the GI tract serves to balance Nature's cycles of work and rest. In his classic treatise about the Sabbath, Wayne Muller beautifully reminds us of life's intrinsic rhythms:

> All life requires a rhythm of rest. There is a rhythm in our waking activity and the body's need for sleep. There is a rhythm in the way day dissolves into night and night into the morning. There is a rhythm as the active growth of spring and summer is quieted by the necessary dormancy of fall and winter. There is a tidal rhythm, a deep, eternal conversation between the land and the great sea. In our bodies, the heart rests perceptibly after each life-giving beat; the lungs rest between the exhale and the inhale. [46, 47]

There is mounting scientific evidence that regular fasting leads to a healthier life. [48, 49] In practice, this can be as simple a change in daily habits as not eating between meals. The reason many popular "diets" work is related to the fasting principle: Keto is a fast from carbohydrates; Vegetarianism and Vegan are fasting from animal products to varying degrees; the Whole 30 is a fast from dairy, wheat, and any processed foods; and a growing number of health experts promote "intermittent fasting" — which means confining their daily intake of food to within eight hours out of each twenty-four, for instance, between 10 am and 6 pm.

Understanding fasting as a part of the natural cycle can help balance the mind/body/spirit. Fasting has been a part of most wisdom traditions for centuries: Moses fasted, Jesus fasted, Buddha fasted, Muhammad fasted. Regular fasting, whether once a week, once a month, or for extended periods — Roman Catholic practices during Lent, Ramadan in Muslim tradition — promotes clarity of body/mind/spirit. It allows the body to detoxify and deeply rest. And when the stomach and intestines are allowed to be clear and quiet, the mind can become more settled. In this attitude of stillness, awareness is keener. Those who practice yoga and/or meditation know that an empty stomach is needed to focus mind and body.

There is no single way to fast; fasting can be adopted for the amount of time and interval that works best for each individual. Some people choose a particular day of the week to fast for ten, twelve, or twenty-four hours. Popular fasting patterns include:

- 5:2 pattern: Calorie restriction for two days/week, preferably not consecutive. No less than 500 calories per day for women and 600 calories per day for men are recommended.

- 6:1 pattern: As described above but calories are restricted for only one day a week.

- Eat-Stop-Eat: A complete fast from solid food for twenty-four hours, one or two times per week.

- 16:8 pattern: Also known as "intermittent fasting," in this pattern, all food is consumed within an eight-hour window, and sixteen hours are fasted every day.

Some people choose much longer fast periods — forty-eight hours or more — which significantly increases the risk of problems: hunger, dehydration, hypoglycemia, headaches, irritability, mood changes, difficulty concentrating, fainting, muscle cramping, and weakness. To reduce the incidence of these, it is advised that fast periods do not exceed twenty-four hours.

A few other tips for fasting safely include:

- Reduce food consumption the day before a fast, so the body can adjust to lower caloric intake.

- Eat a small amount on fast days. The 5:2 pattern allows up to twenty-five percent of normal caloric intake, and the majority of it should be in the form of protein.

- Stay well, hydrated. Because your body gets between twenty and thirty percent of daily fluid intake from food, you will dehydrate easily on a fast. a good rule of thumb is "8x8"— at least eight 8-ounce glasses of water a day while fasting. Thirst is a very individual and reliable indicator, however, so if you are thirsty – listen to your body and drink more!

- Plan activities to avoid boredom but avoid high energy expenditure. Slow walking, gentle yoga/stretching, meditation, reading, light housework, listening to music, or a podcast will help the time go by more quickly.

- Stop fasting if you feel unwell. Feelings of nausea, fainting, being too weak or tired to carry out normal activity are signs that you need food for energy. Be prepared with an energy bar or quick protein snack to break the fast before medical attention may be required.

- Eat plenty of whole foods on non-fasting days: meat, fish, eggs, fruits, veggies, and legumes to keep you well during your fast.

- Do not break a fast with alcohol or a celebratory feast. Doing so can lead to nausea and vomiting, fatigue, and lethargy. Try to ease gently back into a normal eating routine with smaller portions for the first meal or two.

- Consider taking multivitamin supplements if you fast regularly. People on lower-calorie diets tend to be deficient in essential nutrients like iron, calcium, and B vitamins.

Note: Persons with certain medical conditions, such as diabetes, should consult their healthcare providers before adopting a fasting routine. Some people choose a particular day of the week to fast for ten, twelve, or twenty-four hours. It is important to remember that energy levels during fasting may be diminished, and activities need to be structured accordingly on fast days. It might be possible to consider devoting the fasting day to rest, allowing your body/mind/spirit to catch up from the busy-ness of the week, taking time to restore and heal.

Weighty Issues

Obesity and its many related medical problems are epidemics among both adults and children in American society today. [50, 51] More than 70% of Americans are overweight, and 40% qualify as obese. [52] Adding a further element of urgency to an already detrimental condition, during the pandemic of 2020, obesity was listed as one of the many underlying medical conditions that can lead to death from COVID-19. [53, 54, 55, 56]

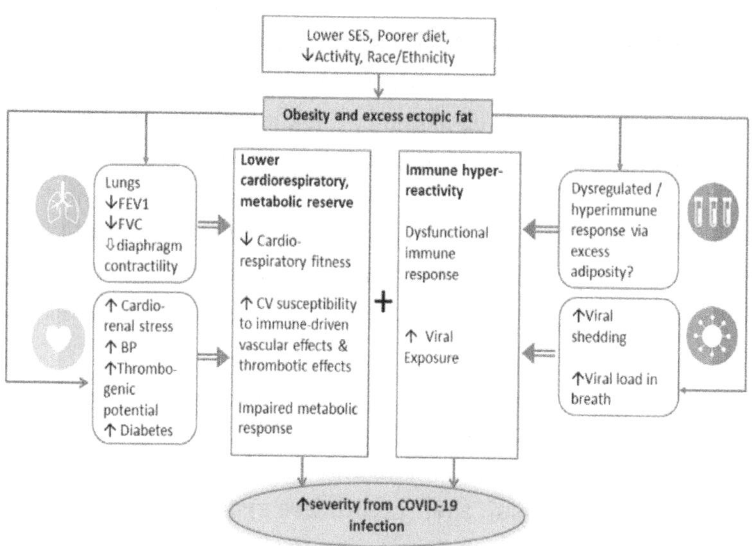

Pathways potentially linking obesity or excess ectopic fat to more severe coronavirus disease 2019 (COVID-19) illness. There are multiple pathways by which obesity (or excess ectopic fat) may increase the effect of COVID-19 infection. These include underlying impairments in cardiovascular, respiratory, metabolic, and thrombotic pathways in relation to obesity, all of which reduce reserve and ability to cope with COVID-19 infection and the secondary immune reaction to it. At the same time, there are several reasons why obese individuals may have amplified or dysregulated immune response, linked both to greater viral exposure, as well as the possibility that excess adipose tissue potentiates the immune response. BP indicates blood pressure; COVID-19, coronavirus disease 2019; CV, cardiovascular; FEV1, forced expiratory volume; FVC, forced vital capacity; and SES, socioeconomic status. Circulation Vol. 142, No. 1 22 Apr 2020:

Leaving aside medical issues, the epidemic of obesity is caused by the choice's individuals make. Every day millions of people try fad diets, medications, and supplements for weight loss to no avail. Many struggle for years to lose weight and keep it off. Statistics say that fewer than 2% of adult dieters who have lost at least five pounds are successful at keeping it off for two years. [57]

> *"By matter we are nourished, lifted up, linked to everything else, invaded by life."*
>
> ~Pierre Teilhard de Chardin

Drs. Chopra and Tanzi write that the biggest single thing Americans need to heal is the belief that the mind and body are somehow separate. They state that the mind of a typical dieter is struggling with what the body is actively doing, which dooms the dieting process to failure. Why don't diets work? Because usually, the mind is operating as if it were disconnected from what the body is actually doing. Decisions are conscious, but habits are not. Habits of a frustrated dieter can often look something like these: [58]

- The body is taking in and processing more calories than it requires.
- The body is coping with overloads of fat, sugar, and salt.
- The body adjusts to toxins in food, water, and air that often have unknown adverse effects.

- The body creates and then must deal with low-level chronic inflammation exacerbated by highly processed fast or junk foods.

- The body is confronting energetic ups and downs related to irregular eating during all hours of the day and night.

For decades, in book after book, Dr. Deepak Chopra has offered the same thinking about achieving a right-sized body. Each person, who he refers to as a bodymind, is naturally equipped to do what the body and mind both want to do; which is to eat normally by paying attention to and following the signals of hunger and satiety. Two neuropeptide hormones, leptin and ghrelin, secreted in a natural biorhythm, are primarily responsible for balancing hunger and satiation. [59] The real truth is this: an individual does not feel like they have had enough to eat when their *stomach* says it is full. They feel like they've had enough to eat when their *brain* says so. However, when one's mind and body are separated — that is, by holding the belief that this is so — a person can override the brain's normal chemical signaling by distorting the mind's relationship to the brain.

The result? Instead of simply listening and responding to the hormonal signals of the body's natural biorhythms governing hunger and satiation, a person's mind can impose other behaviors. Because each individual possesses free will, these behaviors run the gamut from needing to *clean your plate* — even if that means continuing to eat after you are full. To mindlessly snacking at all hours, to *eating your feelings* and consuming excessive sugars and fats, to drinking alcohol. When obesity results from these behaviors, the blame is usually put on the body!

Besides breathing and sleeping, eating is life's most vital activity. We cannot sustain ourselves without eating. According to psychologist and author on mindfulness, Jon Kabat-Zinn. [60, 61] "For the most part, we eat with great automaticity and little insight into its critical importance for us in sustaining life and also in sustaining health." [62] Mindful eating may be an approach to weight management that ends the struggle; adopting a holistic approach — such as viewing each individual as a bodymind — no longer pitches the body as the enemy against the mind, leaving the person to be its victim.

A novel way to break the self-defeating cycle of frustration with failed "diets" is not a stomach-shrinking operation, nor a miracle drug to establish a higher metabolic setpoint. It involves deliberately and consciously changing one's mind about a new goal that is not a desired weight, but the goal of finding and keeping *balance* in the whole bodymind. Over time, poor nutritional choices can lead to actual chemical imbalances in brain circuitry, resulting in strengthening neural pathways associated with impulsive eating and drinking behaviors. Concurrently, the areas in the brain that govern rational conscious decision-making become weakened. [63] To make matters worse, when an individual blames themselves for poor decisions and/or feels like a failure, lower parts of the brain that deal with primitive emotions begin to override the cerebral cortex, which negatively influences decision-making — a vicious cycle.

Food Anthropology research suggests paleo-humans consumed a 1-to-1 ratio of Omega-6 to Omega-3 fats. In current western diets, the ratio has shifted to approximately 16-to-l, in large part due to the 20th-century explosion of Omega-6 dominant vegetable oils in ultra-processed industrial foods. Omega-3 fats are essential, meaning our bodies cannot produce them but are vitally necessary for normal cellular activity. Research has shown their positive effect on various cardiovascular concerns, inflammatory patterns, cognitive development, and psychiatric disorders. [64]

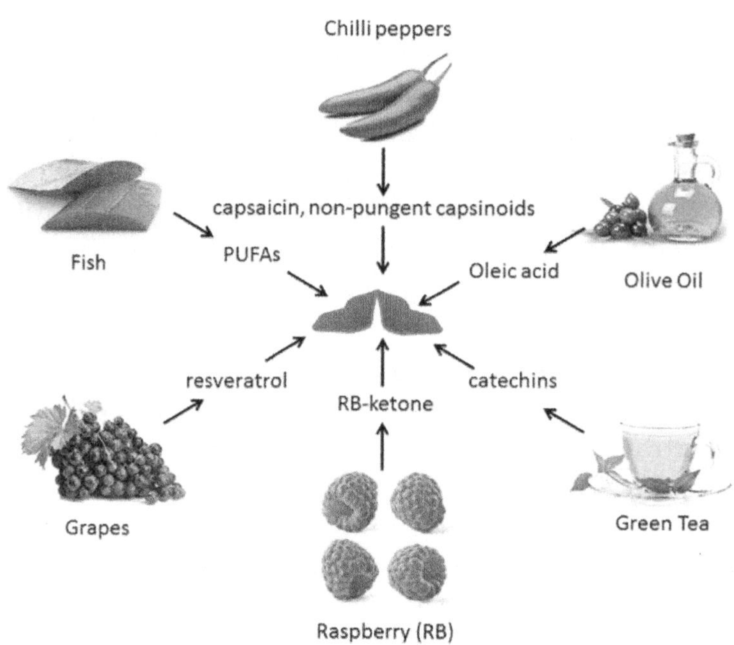

Image Credit and Reference: Srivastava S, Veech RL. Brown and Brite: The Fat Soldiers in the Anti-obesity Fight. Front Physiol. 2019;10:38. Published 2019 Jan 30. doi:10.3389/fphys.2019.00038

Scientific research suggests that white adipose cells — which tend to store fat and become inflamed — may actually be modified into more metabolically-active adipose cells through foods. Certain foods have been shown to activate that process in cell studies. [65, 66, 67, 68]

Body/mind/spirit balance can be restored in many ways; one good decision at a time. Good decisions involve successfully making choices that are self-enhancing, such as:

- not reaching for food as an "emotional fix"
- stopping the energy-draining and futile mental battle of "fighting with yourself." Remember: What you resist, persists.
- ignoring calorie counts and instead improving portion control and nutritional content of food
- focusing on reaching small self-improvement goals, not all related to weight, in a step-by-step fashion
- defining and reaching a turning point

Like journaling, self-inquiry exercises can help an individual examine where imbalances exist in their life and rank them in order of importance: sleep; work, life, and time balance; stress; emotions; relationships, etc. Making choices to empower oneself to deal with the things that bring one out of balance, along with finding ways to restore what equals balance for each individual, opens the way for lasting change in the holistic bodymind. As does making the vital mind shift of *believing* in the healing power and wisdom of the bodymind, which is always seeking *homeostasis*, the medical word for the dynamic balance of all the many processes involved in keeping a human healthy at any age.

In the practice for mindful eating outlined below, an individual can override the brain's 'default' setting of operating via mostly conditioned responses to events and allow communication directly with the higher brain — the pre-frontal cortex responsible for conscious thoughts, decisions, and actions. When pausing to make a conscious choice, an individual's reason for eating should be: *I'm hungry*, **not** - *I am pacifying a feeling'*. If the latter is true, it is important to realize that the feeling will be just as present as hunger. Most often, people are in the habit of racing past the feeling to the food. The goal here is to take time (**PAUSE**) to stop and notice what one is feeling before eating (**OBSERVE**).

The list of possible emotions that may urge one to eat is endless, but here are a few to consider:

Overwhelmed
Tired or exhausted
Pressured
Distracted
Anxious or disturbed
Bored
Restless
Insecure or frustrated
Angry or upset

Taking time before eating to register if one is physically hungry or just pacifying a feeling is a mindful practice anyone can adopt, not just those interested in weight loss. If this mindful pause is practiced faithfully, the time will come when your mind may surprise you by saying something new in response to the usual questions! For instance, "I don't need to eat this." Or "I'm not really hungry, so why eat right now?" or "Maybe I'm thirsty. I'll have a drink first and then see if I still want to eat." The urge to free oneself from a habit is real motivation, so when this unexpected moment arrives, ACT ON IT!

Of course, the bodymind knows if one has been eating to cope with feelings, but it also knows there are other ways to cope. Once this has been recognized, other choices can be made to learn different methods to deal with feelings, and the urge to eat will lessen. This mindful eating practice's eventual goal is allowing the bodymind to regain its natural ability to recognize the body's hormonal signals in a normal biorhythm of hunger and satiation.

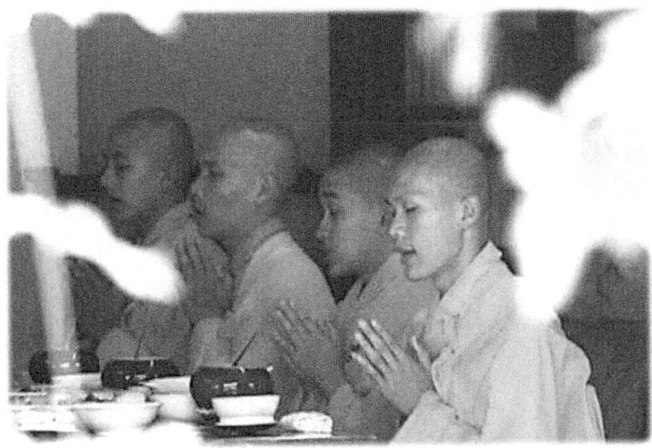

Individual practice for mindful eating [69]

"The next time you eat anything, whether as a meal or a snack, do the following:

Step 1: Pause before you eat the first bite and take a deep breath. Practicing mindfulness, become aware of all that is good in your life, being grateful for this food and other blessings.

PAUSE

Step 2: Ask yourself, "Why am I eating this?"

BREATHE

Step 3: Whatever answer you get, take note of it. Better yet – write it down. You might even start a mindful eating journal.

OBSERVE

Step 4: Make a *conscious* choice to eat or not eat.

RESPOND

Mindfulness for veterans

Post-traumatic stress disorder (PTSD) affects 23% of veterans returning from Afghanistan and Iraq. Left untreated, PTSD is associated with high rates of other disorders, disability, and poor life quality. [70, 71, 72] Evidence suggests that mindfulness-based stress reduction (MBSR), an intervention that teaches individuals to attend to the present moment in a non-judgmental, accepting manner, can reduce depression and anxiety symptoms.

By encouraging acceptance of thoughts, feelings, and experiences without avoidance, mindfulness-based interventions target experiential avoidance, a key factor in the development and maintenance of PTSD, and may be an acceptable type of intervention for veterans who have poor adherence to existing treatments for PTSD, according to a study done by the Minneapolis Veterans Administration.

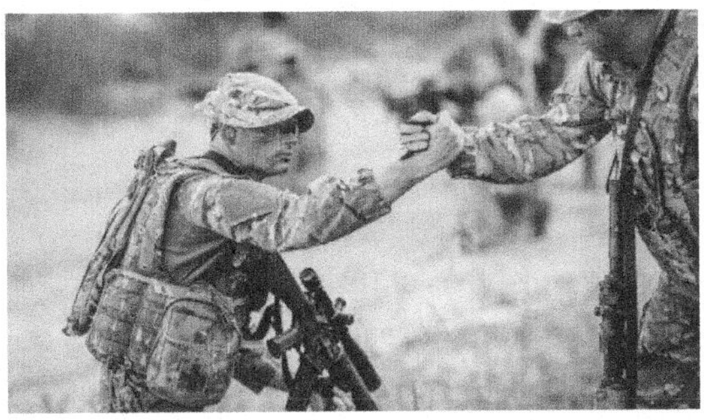

In a study done by the Salt Lake Veterans Health Administration in 2020, 185 military veterans surveyed their interests, beliefs, knowledge, and mindfulness practice. Thirty percent practiced mindfulness in the past year, mainly for stress, posttraumatic stress disorder, sleep, and depression. Over seventy-five percent who practiced reported perceived benefit. Veterans rarely reported negative beliefs about mindfulness; 56% perceived an understanding of mindfulness, and 46% were aware of Veterans Health Administration mindfulness offerings. In all, 55% were interested in learning about mindfulness, 58% were interested in learning how it could help, and 43% were interested in combining mindfulness with a pleasurable activity.

A diet for the mind

In the 21st century, we are faced with an overwhelming array of technological devices that supply a constant stream of opinions, comments, news, information, misinformation, marketing ploys, solicitations, and even humor. This never-ending barrage of information can be a source of stress and anxiety; conditions known to increase risk factors for serious illnesses. A few examples of research about health sequelae associated with media overload are included here:

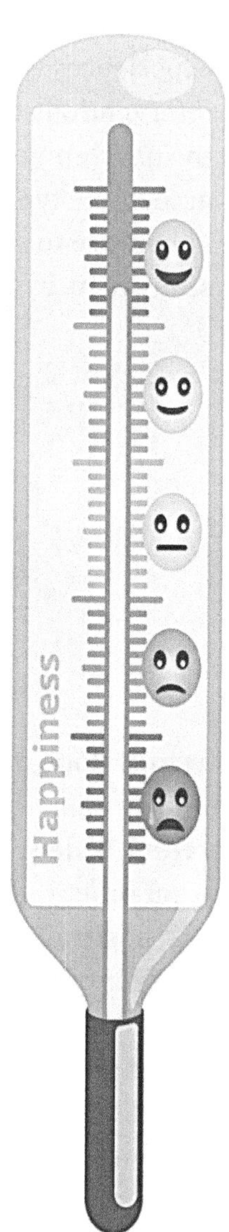

Much of the news we receive is slanted in a negative or fearful direction. Research out of the College of London published in *Alzheimer's & Dementia* found 'repetitive negative thinking' (RNT) is linked to subsequent cognitive decline as well as the deposition of harmful brain proteins linked to Alzheimer's. [73]

"The way that news is presented and how we access news has changed significantly over the last 15 to 20 years," says Graham Davey, a professor emeritus of psychology at Sussex University in the UK editor-in-chief of the *Journal of Experimental Psychopathology.* [74, 75]

> *"Every illness involves stress, either as a cause or as a result."*
>
> ~Deanna Minich, PhD author of *The Rainbow Diet*

"These changes have often been detrimental to general mental health." Davey says today's news is "increasingly visual and shocking" and points to the inclusion of smartphone videos and audio clips as examples. These bystander-captured media can be so intense that they can cause acute stress symptoms — like problems sleeping, mood swings, or aggressive behavior — or even PTSD, he says. [76] Davey's research has shown that negative television news is a significant mood-changer, and the moods it tends to produce are sadness and anxiety. "Our studies also showed that this change in mood exacerbates the viewer's worries, even when those worries are not directly relevant to the news stories being broadcast," he says. [77]

A 2012 study done at Harvard showed that social media use activates the brain's parts associated with pleasurable sensations; the same pleasure that we get from eating food, getting money, or even having sex. [78] Kids today register for their first social media accounts at an average age of 11.4 years. [79]

According to a 2015 study by Common Sense Media, the typical American teen spends about nine hours per day, or sixty-three hours per week) on personal electronic media — not including technology used in schools. The majority of teens check their devices hourly, at least, and most feel compelled to respond to texts and other messages almost immediately. [80]

Mental health and childhood development experts express serious concerns about the damage this kind of addiction to screen time is doing to children. One in ten youths today carries a diagnosis of ADHD; a condition that has soared in incidence since 2000. [81] "I believe the increase in ADHD diagnoses has everything to do with the amount of time our children are spending in front of screens," says Thomas Kersting, licensed psychotherapist and author of *Disconnected: How to Recover Our Digitally Distracted Kids.* Today, many teens exhibit antisocial behaviors like struggling to make eye contact in conversation, poor coping skills, and difficulty forming friendships in person.

> *"Opportunities to find deeper powers within ourselves come when life seems most challenging."*
>
> ~ Joseph Campbell

Another effect the overuse of electronic devices may have on teens is the proper growth and development of the prefrontal cortex, which is not complete until most people have reached their mid to late twenties. [82] This brain area plays a significant role in judgment, willpower, decision-making, and critical thinking ability. "There is a biochemical reaction taking place when you get a text or notification. The reward center in the brain lights up with the presence of chemicals like dopamine and serotonin," says Dr. Larry Rosen, professor emeritus in the Psychology Department at Cal State University, Dominguez Hills. [83, 84] A research psychologist and author of *The Distracted Mind: Ancient Brains in a High-Tech World,* Rosen sees an increase in anxiety among younger users who might want to turn off their phones but feel pressure not to disappoint their friends, real and virtual, when they do so.

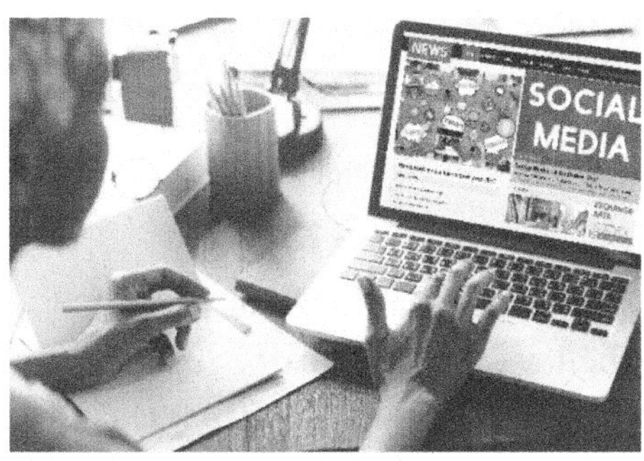

When there is an endless supply of information, stimulation, virtual connection, and entertainment at your fingertip's night and day, there is no need for anyone to be bored. Dr. Kersting says that is a bad thing: "Boredom is the Miracle-Grow for the mind and your emotional well-being. It's a form of mindfulness that we can all use to reflect and build creativity. We have to teach our kids to embrace boredom, not avoid it." [85]

According to eMarketer research done in 2019, adults in the U.S. spend twelve hours and nine minutes per day using some form of electronic media. This figure includes all digital media platforms, television, and radio. In contrast, worldwide data from 2020 states that the average time an adult spends on social media amounts to 144 minutes (two hours and twenty-four minutes) per day. Notably, this figure has risen by one hour/day, or 62%, since 2012. Obviously, if this is an average, there are many countries that exceed this number and also many others where time spent with electronics is less.

Among 1,000 young adults born in the U.S. after 1994 (Generation Z), 91% are daily social media users, with 51% reporting "almost constant" use in a 2017 report released by Origin, the in-house research group arm of the marketing agency Hill Holliday. Only twenty-nine percent of this group uses television daily. Although 75% of them thought social media had more benefits than drawbacks — like making it easier to connect with friends —68% of this group said they were anxious, depressed, and saddened by social media; with 22% feeling like they were *missing out*, twenty-nine percent feeling insecure and 72%, reporting lowered self-esteem. 72% of these Gen Z'ers agreed that people their age were "too distracted" by electronics.

The research findings noted here only serve to confirm what the authors of Empty Plate believe wholeheartedly to be true: Social media is not going anywhere anytime soon – at least not until eating food becomes unpleasurable. The brain's chemical changes that accompany social media use interrupt and disrupt the workings of the mind. Consuming excessive amounts of this *mental food* can lead to mental disorders in users of all ages and make mindfulness much more elusive and challenging to achieve.

Along with Dr. Bruce Lipton, Dr. Deepak Chopra, and Dr. Rudolph Tanzi, thought leaders in human science today propose that the location of the 'mind' is everywhere, with innate intelligence imbuing every cell in the body. [86] It might even be said that the bodymind's innate intelligence, as featured in the *information superhighway* that delivers chemical messages to and from every cell in our bodies, is *more mindful*— than our conscious behavior choices. If an individual chooses to engage in 'mindless' behavior, like eight to twelve hours of electronic media use each day, the effects are far-reaching. [87, 88]

The science of psychoneuroimmunology (PNI) studies the interaction of mental activity with the functioning of the immune system. A harmful activity of the mind that almost everyone can relate to is worry. Worry qualifies as a mindless behavior in many ways. It can become obsessive; it leads to states of anxiety and distress; it is generated by lower brain regions and blocks access to thinking that produces rational solutions to problems. And worry is rarely, if ever, capable of providing a solution for what is being worried about.

Yet, despite its futility, worry is all-pervasive in American society today. Turbulent politics, pandemic disease and mass fatalities worldwide, social unrest, protests, increasing violence, and mental illness in our society contribute to anxiety in the present and worrying about the future. Chronic and seemingly uncontrollable worry are forms of self-created stress. Stress has been extensively studied in PNI. Chronic stress can compromise the immune system and has been associated with severe infections, as well as worse prognoses for cancer, heart disease, and HIV-AIDS.[89, 90]

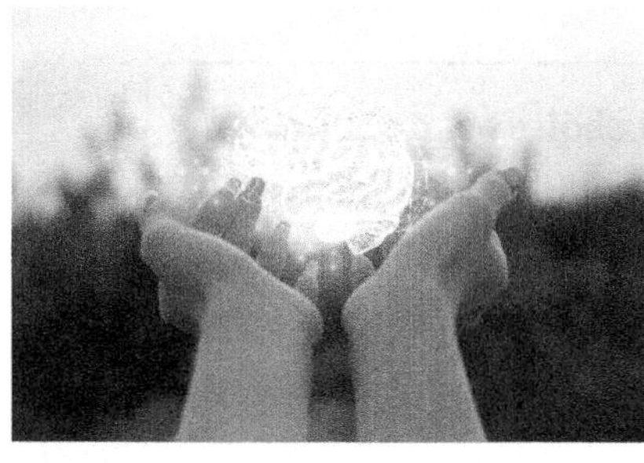

When the mind — through positive thoughts, beliefs, and emotions — directs the body to improve one's health, it is called the *placebo* effect. In contrast, the *nocebo* effect occurs when the bodymind is subjected to the damaging effects of negative thoughts, fearful emotions and beliefs.

During the pandemic of 2020, *nocebo* suggestions were being supplied in mega-doses by most media sources. According to Dr. Bruce Lipton, our positive and negative beliefs impact physical health and all aspects of our lives. "Your beliefs act like filters on a camera, changing how you see the world. And your biology adapts to those beliefs. When we truly recognize that our beliefs are THAT powerful, we hold the key to freedom." [91, 92, 93, 94]

Tammera and Kathleen both practice conscious restraint in exposure to negative and alarmist media in our *diet of the mind.* Our expert recommendation to you, dear reader, is to thoroughly consider the effects of what you are allowing into your holistic consciousness today on your body/mind/spirit. Now more than ever, it is essential to be selective about, periodically abstain from, and even disengage altogether from media sources that are negatively influencing our well-being. Just as we can commit to making conscious choices about the food we allow our bodies to consume, we can monitor what we choose to allow our minds to absorb and thus enter our bodymind consciousness.

> *Principle 4*: Behavioral choices can support or compromise innate cellular intelligence.

The Power of Slowing Down

Do you remember what you ate for lunch yesterday (if you ate lunch, that is)? Can you describe the colors, flavors, smells, and textures of the food you ate? Do you remember how hungry you were before you ate? Could you rate the feeling on a scale of 1 to 10? Or can you remember how full or satisfied you felt after you were finished eating? Chances are pretty good that you cannot, and you would not be alone. Modern times are filled with fast foods, drive-throughs, and on-the-go-meals — we eat lunches at our desks or in meetings, and dinners are eaten on the couch in front of at least one screen.

As discussed earlier, mindful eating can help an individual rediscover what their body is *telling* them at any moment. It is a way of eating that truly supports overall and holistic well-being. Since eating is something most people usually do a number of times each day, mindful eating can be another tool to polish awareness skills and invite more moments of mindful presence into daily life. *Being fully aware in the moment* is the first tenet of the Buddhist practice of mindfulness. It involves getting rid of distraction and making a meal the object of your full attention. While eating, consciously place your focus and full attention on the food — noticing all the sensations that are involved: flavors, colors, smells, form, textures. Savor each bite, one by one. Did your grandmother ever tell you to chew your food 100 times? Kathleen's did! Maybe that's a slight exaggeration of this process, but it does slow a person down!

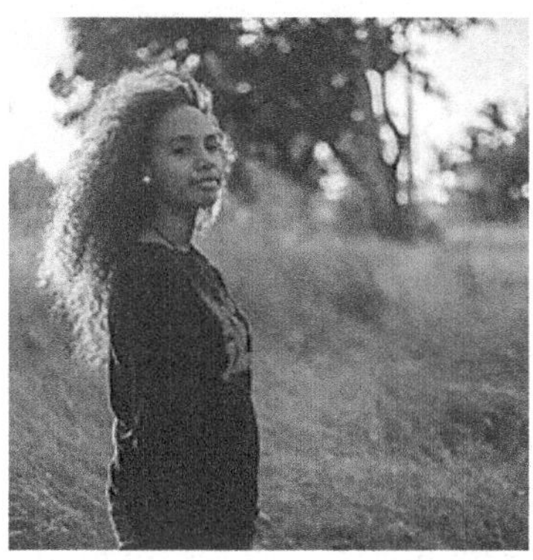

Avoiding judgment is another key component of mindfulness, and this includes mealtimes. Don't be tempted to listen to the *monkey mind* chattering away during a meal, making unwanted associations or accusations, and labeling foods as *good* or *bad.* These judgmental labels come from the ego and not from the bodymind. They can set up guilty feelings about eating, which takes away from the ability to enjoy being present. If the mind succeeds in wandering into judgment, one can practice just noticing that is happening and observe it — "Look at that! Isn't that interesting?" — and gently bring the focus back to noticing the food itself and what feelings may exist in the moment.

Another mindful technique is to pause and deliberately assess hunger and fullness cues before, during, and after a meal. [95] Using the 1 to10 scale — with zero being famished and ten feeling stuffed full — a person can ask his or herself where they want to be both before and after eating? If an individual is feeling famished when they begin, it is more likely that overeating will result. If one begins at around three and can learn to feel comfortable completing a meal when feeling around six or seven, their food intake will be in more reasonable portions.

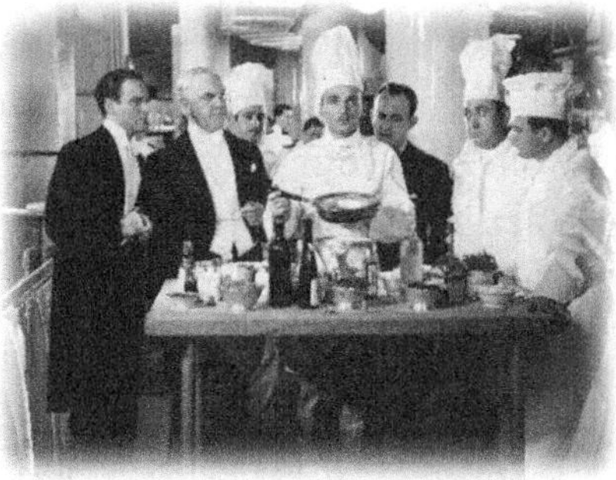

Checking in with a physical hunger level measure when wanting to eat something helps one learn to recognize that the bodymind may indeed need something, but it may not be food. If an individual finds his or her measuring at six before eating, there may be something else they are *hungry* for. Maybe they are bored, or stressed, or procrastinating, or sad, or feeling lonely or disconnected. As mentioned in the mindful eating practice outlined earlier in this chapter, realizing those other needs as different from the physical body's actual need for food/fuel is a big part of mindful eating. Maybe what is needed after dinner is not a scoop of ice cream for dessert, but sweetness is what is craved. Spending some quality time with a spouse, a friend, or your children may fill that emotional need for sweetness in your life.

Five proven benefits of eating slowly [96]

- *You can eat anything you want.* No foods are off-limits, says Meredith Milton, a Seattle-based nutritionist and mindful eating coach. Whether it's a burger that you realize is fatty and salty or a sweet piece of cake, you realize how the food really tastes when you are fully present. You may find that you enjoy the food more while wanting less.

- *Your taste buds may change.* When you slow down and truly tune in to taste preferences, prepare yourself to learn how much better real, not processed, foods taste.

- *You may lose weight.* Learning to listen to your body's hunger and satiety cues can help you reach a healthy, right-sized body. However, mindful eating is best approached from a perspective of self-care and health improvement versus a weight-loss strategy.

- *Your digestion improves.* Mindful eating can work wonders for common GI problems like flatulence and bloating. Chewing your food more slowly helps digestion because saliva contains important enzymes. Also, mindful eating may help discover food intolerances that are responsible for digestive issues.

- *You will have learned a new skill for life.* Remember the "mindfulness muscle" that was mentioned as this chapter began? Once you develop the skill of mindful eating, you have the "muscle memory" for it. Of course, no one eats every single meal mindfully, but it is a skill that you can always come back to and practice again and again in diverse settings.

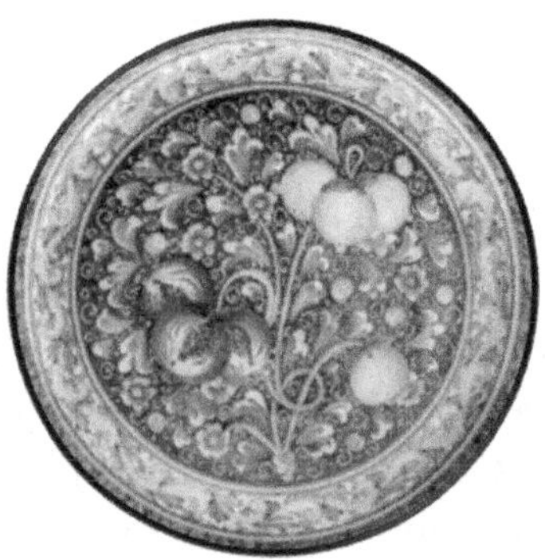

Eating a mindful meal: the whole experience

1. Begin by banning distractions. No television, no phone, no computer, no reading a book or magazine, no open door for the neighbors to interrupt your meal.

2. Take at least one long, slow, deep breath. More if you like it!

3. Become aware of how you are feeling at the moment. Are you stressed? Rushed? Tired? Remember not to judge the feeling, just to notice it. Try to relax your body-mind and use your breath to exhale any tension away from what is present, right here and right now. How hungry are you? Use the 1 to 10 scale.

4. Smile to yourself and spend a few moments giving thanks for the nourishment that is before you. Give thanks for those who prepared it; those who grew, harvested, and transported it to your area; and for the Earth itself that has produced it.

5. Become aware of *seeing* the food as if you've never seen it before! Let that bowl of steaming soup or juicy sandwich become *real* to you. Notice the food's temperature, smells, colors, shape, form, and any noises it might make.

6. The next step is intending to reach for the food. *Become aware of this.* The power of conscious intention drives the body into action, in this case — to reach for the food. When you are ready, mindfully reach out and make contact with the food. Pay attention to this whole process, the moving of your arm and hand, the initial touch on contact — feeling the sensations of apple or sandwich. Be aware of raising your arm as you lift the food to your mouth and of your mouth opening. As you place the first bite or spoonful into your mouth, you may want to close your eyes. Be exquisitely aware of the touch, texture, temperature, and taste of the food on your tongue and the burst of sensations that light up your mouth as you begin to chew.

7. Carefully notice each phase of the eating process: as the food comes toward your mouth, notice it opening and closing again, notice your arms raising and lowering. Enjoy all the sensations of chewing and tasting the food in your mouth. Chew slowly and thoroughly, then swallow and notice what that feels like. If you have the time, pause for a mindful breath before going on to the next mouthful.

8. Put your eating utensil down between bites to *SLOW DOWN.* You can also try eating with chopsticks or using your non-dominant hand to help slow a meal's pace.

9. Notice any feelings of unease or compulsiveness that might encourage you to shovel in another mouthful even before you have finished the one before it. Mindfulness can help you begin to understand that you can take control over forces that all too often unconsciously control eating behavior. Watch how the desire for more arises, leading to the intention for another bite.

10. Pause about a third of the way through the food on your plate and ask yourself: Do I feel satisfied? Do I need to continue eating? Do I feel like I've had enough? Use a 1 to 10 scale. Does the food still taste as good, or am I losing interest?

11. Continue to eat mindfully if you are still hungry, repeating steps eight through ten. Pause again to check hunger levels after eating another one-third of your food.

12. No matter how much food remains on your plate, when you feel satisfied, simply stop eating.

When individuals learn to eat mindfully, they become more in tune with both the food and the body. A deep awareness of knowing about what is eaten grows, including a greater understanding of what is beneficial for the bodymind and what is not. With practice, one becomes unmistakably aware of the signals the body is sending to stop eating, making it harder to overeat. As mentioned earlier, consistent mindful eating can help break unconscious, compulsive eating habits, and eliminate food addictions.

How much an individual can learn about themselves by eating a meal mindfully can be quite a surprise. By slowing down and noticing the process of eating as an activity, we may begin to recognize and thus gain the power to transform old, limiting patterns of thinking and behavior that are self-sabotaging. Seen mindfully — that is, with compassion and without judgment, these insights may offer valuable understanding into how we assimilate other things into our lives.

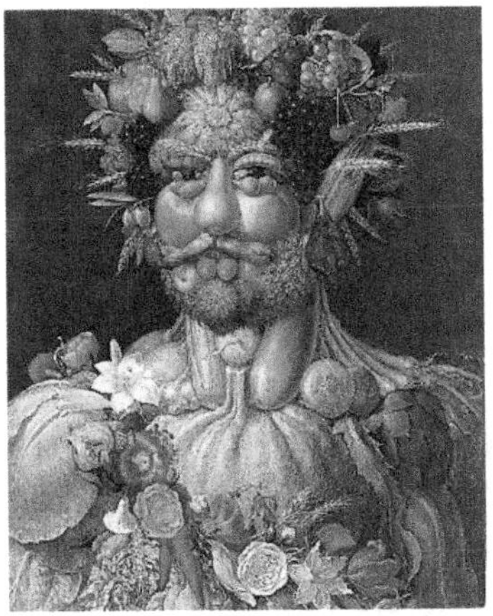

For example, are the life choices we make really nourishing us? How well are we chewing and assimilating the information we put on our empty plates in other areas of life? Are we suffering from *information indigestion*?

The same feeling of neediness that leads one to reach for another bite while the mouth is still full may offer some insights into conditioned patterns that can prevent an individual from fully savoring complex relationships in their work or with family. Keeping in mind that we nourish ourselves in many ways and striving for the balanced body-mind that allows health to flourish, we can create new patterns that promote sustainable health and self-development in our lives.

> *"Spirit and body go hungry when the outcome takes precedence over love."*
>
> ~Haven Trevino [97]

Mindfulness lessons: prayer and spirituality

In many of the world's wisdom traditions, prayer is a way to express faith, hope, love, and gratitude. Taking time to reflect and contemplate important issues to you can also be a form of prayer. Confucius, Lao Tzu, Jesus, Buddha, and Muhammad all took time alone to pray, meditate, and practice what we call mindfulness today. His Holiness, the Dalai Lama meditates for at least 3 hours per day (and has for decades), and the Pope spends time daily in solitary prayer. Most spiritual traditions recommend some form of distancing oneself from the world's attractions and distractions as a regular practice. No matter what beliefs an individual holds, there is room on the empty plate for helpings of wisdom from time-honored teachings.

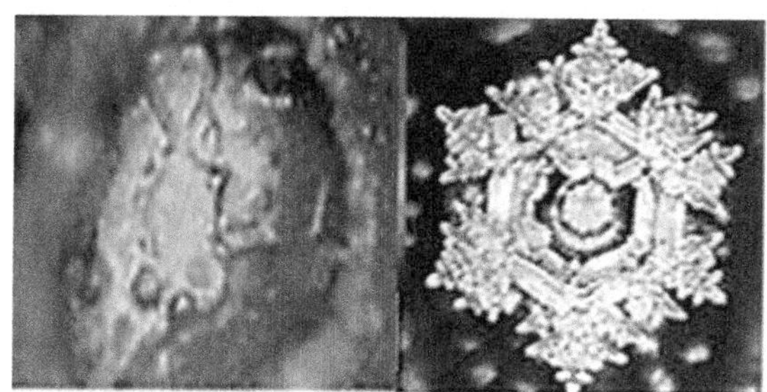

Before Buddhist Prayer — After Buddhist Prayer

Blogspot.Com Image

BUDDHISM: *Meditation*
About 2,500 years ago, the Buddha wandered around India, seeking to ascertain the meaning of life and trying out many different established meditation techniques. Not satisfied with any of them, he developed the practice now thought of as mindfulness — being attentive to the present moment. Over time, as his followers developed the religion named after him, qualities like compassion, empathy, and gratitude emerged as

foundational for Buddhist practice, which focuses on all other beings' welfare. Dr. Mark Muesse, professor of religious studies at Rhodes College, describes integrating meditation into daily life this way, "Mindfulness is intended to be something you do all day long." [98, 99] The more a person practices, the easier these attitudes become.

CHRISTIANITY: *Attentiveness*

Although the word mindfulness may not be used very often in Christian theology, attentiveness is a recurring theme. Jesus said, "...the kingdom of God is within you." [100] He may have been saying it is important to look within oneself to find love, peace, and justice — qualities that are considered godlike. The practice of Christian contemplative prayer does not involve petitioning a deity for anything; it calls for sitting silently in a reflective experience that creates interior space to discover God's presence. Dr. Muesse says, "Every Christian prayer should have some element of giving thanks or reflecting gratitude." Whether this involves giving thanks for food, family, or any other blessings in an individual's life, the practice of gratitude amplifies good intentions. Recall what happened to the water in Emoto's experiments when exposed to the energy of a blessing or grace before meals or a heartfelt, "Thank you."

Christianity also emphasizes the idea of shared responsibility, whether that means donating financially or working within the community. "The earliest Christians embraced this sense of taking care of others - and that humans are here on Earth to take care of the world and each other," says Dr. Muesse. [101, 102] These words provide a mindfulness lesson in themselves.

HINDUISM: *Mantra*

Hindu practices include mantra and yoga; the aim of both is to focus the mind and achieve unity of mind, body, and spirit within oneself. The technique of mantra involves silently repeating or chanting out loud a single word or phrase. Kathleen's initial meditation training was focused on attention to the breath. It did not include mantra, in contrast with Transcendental Meditation, which is based on the individual receiving a personal mantra from the teacher. Seven years into her daily meditation practice, mantra was introduced to her by Dr. Deepak Chopra, whose teachings are heavily influenced by his Hindu upbringing. When teaching meditation classes, Kathleen calls mantra *a magic carpet for the mind*. Similar to the cadence of repeated prayers used in reciting a rosary or mala, mantra lulls the mind into a calm and relaxed state that is impervious to distraction.

Yoga requires attentiveness to both the body and the breath. *Pranayama*, or controlled breathing techniques, are time-tested Ayurvedic techniques to calm the central nervous system and create healing in the body/mind/spirit. Mantra is very individual and personal; with a little effort, anyone can find a mantra that speaks to them and has meaning. Regular use can help create the best qualities one desires positivity, generosity, patience, self-compassion, or anything else.

ISLAM: *Intention*

> Muhammad said that the main problem with human beings is we forget. Much about Islam is about trying to make us remember and become aware of what is true, Dr. Muesse explains. [103]

Devout Muslims pray five times a day, a practice called *salat*. This observance involves movement, like yoga, and recitation of passages from the Quran, like mantra. Ramadan, the lunar month-long holiday that involves fasting from anything offensive as well as from eating, drinking alcohol, and smoking, is a way to turn people's focus away from worldly pleasures and focus on the inner self. Fasting helps one become aware of how much eating is a part of daily life, as well as allowing the room to realize that not everyone has enough food, which helps develop empathy and compassion. A person does not need to kneel and pray five times in order to have a mindful day. But learning to set an intention for the day in the morning, and revisiting that intention regularly throughout the day, and then reflecting on it again before sleep — with self-compassion and gratitude — is a mindfulness practice that anyone can adopt.

JUDAISM: *Unplugging*

Every week, observant Jews celebrate the Sabbath (*Shabbat)* from sundown on Friday evening until after nightfall on Saturday by withdrawing from electronic devices, staying at home, saying, or singing blessings before meals. And asking at the end of the day that anyone they have offended forgives them as well as forgiving anyone who has offended them. The importance of the Sabbath concept is that it offers a regularly scheduled time to rest, refresh, and connect to the larger Universe, which can help individuals find a deeper sense of meaning in their lives. Anyone can adopt a *device-free* time each week — maybe just a portion of a day — to disconnect from technology, refresh and reconnect with themselves during some peaceful and undisturbed time as a mindfulness practice. After attending a *five-day* silent retreat on her last birthday, Kathleen has adopted the practice of silence one day a week. Her definition of *silence* includes refraining from conversations and other personal interactions, silencing the cellphone, and no computer or television input. These exclusions allow her more time for solitude, meditation, Reiki practice, yoga, writing, and time spent outdoors.

> *Principle 5*: The power of conscious intention drives action.

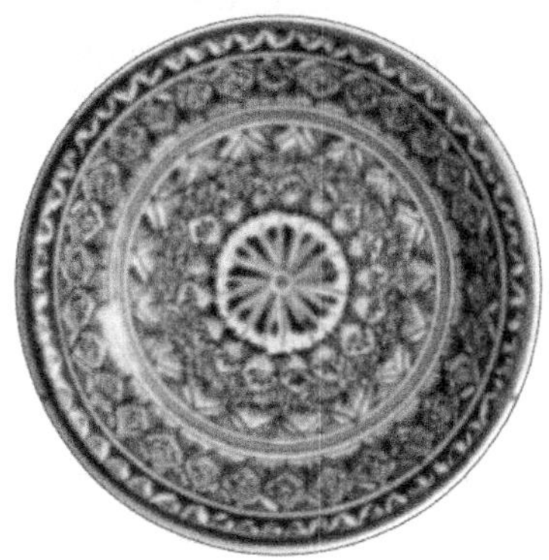

Blessing food with grace:
The benefits of gratitude

Archaeological evidence shows that the Neanderthals in Europe and Southwest Asia had a system of religious beliefs and performed rituals such as funerals. Our cultures have evolved and developed in specific environmental contexts, enabling their communities to not only survive but to flourish in unique and dynamic ways.

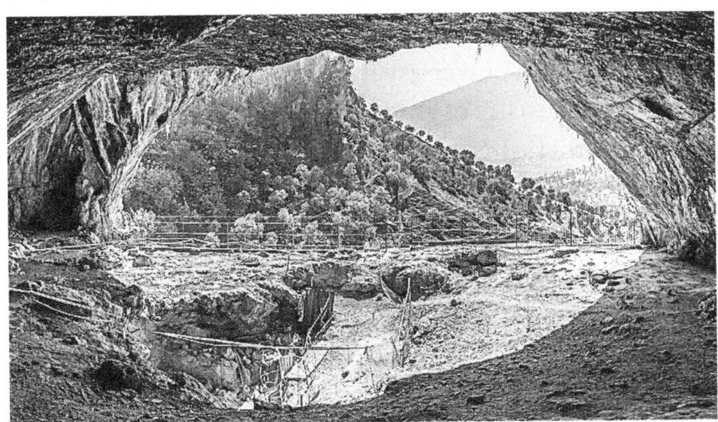

Shanidar Z (Flower Burial) Cave northern Iraq, University of Cambridge

But what exactly is culture? Culture is a broad term that encompasses the full range of learned human behavior patterns. Behaviors, like eating, are often linked to survival. Rather than physical transformation, cultural creativity became the central way humans coped with the demands of nature. Homo sapiens' unique aptitude for creativity allowed for symbolic expression, particularly in cultural and spiritual contexts, such as artwork and burial rituals. This creative activity is the hallmark of the subspecies *Homo sapiens sapiens* — which, translated literally from the Latin, means wise wise human. This is who we are today, a subspecies that is distinguished from others by its intellectual abilities.

The ancient ritual act of blessing food or saying "grace" before it is eaten brings about a heightened state of presence and mindfulness within those preparing to partake. Emoto's groundbreaking work demonstrated that the miraculously, powerful energetic qualities of joy, love, and gratitude caused beneficial physical changes in the molecules of water contained in the food. Expressing gratitude over a meal allows one to pause, breathe, appreciate and be more present to themselves and others, the food itself, the setting, the larger environment, and sometimes to a power greater than themselves. An amazing characteristic of gratitude is that it multiplies when shared with others. Instead of diminishing its power to transform both ourselves and our food, gratitude is amplified when shared within a group of people. Often families will hold hands to physically connect as they share in blessing the food that will be eaten together. As a sincerely cultivated state, gratitude imbues each person with undistracted presence, and everyone can then eat mindfully and enjoy the food more. Appreciation and gratitude turn every meal into a holy time of rest, recovery, and joy. [104, 105]

According to the poet Mark Nepo,

> The goal of all experience is to remove whatever might keep us from being whole. The simplest and deepest way to make who we are at one with the world is through the kindship of gratitude. Sometimes, just giving thanks for the mystery of it all brings everything and everyone closer, the way suction pulls streams of water together. So, take a chance and openly give thanks, even if you're not sure what it is for, and feel the plenitude of all that is living brush up against your heart. [106, 107]

Our plate is now covered with nourishment for the body (food and sustainability) and the mind (mindfulness); we move forward into those elements that add flavor and spice to our life.

"My mind goes to nourishment —
of the body, yes – but also the other kind.

How often it seems I have to be in trouble before I will let in the compassion, I need to live a human life.

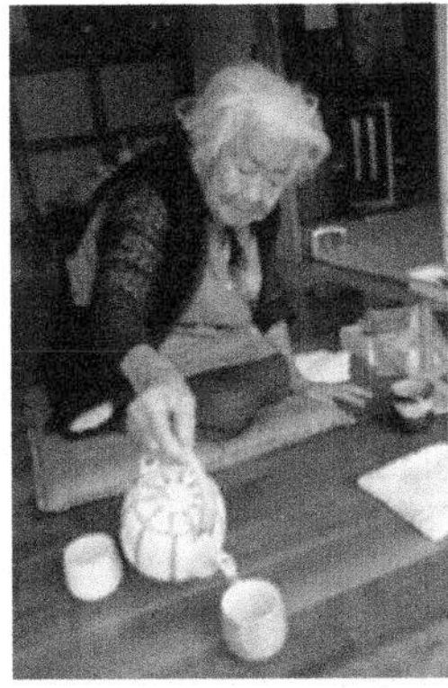

When I discover in myself, finally, a deep willingness to receive nourishment, something has to change in me.

In some alchemical way, I know I will have become the nourishment I sought in the first place."

~Excerpt, "Breakfast" by Gunilla Norris [108]

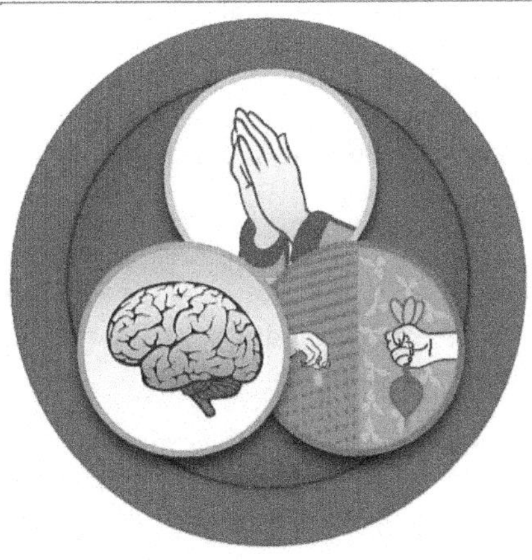

---

1. Tzu, L. Tao Te Ching

2. Emoto, M. (2005) The Hidden Messages in Water.

3. Kabat-Zinn, J. (1990). Full Catastrophe Living: Using the wisdom of your mind to face stress and illness. New York: Dell Publishing.

4. Kabat-Zinn, J. (1990). Full Catastrophe Living: Using the wisdom of your mind to face stress and illness. New York: Dell Publishing.

5. Killingsworth MA, Gilbert DT. 2010. A Wandering Mind Is An Unhappy Mind. Science 330(6006):932

6. Good DJ, Lyddy CJ, Glomb TM, Bono JE, Brown KW, et al. 2016. Contemplating mindfulness at work: an integrative review. J. Manag. 42:114–42

7. Sibinga EMS, Webb L, Ghazarian SR, Ellen JM. 2016. School-based mindfulness instruction: an RCT. Pediatrics 137(1):1–8

8. (2017) https://health.clevelandclinic.org/science-clear-multitasking-doesnt-work/

9. PLOS. (2020, September 2). Heavy electronic media use in late childhood linked to lower academic performance: Findings could help guide parents, teachers, clinicians in planning kids' screen time. ScienceDaily. Retrieved September 4, 2020 from www.sciencedaily.com/releases/2020/09/200902152150.htm

10. https://www.nytimes.com/2006/03/31/health/longawaited-medical-study-questions-the-power-of-prayer.html

11. "Eliciting the Relaxation Response," Benson-Henry Institute for Mind-Body Medicine, Massachusetts General Hospital. Accessed October 3, 2020, https://www.massgeneral.org/bhi/basics/eliciting_rr.aspx.

12. Davidson, R.J. et al. (2003). "Alterations in Brain and Immune Function Produced by Mindfulness Meditation", Psychosomatic Medicine (65, no.4), pp.564=570.

13. Macdonald, A. (Nov.10, 2010) "Using the Relaxation Response to Reduce Stress", Harvard Health Publications. https://www.health.harvard.edu/blog/using-the-relaxation-response-to-reduce-stress-20101110780

14. https://www.nytimes.com/2006/03/31/health/longawaited-medical-study-questions-the-power-of-prayer.html

15. Baylor University. "Mindfulness Combined With Hypnotherapy Aids Highly Stressed People, Study Finds: 'Novel Intervention' May Be As Effective -- Or More So -- As Existing Treatments." Sciencedaily. Sciencedaily, 15 June 2020. Www.Sciencedaily.Com/Releases/2020/06/200615184150.Htm

16. Mindfulness—Classes & Training in Mindfulness Based Stress .... https://healthcare.utah.edu/wellness/services/mindfulness.php

17. European Society of Cardiology. (2020, August 24). Yoga linked with improved symptoms in heart patients. ScienceDaily. Retrieved August 25, 2020 from www.sciencedaily.com/releases/2020/08/200824092010.htm

18. DOI:10.3389/fpubh.2016.00057NationalCenterfor Complementary and Integrative Health: Ayurvedic Medicine: In Depth: https://www.nccih.nih.gov/health/ayurvedic-medicine-in-depth

19. Chokoisky, S. (2015). Sex, Love and Dharma.

20. European Society of Cardiology. (2020, August 24). Yoga linked with improved symptoms in heart patients. ScienceDaily. Retrieved August 25, 2020 from www.sciencedaily.com/releases/2020/08/200824092010.htm

21. Chokoisky, S. Sex, Love and Dharma

22. Chokoisky, S. Sex, Love and Dharma

23. Guha, A. (2006). University of Connecticut Library Open Commons, Ayurvedic Concept of Food and Nutrition

24. Chokoisky, S. Sex, Love and Dharma

25. Leggett, D. (2017). Qi Nutrition, The Energetics of Food-4 http://www.meridianpress.net/articles/energetics-of-food-4.html

26. Payyappallimana, U. & Venkatasubramanian, P. (2016). ResearchGate, Exploring Ayurvedic Knowledge on Food and Health f or Providing Innovative Solutions to Contemporary Healthcare

27. DOI:10.3389/fpubh.2016.00057NationalCenterfor Complementary and Integrative Health: Ayurvedic Medicine: In Depth: https://www.nccih.nih.gov/health/ayurvedic-medicine-in-depth

28. Svoboda RE. Ayurveda's role in preventing disease. Indian J Med Sci. 1998;52(2):70-77.

29. Energetics of food, Qi nutrition by Daverick Leggett: http://www.meridianpress.net/articles/energetics-of-food-4.html

30. Payyappallimana, U. & Venkatasubramanian, P. (2016). ResearchGate, Exploring Ayurvedic Knowledge on Food and Health f or Providing Innovative Solutions to Contemporary Healthcare DOI:10.3389/fpubh.2016.00057

31. Energetics of food, Qi nutrition by Daverick Leggett: http://www.meridianpress.net/articles/energetics-of-food-4.html

32. S., D., N V, R. & Mishra, A. Traditional methods of food habits and dietary preparations in Ayurveda—the Indian system of medicine. J. Ethn. Food 6, 14 (2019). https://doi.org/10.1186/s42779-019-0016-4

33. Chopra, D. Perfect Health

34. Guha, A. (2006). University of Connecticut Library Open Commons, Ayurvedic Concept of Food and Nutrition

35. Payyappallimana, U. & Venkatasubramanian, P. (2016). ResearchGate, Exploring Ayurvedic Knowledge on Food and Health f or

Providing Innovative Solutions to Contemporary Healthcare DOI:10.3389/fpubh.2016.00057

36. S., D., N V, R. & Mishra, A. Traditional methods of food habits and dietary preparations in Ayurveda—the Indian system of medicine. J. Ethn. Food 6, 14 (2019). https://doi.org/10.1186/s42779-019-0016-4

37. Norris, G. Becoming Bread, p. 29

38. What Is the Ayurvedic Diet? Benefits, Downsides, and More by Rachael Links, MS, RD 2019

39. Love Doesn't Sit There Like a Stone. https://www.lovequotes.net.in/love-doesnt-sit-there-like-a-stone/

40. Norris, G. Becoming Bread, p. 29

41. Levy, J&M. Luminous Mind, Pp.102-103

42. Chokoisky, S. Sex, Love And Dharma

43. Muller, W. Sabbath: Finding Rest, Renewal, And Delight In Our Busy Lives.

44. Harvie, M. & Howell, A. Potential Benefits and Harms of Intermittent Energy Restriction and Intermittent Fasting Amongst Obese, Overweight and Normal Weight Subjects, Behavioral Sciences,2017, Mar,7(1), 4. Doi:10.3390/bs7010004

45. Link, R. (July 30, 2018) Https://Www.Healthline.Com/Nutrition/Fasting-Benefits

46. https://www.healthline.com/health/obesity-facts

47. Sabbath: Finding Rest, Renewal, and Delight in Our Busy https://www.barnesandnoble.com/w/sabbath-wayne-muller/1102516406

48. Chopra, D. & Tanzi, The Healing Self

49. Muller, W. Sabbath: Finding Rest, Renewal, And Delight In Our Busy Lives.

50. Kabat-Zinn, J. (1990). Full Catastrophe Living: Using the wisdom of your mind to face stress and illness. New York: Dell Publishing.

51. Chopra & Tanzi, Super Brain

52. Cernohous, Sarica; The Funky Kitchen, the missing link in your nutrition and wellness: 2017 Living Wellness, Flagstaff, AZ

53. Srivastava, S., & Veech, R. L. (2019). Brown and Brite: The Fat Soldiers in the Anti-obesity Fight. Frontiers in physiology, 10, 38. https://doi.org/10.3389/fphys.2019.00038

54. https://www.healthline.com/health/obesity-facts

55. Chopra, D. & Tanzi, The Healing Self

56. The JAMA Network Journals. "Mindfulness-Based Stress Reduction Therapy Decreases PTSD Symptom Severity Among Veterans." Sciencedaily. ScienceDaily, 4 August 2015. Www.Sciencedaily.Com/Releases/2015/08/150804142744.Htm

57. Tracy Herrmann , William R Marchand, Brandon Yabko , Ryan Lackner, Julie Beckstrom , Ashley Parker. Veterans' interests, perceptions, and use of mindfulness. National Library of Medicine 2020 Jul 31;8:2050312120938226.
doi: 10.1177/2050312120938226 PMID: 32821386 PMCID: PMC7406919

58. Johnston, W. & Davey, G. (2011) British Journal Of Psychology, The Psychological Impact Of Negative News Bulletins: The Catastrophizing Of Personal Worries. Https://Doi.Org/10.1111/J.2044-8295.Tb02622.X

59 . Brown, L. (May 12, 2012) Marketing.Wtwhmedia.Com/New-Harvard-Study-Shows-Why-Social-Media-Is-So-Addictive

60. Mindfulness with Meals | Oregon Holistic Nurses Association. https://www.oregonholisticnurses.org/mindfulness-with-meals/

61. Shaffer, A. (2017) The Power Of Mindfulness, Generation Tech, Pp. 42-45

62. Kabat-Zinn, J. (1990). Full Catastrophe Living: Using the wisdom of your mind to face stress and illness. New York: Dell Publishing.

63. Society for Neuroscience. "Loneliness alters your brain's social network: Feeling disconnected from others is reflected by how the brain represents relationships." ScienceDaily. ScienceDaily, 15 June 2020. www.sciencedaily.com/releases/2020/06/200615140904.htm

64. Lipton, B. The Biology of Belief, Killingsworth MA, Gilbert DT. 2010. A wandering mind is an unhappy mind. Science 330(6006):932

65. Srivastava, S., & Veech, R. L. (2019). Brown and Brite: The Fat Soldiers in the Anti-obesity Fight. Frontiers in physiology, 10, 38. https://doi.org/10.3389/fphys.2019.00038

66. https"//www/broadbandsearch.net/blog/average-daily-time-on-social-media

67. Florida Atlantic University. (2020, September 9). Mindfulness with paced breathing and lowering blood pressure. ScienceDaily. Retrieved September 29, 2020 from www.sciencedaily.com/releases/2020/09/200909100214.htm

68. Hughes, L. (2017) Mindfulness, The Power Of Slow Eating

69. Trevino, H. (1999). The Tao of Healing, verse 75

70. Yoga shown to improve anxiety, study shows. ScienceDaily. Retrieved August 19, 2020 from www.sciencedaily.com/releases/2020/08/200812144124.htm

71. Mindfulness-based stress reduction therapy decreases PTSD ....
https://www.sciencedaily.com/releases/2015/08/150804142744.htm

72. The JAMA Network Journals. "Mindfulness-Based Stress Reduction Therapy Decreases PTSD Symptom Severity Among

Veterans." Sciencedaily. Sciencedaily, 4 August 2015. Www.Sciencedaily.Com/Releases/2015/08/150804142744.Htm

73. Washington University School of Medicine. (2020, September 14). Immune system affects mind and body, study indicates: Immune cells produce molecule that influences vigilance, alertness in mice. ScienceDaily. Retrieved September 29, 2020 from www.sciencedaily.com/releases/2020/09/200914131915.htm

74. University of Konstanz. (2020, September 18). Ten minutes of massage or rest will help your body fight stress. ScienceDaily. Retrieved September 29, 2020 from www.sciencedaily.com/releases/2020/09/200918104305.htm

75. Is Constantly Reading the News Bad For You? | Time. https://time.com/5125894/is-reading-news-bad-for-you/

76. TFI Daily News - Is It Bad for You to Read the News https://news.tfionline.com/post/170490429702/is-it-bad-for-you-to-read-the-news-constantly

77. Johnston, W. & Davey, G. (2011) British Journal Of Psychology, The Psychological Impact Of Negative News Bulletins: The Catastrophizing Of Personal Worries. Https://Doi.Org/10.1111/J.2044-8295.Tb02622.X

78. Brown, L. (May 12, 2012) Marketing.Wtwhmedia.Com/New-Harvard-Study-Shows-Why-Social-Media-Is-So-Addictive

79. Shaffer, A. (2017) The Power Of Mindfulness, Generation Tech, Pp. 42-45

80. NYU Langone Health / NYU School of Medicine. (2020, August 12). Yoga shown to improve anxiety, study shows. ScienceDaily. Retrieved August 19, 2020 from

81. Norton, A. Journal Of Clinical Psychiatry (Dec,8, 2015) Https://Www.Webmd.Com/Add-Adhd/Childhood Adhd/News

82. Kalil, Carolyn. "SELF-DISCOVERY: Inside-Out Approach to Life and Work." Career Planning and Adult Development Journal, vol. 32, no. 4, Career Planning and Adult Development Network, Dec. 2016, p. 9.

83. Society for Neuroscience. "Loneliness alters your brain's social network: Feeling disconnected from others is reflected by how the brain represents relationships." ScienceDaily. ScienceDaily, 15 June 2020. www.sciencedaily.com/releases/2020/06/200615140904.htm

84. nutrition-even-though-the-reward-center-in-the-brain .... https://don.essaysmiths.com/nutrition-even-though-the-reward-center-in-the-brain-lights-up-in-response/

85. Lipton, B. The Biology of Belief, Killingsworth MA, Gilbert DT. 2010. A wandering mind is an unhappy mind. Science 330(6006):932

86. Chopra & Tanzi, The Healing Self

87. Lipton, B. The Biology of Belief, p.157

88. Florida Atlantic University. (2020, September 9). Mindfulness with paced breathing and lowering blood pressure. ScienceDaily.

Retrieved September 29, 2020 from
www.sciencedaily.com/releases/2020/09/200909100214.htm

89. Hughes, L. (2017) Mindfulness, The Power Of Slow Eating
90. Emotionally Exhausted: 7 Serious Signs of Burnout That https://www.elevatecounseling.com/blog-post/emotionally-exhausted-7-serious-signs-of-burnout-that-require-your-immediate-attention
91. Trevino, H. (1999). The Tao of Healing, verse 75
92. Washington University School of Medicine. (2020, September 14). Immune system affects mind and body, study indicates: Immune cells produce molecule that influences vigilance, alertness in mice. ScienceDaily. Retrieved September 29, 2020 from www.sciencedaily.com/releases/2020/09/200914131915.htm
93. University of Konstanz. (2020, September 18). Ten minutes of massage or rest will help your body fight stress. ScienceDaily. Retrieved September 29, 2020 from www.sciencedaily.com/releases/2020/09/200918104305.htm
94. Why Change Beliefs? – Awaken. Dream. Believe.. https://theuniverseisadreammachine.com/why-change-beliefs/
95. Hughes, L. (2017) Mindfulness, The Power Of Slow Eating
96. Risher, B. (2017) Mindfulness, World View, p. 25
97. Trevino, H. The Tao of Healing, verse 75
98. NYU Langone Health / NYU School of Medicine. (2020, August 12). Yoga shown to improve anxiety, study shows. ScienceDaily. Retrieved August 19, 2020 from www.sciencedaily.com/releases/2020/08/200812144124.htm
99. Risher, B. (2017) Mindfulness, World View, p 25
100. Ibid
101. Ibid
102. NYU Langone Health / NYU School of Medicine. (2020, August 12). Yoga shown to improve anxiety, study shows. ScienceDaily. Retrieved August 19, 2020 from
103. Risher, B. (2017) Mindfulness, World View, p 25
104. Paleolithic societies by Eman M. Elshaikh: https://www.khanacademy.org/humanities/world-history/world-history-beginnings/origin-humans-early-societies/a/what-were-paleolithic-societies-like
105. Paleolithic societies by Eman M. Elshaikh: https://www.khanacademy.org/humanities/world-history/world-history-beginnings/origin-humans-early-societies/a/what-were-paleolithic-societies-like
106. Nepo, M. (2016) The Little Book of Awakening, p.130-131
107. November 26 – The Kinship of Gratitude – Mark Nepo, The https://kitt.global/november-26-the-kinship-of-gratitude-mark-nepo-the-book-of-awakening/
108. Norris, G. (2001) Being Home

Chapter Four
Color, Sound & Health

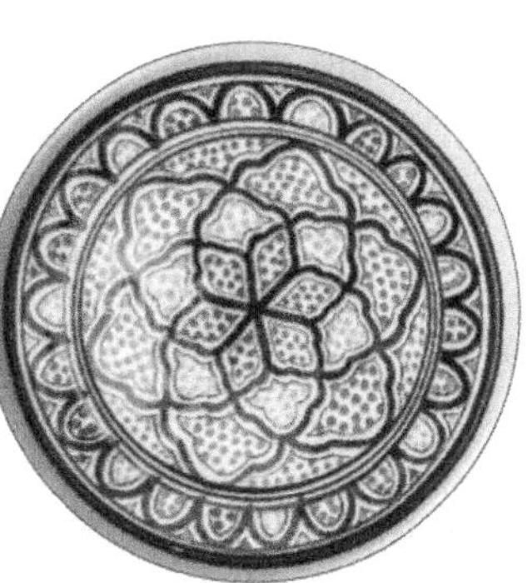

"My study of colorful carotenoids and phytonutrients in graduate school had shown me that there is an important 'color connection' in nutrition science... I began to realize that color, nutrition, and life issues were intertwined, ... I started to see correlations rather distinctly."

~Deanna Minich, PhD
author of *The Rainbow Diet*

Artists are not the only ones drawn to color; humans and animals alike use color and sounds as signals. A blossom of crimson, the glow of new green, or the aqua of water in nature attract wildlife. For the human passerby, attention can be drawn by the plates in cupboards, art on the walls, and vibrant glass vases catching the sunlight. Art, in all its forms, reflects the depth and vibrancy of color found in Nature. Color and sound take us on a journey into the world of frequencies. Light and sound both travel in waves and on specific frequency bands, being seen and heard in diverse ways by humans and animals. [1,2]

Principle 1: Color has definitive and measurable effects on the mind, body, and spirit.

Color and sound are the seasonings added to the plate filled with our food, sustainability, and mindfulness meal. Just as rosemary, oregano, ginger, and garlic add dimensions of flavor to traditional dishes, so to do color and sounds add dimensions to the human journey. These seasonings add a depth of flavor and connection to culture, origins, nature, and beyond. How Nature has used color to attract both animals and humans to nourishment is one example. The vibrancy of color passing through the retina of the eye signals the brain, which creates chemical signals tuned to seek out nutrients. [3, 4, 5, 6] The magic of this process goes beyond merely keeping one alive to sustaining health and regenerating cells, which is the key to retaining youthful energy and lifelong vitality.

In the modern world, the color packaging of produce, meats, and countless food-related products attracts shoppers' visual attention. The color of foods in their natural and processed forms signals the brain to stimulate hormone production in preparation for food digestion. In 2018, researchers at the Max Planck Institute of Psychiatry demonstrated scientifically for the first time: that the mere sight of delicious food stimulates the appetite. [7]

> *Warning:* Avoid looking at pictures of appetizing food as it will make you hungry!" Dieticians could be making recommendations along these lines in the future. It has long been known that, in addition to the

> physiological regulatory circuits for the maintenance of a sufficient energy status for the body, external stimuli like smell or the sight of food also influence our feelings of hunger and our resulting eating behavior. The danger that the exposure to such images will result in the consumption of food that is not needed to maintain the body's energy status is particularly high in our advertising-dominated society, said Axel Steiger.[8, 9]

In preparation for digestion, the stomach begins to activate hydrochloric acid, and the pancreas produces bile to transport enzymes and insulin for regulating blood sugars vital for the brain.

> There have been important new insights into how people perceive food flavors, said Terry E. Acree, Ph.D. Years ago, taste was a table with two legs — taste and odor. Now we are beginning to understand that flavor depends on parts of the brain that involve taste, odor, touch, and vision. The sum total of these signals, plus our emotions and past experiences, result in the perception of flavors, and determine whether we like or dislike specific foods.[10, 11]

Food manufacturers are well aware of how Nature utilizes color seasonally, which lends itself to seasonal food sales increases. A result: one-pound bags of M&Ms evaporating off the shelves at Halloween.[12]

Color is often used to describe emotions: "seeing red" with anger or rage, "green with envy," "happy as sunshine," sad or "feeling blue," "white as a sheet with fear," and "tickled pink with joy or excitement." Color can influence various human behaviors such as object recognition, identifying facial expressions, and categorizing stimuli as positive or negative. Researchers have found yellow and white are associated with positive emotions. [13, 14]

Color your world

In humans, color perception relies on banks of specialized receptor cells, the rods, and cones in the retina. The cone cells' job is to absorb the light of different wavelengths and pass the information on to the brain's visual cortex. The cortex is where these signals of color information can be interpreted. The visible light spectrum, the colors we attribute to a rainbow, is broad, so the most effective means of discerning color is not one type of generalized eye cone. Rather, it is a collection of three specialists, each perfectly tuned to absorb one or two specific color wavelengths. One cone excels at detecting red and associated wavelengths. Another is tuned to blue and related wavelengths. And the third optimally perceives the light wavelengths of two colors: purple and yellow. The perfectly designed human eye can detect these colors and send a signal pulsing to the brain. The two colors viewed by cone three are complementary colors, as different as possible. The combining of yellow and purple (complementary colors on an artist's color wheel) makes each color more vivid to the eye.

Human eyes are so sensitive to these color wavelengths that the cones can get oversaturated, and the stimulus pours over onto the other cone cells. Anyone who has taken art may have done the following experiment — if you stare for several minutes at a color block of yellow and then shift the gaze to a white sheet of paper, you will see the white as violet for a moment.

This phenomenon — the colored after image — occurs because there is an active interchange between purple and yellow pigments, which Mother Nature knew before human scientists, as demonstrated by the vivid and dramatic color arrays of alpine meadows and forest roadsides. As it turns out, dramatic yellow goldenrod and royal purple asters appear very similar to bee eyes and human eyes. Their striking contrast makes them the most attractive target for bees in the whole meadow when growing together. [15]

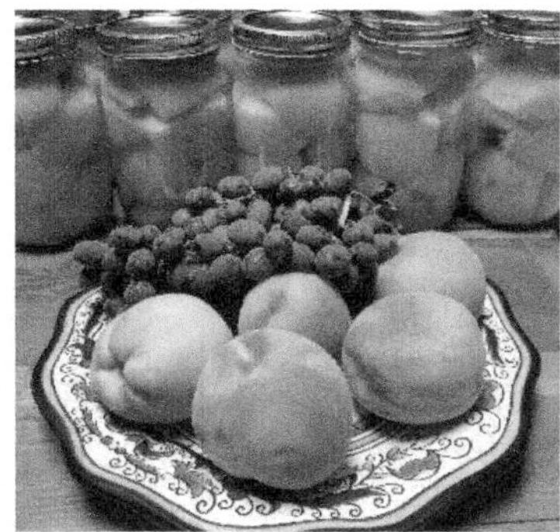

For decades researchers and medical experts believed infants could only see in black and white with shades of grey. Alice Skelton, doing visual color research at the baby lab at the University of Sussex, working with three-month-old infants in 2017, revealed color and visual acuity happen much sooner than initially thought. [16] With modern technology, researchers can track the corneal reflection and position of an infant's eyes. At birth, everything is a blur, with visual acuity around 5% of an adult. Stereoscopic vision develops, with babies unable to perceive depth until several months old. At the same time, faces are only discernable at a distance, similar to that between a mother's face and her breast. "The early stages of learning to see color and basic forms happen relatively quickly," says Alex Wade, professor of psychology at the University of York, and an expert in visual processes. By the age of six months, babies have more or less adult levels of visual acuity. [17]

Exploring color's untapped potential

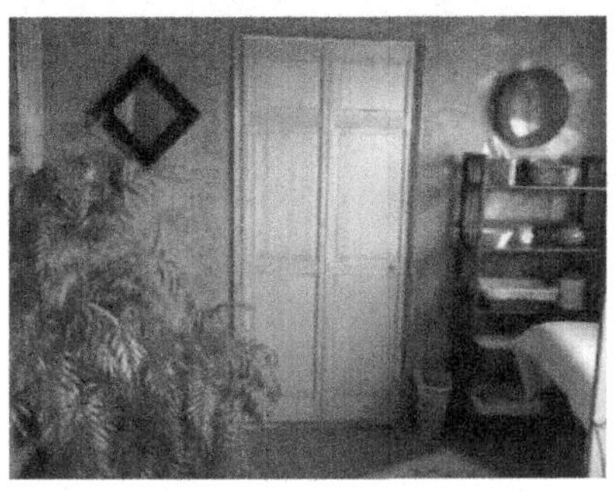

Twenty years ago, Tammera began challenging herself to use color in her work environment; the goal was to elicit comfort, calm, and clarity of mind. Surprisingly, she found that color has untapped potential for clinical health environments and home use. Routinely, she saw clients who arrived all wound up, tense, and unfocused. She observed them as they unwound in her office space, relaxed, and became open to suggestions and making diet and lifestyle changes.

> *Principle 2*: Color and Sound take us on a journey into the world of frequencies.

Tammera quickly learned colors she had always shied away from in her wardrobe actually, had the most significant benefit when used as wall colors. Increases in productivity and mental clarity were the most noticeable benefits. Apricot, peach, and sage green, to this day, are part of the Holistic Nutrition for the Whole You office color pallet. How color affected clients, co-workers, and Tammera, inspired her to look deeper into how humans respond to color in their environment, especially in food.

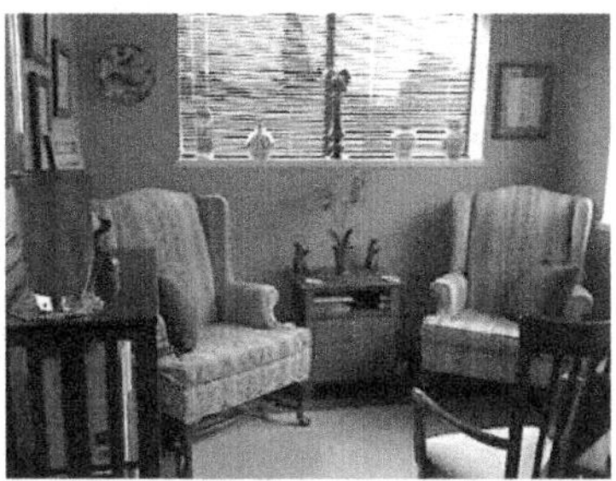

Deanna Minich, Ph.D., author of *The Rainbow Diet,* and a leading expert in the area of color and food, published a literature review in 2019.

> *A Review of The Science of Colorful, Plant-Based Food and the Practical Strategies for "Eating the Rainbow."* Dr. Minich found: "Moreover, a report based on food consumption data from the *National Health and Nutrition Examination Survey (NHANES)* conducted in 2003-2004 and 2005-2006 found eight out of ten Americans fall short in every color of phytonutrients (referred to as a *phytonutrient gap*), especially in the color category of purple/blue foods (88% of people neglected to meet their daily serving)." [18, 19]

Why are blue and dark purple foods selected least among western consumers? Part of the answer is due to the limited availability of purple and blue foods as related to the regional area of production and harvest season.

Darker and more highly colored fruits and vegetables are more nutrient-dense than their pastel relatives. Dr. Minich's good advice to *eat the rainbow* includes these many benefits:

- RED foods like tomatoes, cherries, ruby grapefruit, persimmons, red cabbage, and rhubarb are rich in anthocyanins and lycopene — a powerful antioxidant with many health benefits.

- Foods that are ORANGE — carrots, pumpkin, and other squashes, oranges, and sweet potatoes' — contain carotenoids that the body converts to Vitamin A.

- YELLOW foods are good sources of Vitamin C: bananas, pineapple, lemons/limes, mangos, corn, yellow squash, and potatoes. They promote collagen production needed for skin, hair, nails, bone, and dental health.

- GREEN foods, the darker the better, are full of B vitamins and other vital compounds that reduce the risk of many cancers by boosting enzymes that defuse carcinogens. Some of the most nutritious are kale, broccoli, cauliflower, mustard and collard greens, arugula, spinach, asparagus, and alfalfa sprouts.

- BLUE and PURPLE foods contain a dynamic combination of polyphenols, flavonoids, tannins, bitter compounds, and vitamins, all necessary for humans' sustainable health. Look for blueberries, blackberries, elderberries, huckleberries, currants, plums, purple grapes, eggplant, and radicchio.

Tammera found a kindred voice of mindfulness and common sense in Dr. Minich's spoken words and writings. Her grounding in science and love of color adds to her personal vibrancy and provides a rare third dimension and a broader lens of perspective on nutrition. In her book the *Rainbow Diet*, Dr. Minich shares,

> Unlike most traditional restrictive *diets*, the *Rainbow Diet* is about finding the foods, supplements, and eating styles that fit your unique, personal physiology and psychology .... I've never believed in the *one-diet-fits-all" approach.* [20, 21]

> *"Food is Information. Color is Inspiration."*
>
> ~Deanna Minich PhD
> author of *The Rainbow Diet*

For decades, Tammera has shared this same opinion on diet in her writing and clinical work. A palpable sigh of relief is often heard from clients when they hear she is not repeating the newest popular diet spiel; individual likes and needs are possible with food recommendations.

Mindfully choosing to *eat the rainbow* helps the body fight chronic, low-level inflammation that is the result of toxins produced by digesting highly processed foods. Although the process is gradual, low-level chronic inflammation is linked to a growing number of illnesses and medical disorders. [22] Body wide cell renewal and restored balance are the goals;

these are the keys to lifelong wellness. Individuals can focus on eating those foods that have nurturing, calming, healing, and balancing effects on their own bodymind as a whole. On day eight of his Twenty-One Day Meditation program focused on Youth and Energy, Dr. Deepak Chopra's comments on an anti-inflammatory diet included.

> You can't tell, when you eat them, which foods are inflammatory – but your cells can! ... The anti-inflammatory diet is what our cells would ask for if they could talk directly to us. — This is the type of food our bodymind needs for its energy, balance, and maintenance, but most of us haven't been listening. [23]

Each person has a favorite color. When a person wears specific colors, they are reflecting their temperament, mood, or an unconscious attempt to balance emotions. Blue is seen as the safest political color choice around the world since it has numerous positive connotations. Blue is considered soothing and peaceful in North America and Europe, representing trust, security, authority. In Ukraine, blue signifies *good health*. [24, 25]

When Tammera recently learned of her own genetic link to Romania and Ukraine and the cultural symbology of the color blue, [26] she reflected on her earlier words in *Our Journey with Food*, "our cells carrying the memories of our ancestors." [27, 28]

Researchers are learning more about how color is a powerful psychologic and communication tool and how it can be used to signal action and even influence physiological reactions. Specific colors have been associated with increased blood pressure, increased metabolism, and eyestrain, while others improve wound healing.

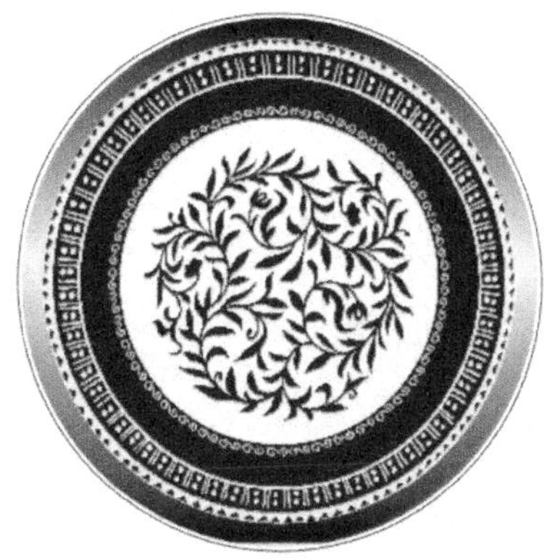

Is it possible colors draw us back to traditional foods and cultural connections? We may never know the answer to that question, but it is fun to ponder.

Let the Light Shine

In 1666, English scientist Sir Isaac Newton discovered when white light passes through a prism it separates into all of the visible colors. Newton found each color is made up of a single wavelength and cannot be separated any further into other colors. He further learned that light wavelengths can be combined to form additional colors. For those who are not color savvy, here is another fascinating aspect of color: some colors, such as green and magenta (red), cancel each other out when mixed, resulting in white light. [29, 30]

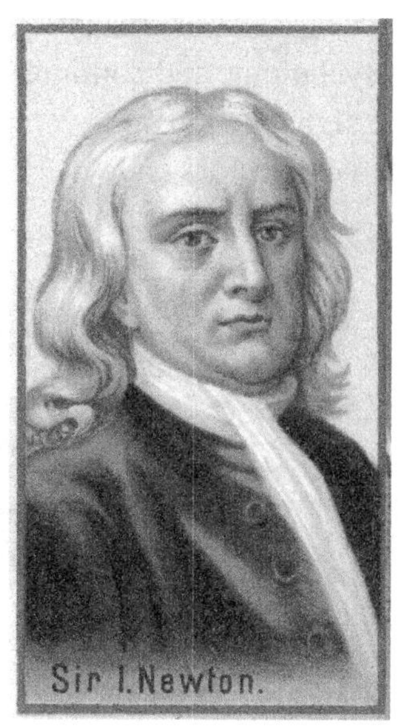

The entire light spectrum contains all electromagnetic frequencies of energy, from the zero-point field — frequency slowing down — all the way to matter. As energy increases, the frequency of light waves speeds up, and their wavelengths decrease. The converse is also true: as energy decreases, the frequency slows down, and the wavelengths increase. Light is measured in nanometers, each one equal to one-billionth of a meter. The light spectrum visible to humans — where we perceive the colors of the world around us — makes up less than one percent of all the existing frequencies of light and is located pretty much in the middle range of frequency at around 500 nm. Light in the infrared frequency band has a slower frequency; the wavelengths are longer than light in the ultraviolet frequency band, where the wavelengths are shorter. The color red has a slower frequency (450 cycles/second) and has longer wavelengths than the color blue (650 cycles/second). [31, 32]

Color is critical for survival in nature, so much so that unlike humans, birds' eyes have a fourth color cone that can detect ultraviolet light. To find food, dazzle mates, escape predators, and navigate diverse terrain, birds rely on their excellent color vision. Humans can see only one *nonspectral* color — purple; birds can theoretically see up to five. [33]

> *"To me, the rainbow was a profoundly hopeful symbol, separating the white light of appearances into its multiple spectrum and revealing a hidden dimension. It reminded me of my belief that it was the mission of science to pierce through the layers of everyday reality and penetrate to the truth."* [34]
>
> ~Candace B. Pert, *Molecules of Emotion: The Science Behind Mind-Body Medicine*

The understanding of how color can affect health is called *Color Psychology*. Without being aware of color's effect on health, individuals may be missing out on ways to improve responses and reactions within their surroundings. [35, 36, 37] For individuals who are light sleepers, the color on bedroom walls and accents may make a positive or negative difference in sleep quality. Exposure to blue light at night has been found to change sleep patterns. So, all those little indicator lights on electronics and surge protectors are problematic to health, especially in bedrooms.

And when it comes to blue light, it isn't just those little indicator lights that disrupt a person's ability to go to sleep. [38] A 2017 study looked at the light from electronic devices. "The short-wavelength blue light, emitted by the screens we watch, damages the duration, and even more so, the quality of their sleep." [39] The same study also said watching screens that emit red light does not alter sleep, and after red light exposure, normal sleep patterns resulted. "The light emitted by most screens — computers, smartphones, and tablets — is blue light that damages the body's cycles and our sleep," explains Professor Abraham Haim from the University of Haifa. [40, 41]

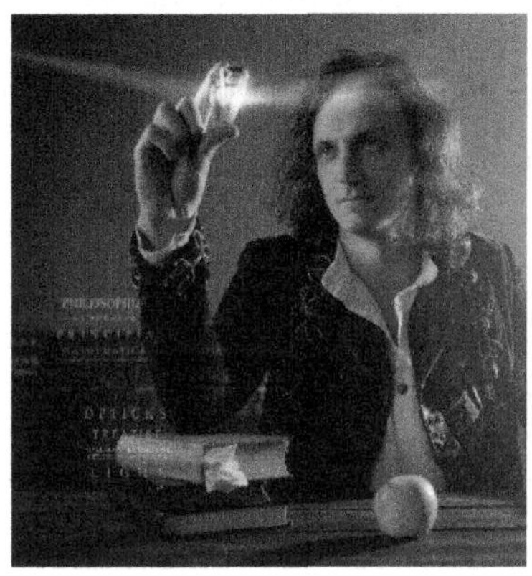

Colors affect mental processes and can change people's moods. [42] Colors like yellow have been found to brighten a person's mood, while black is associated with being somber or depressed in western culture. Each color has a different effect, so in *Color Psychology*, mental conditions determine the colors used. [43, 44]

The University of Arizona is actively studying colored LED light's effects on health. Researchers have found green light reduced the frequency, duration, and intensity of migraine headaches. [45] Migraine frequency was reduced by 60% after ten weeks among the members of an ongoing study. In addition to green light, researchers are looking at the effects of blue lights on mild traumatic brain injuries (mTBI).

Daily exposure to blue wavelength light each morning helps to re-entrain the circadian rhythm so that people get better and more regular sleep. "This is likely true for everybody, but we recently demonstrated it in people recovering from mild traumatic brain injury, or mTBI," said William D. "Scott"

Killgore, psychiatry professor in the College of Medicine – Tucson, and lead author on a study published in the journal *Neurobiology of Disease.*[46]

Keep in mind, while blue light exposure in the morning helps mTBI individuals reset their clock, it can also be a disruptive color for people with insomnia or sleep disturbances. Effects on children have not been well studied, but it makes sense that blue light should be minimized in their bedrooms to encourage healthy circadian rhythms of wake and sleep.

> According to a study published in *PLOS Biology*[47] in 2016, Light shining into our eyes not only mediates vision but also has critical non-image-forming functions such as the regulation of circadian rhythm, which affects sleep and other physiological processes. As humans, light generally keeps us awake, and dark makes us sleepy.[48]

In the UK, there are currently around 12 million people aged over 65: in fifty years, this will increase to approximately 20 million, and all will have some degree of visual decline because of retinal aging, according to Professor Glen Jeffery at University College London Institute of Ophthalmology.[49] As individuals approach 40 years of age, cells in the eye's retina begin to deteriorate. This aging speed is determined by the retinal cells' mitochondria and its ability to produce energy — and boost cell function — which begins to decline. However, researchers say that staring at a deep red light for three minutes a day can significantly improve declining eyesight.[50, 51]

Children are especially susceptible to changes in sleep patterns that affect behavior and focus — poor sleep patterns set children up for a host of health problems later in life. Children's sleeping behavior is being looked at closer in a study at Arizona State University. The use of media in the form of phones, tablets, computers, and TVs, in the hour, preceding bedtime impacts how kids sleep, especially children who struggle to self-regulate their behavior. Out of 537 children in the study, those who scored low on effortful control slept the least amount of time when they consistently used media before bed. [52] These children slept approximately forty minutes less per night than the children who did not use devices in that same hour. The second group gained thirty-four minutes of sleep per night — which adds up to more than four hours a week and sixteen hours a month. [53, 54]

Potential benefits from color therapy

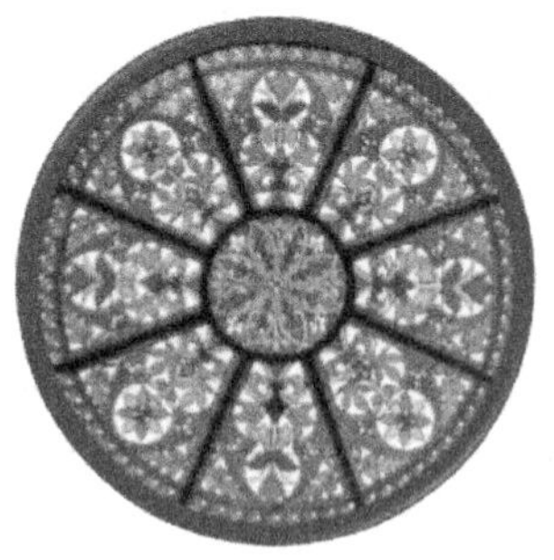

The color around us doesn't have to be some shade of white. Try changing your environment gently with soft color hints to white paint until you learn what tones resonate best with vision and personal energy. If an individual is color blind in the red and or green spectrums — have someone who can see the colors help select and use natural lighting to be sure the color is what you want. Interior lighting can have a blue, yellow, or harsh white frequency, which alters the eyes' perception of the paint samples' actual color.

Experts have found that while color can influence how individuals feel and act; these effects are subject to personal, cultural, and situational factors, making color therapy unique to an individual's traditions and culture. While Latin Americans may do well with bold color, Norwegian or Finnish individuals may find the colors agitating or exciting resulting in anxiety.

Color therapy: colored paint, lights, and art can improve sleep patterns, PTSD, depression, anxiety, migraines, alertness, and concentration.

> ***Green*** improves feelings of sadness, hopelessness, or depression. Green enhances emotions: love, joy, and inner peace. Green increases wisdom and facilitates change and independence. [55]
>
> ***Blue*** encourages the expression of feelings and inner truth. Blue can also be associated with wisdom, creativity, loyalty, and spirituality. The primary color blue is used for meditation and relaxation. [56]
>
> ***Yellow*** is the easiest color for the human eye to see. In tradition and common sense, it is the color of happiness and hope, positivity, energy, and optimism. Yellow encourages action by increasing feelings of happiness and energy. [57]
>
> ***Orange*** signifies abundance, pleasure, well-being, and sexuality. It revitalizes you and gives you increased mental energy. It can increase the

feeling of connectedness between your mind and body. [58]

Red influences emotional issues like financial security, independence, and physical survival. Red is associated with courage, strength, vitality, alertness, sexuality, and pioneering spirit. In 2017 researchers reported on the use of red and infrared light for noninvasive wound healing. [59]

Purple is most strongly associated with beauty, spirituality, and bliss. [60]

"Science and art, matter and spirit, indigenous knowledge and Western Science — can they be goldenrod and asters for each other? When I am in their presence, their beauty asks me for reciprocity, to be the complementary color, to make something beautiful in response." [61]

~ Robin Wall Kimmerer, PhD
author of *Braiding Sweetgrass*

Where tradition meets science

Along with color, music also plays a central role in traditional health care, holistic care, and the ever-present marketing of industrial food products. When shopping for food, even at farmer's markets, there is music that adds to that historic feel of the *middle-ages village marketplace* or "fair." The flash of color banners, smells of sweet and savory foods, and familiar tunes all change brain chemistry, stimulating dopamine, which elevates feelings of pleasure and mood. [62, 63] The historical experience hidden in our DNA of a farm market or fair can have individuals buying those delectable treats while humming along with the musical performer. In today's world, the colors displayed and music played over the grocery store's speaker system are carefully selected by marketing and human behavior experts to guide selections that end up in the shopping basket or cart. [64, 65]

Principle 3: Celebrate your history by including music, art, and creative pursuits that resonate with your DNA and culture.

The ancient cultural healthcare systems of *Ayurveda, Indigenous,* and *Traditional Chinese Medicine* (TCM) have music and color connections with specific health conditions, organ systems, and life cycles. [66, 67] Interestingly, color and sound are combined in a collection of music listed as *Therapeutic Music of the Yellow Emperor's Classic Internal Medicine.* [68] And the theory of the *Five Elements*, also known as the *Five Evolutional Phases*, it is an arrangement of all aspects of the phenomenological world into categories of fire, water, wood, earth, and metal, first developed in the Zhou.

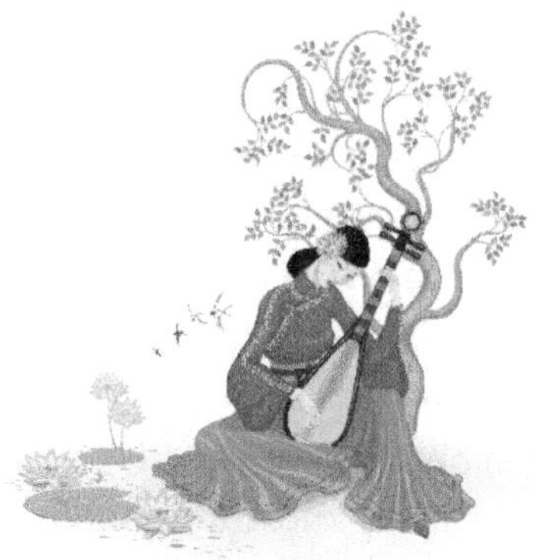

The earliest TCM theories of health/illness and medical treatment, astrology and divination techniques, and musical tonality and composition theories were all unified through a mutual basis on the *Five Element & Yin Yang* theory. [69]

Looking for common ground between art and science is increasingly popular. Science has a long history of employing art to present visual images of anatomy and complex chemical and DNA structures. So, when composer Michael Zev Gordon began playing with music and DNA, it didn't take long for whole scores to be written based on the amino acid chains formed by *Adenine, Thymine, Cytosine,* and *Guanine.*

Music, of all the arts, has the deepest links with scientific thought during Zev Gordon's work forming music from DNA sequencing. "The more the words, music, and science could be integrated, the more powerful the piece would be." Gordon looked to science and nature for another image: the *Fibonacci series* and the associated *golden section.* [70] What is music without the power of words? Ruth Padel joined Zev Gordon and contributed more than twenty-three poems to form the opening runs. [71]

A *National Geographic* article from 2008 further illustrated DNA can be "heard" through music. [72] Geneticist theories suggest humans are made up of approximately 97% "junk DNA." But consider the limited understanding scientists possess about human DNA at present; what if this supposed excess DNA isn't junk at all but contains stored information from past generations? Is "junk" DNA actually storage space for "information" passed down through ancestors as well as "input" from the environment? These are questions we will leave for the evolutionary theorists to work out.

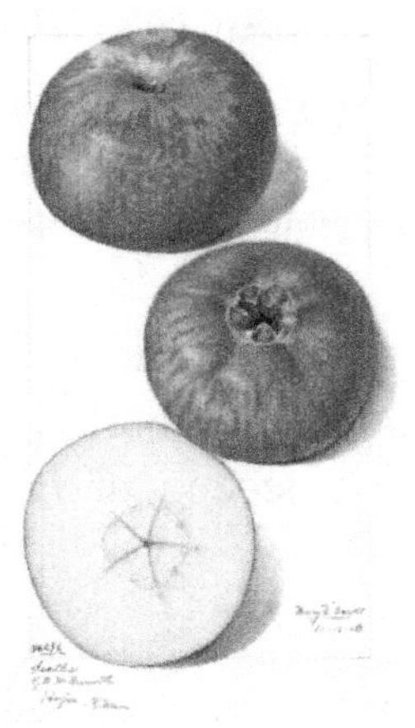

USDA Botanical Illustration 1917

Mystery of tiniest
difference, invisible,
unknown/
Flight of the tiniest
humming-birds, in sequence/
Crimson wings above an
unknown sea/
in autumn wind. The mystery of migrating. [73]

Music is a significant part of indigenous peoples' culture, history, and lifestyle worldwide from the moment of birth through to death. Many indigenous stories from around the world recount the meaning of *birth songs*. One such tale tells of an African tribe where the mother goes away from the tribe for a period of time during pregnancy. She waits for the *song* of the child before she rejoins the rest of the village. That song is sung over the child his/her entire life, and upon their death, it is never sung again. [74] Who has not experienced remembering a lullaby or tune from early childhood memories? Treasured musical memories can flood us with feelings of comfort, love, and safety.

Sounds that soothe, heal, and connect

Sound of all kinds surround humans; the human ear can hear some; many are outside of the conscious hearing range. There is little doubt that sound affects people; it can irritate, energize, calm, or inspire. The sound of music and the human voice can move individuals from the depths of despair to find hope and connection. Rhythm and melodious sounds and words can bring a person to their feet in celebration, to their knees in prayer, or to tears of joy or longing. No other medium has such a profound capacity to affect humans.

> *Principle 4*: Sound is an organizing force of nature.

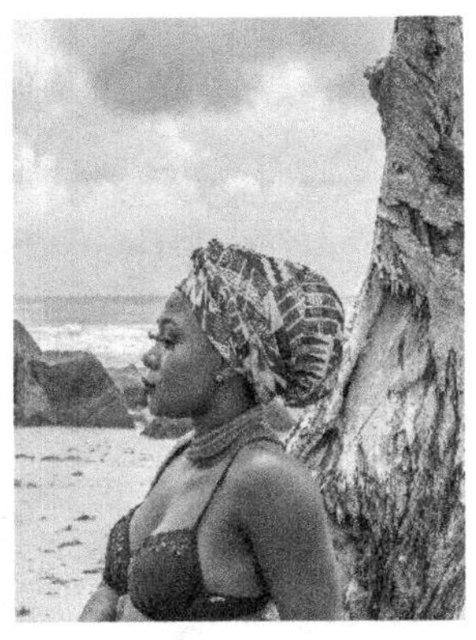

Traditional Gullah music, a blend of gospel, jazz, and rhythm and blues, has been described as *honey for the soul* by listeners. This flavorful blend of traditional music comes from the African American culture of the Lowcountry region of Georgia, Florida, and South Carolina, in both the coastal plain and the sea islands. The sounds, words, and energy of modern Gullah or Geechee music still retain flavor, rhythm, and West African movements and the blended words from over thirty-one African languages. Gullah's sounds' resurgence is preserved by a small handful of African American descendants and musicians like those in the *Ranky Tanky* band, which received a Grammy Award in 2020 for best regional roots album. [75,76] As with most traditions, food is an integral part of the Gullah culture's flavor and story. The native island Gullah people adhere to their ancestors' customs through the sewing of sweetgrass baskets, the weaving of casting nets, and preparation of traditional Gullah food seasoned generously with their ancestors' music. [77]

> *"DNA is our music of life."*
>
> ~Elizabeth Lipski, PhD
> author of *Digestive Wellness*

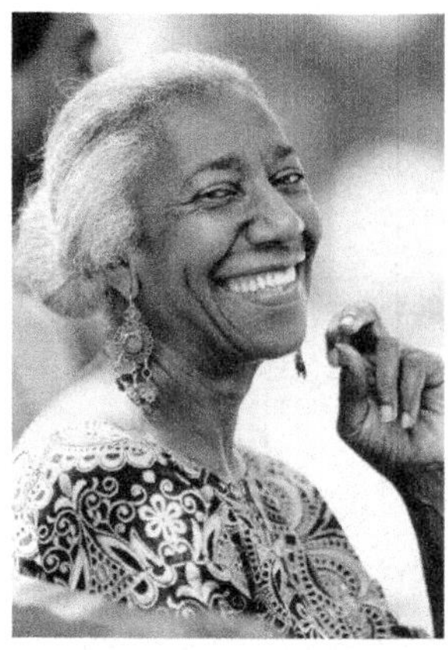
Edna Lewis 1916-2006

Edna Lewis was preserving traditional African American food and culture decades before bands like *Ranky Tank* were even dreamed up. [78] She was born in 1916 in Freetown, Virginia; a community founded in part by her grandfather, an emancipated slave. Her love of the traditional Southern fare that she championed was cultivated there, where her family produced everything they consumed except sugar. [79] Edna, a globally renowned chef at Café Nicholson in Manhattan, New York (1948), provided a model for African Americans on being proud of the culture, foods, art, and music that make up their DNA and connection to history, family and agriculture. Edna quietly argued against *anti-slave food* movements from celebrities with traditional foods and music and is known for saying, *all true paths of self-discovery led home*. Before *farm-to-table* was popular, Ms. Lewis taught it to all, through how she lived her life; countless individuals are now able to travel the path home through traditional African American foods that connect them to their country, culture, and history. [80]

Traditional Celtic music is another example of music's importance in sustaining cultural identity. It began as an oral tradition and has been passed on from generation to generation by listening, learning by ear, and without formally writing the tunes on paper. This custom is still encouraged today. *Fleadh Cheoil na hÉireann* (the Music Festival of Ireland), the world's biggest traditional Irish music celebration, with more than 400,000 attendees each year, celebrates what some say is a 2,000-year-old tradition. [81]

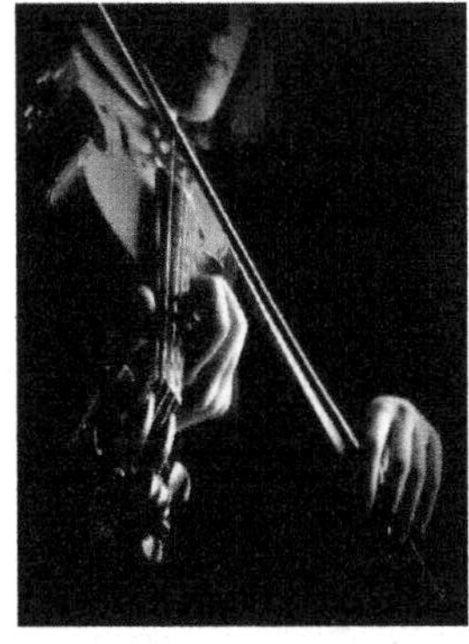

Cultural or traditional music sounds are a vital flavor; connecting, nourishing, and sustaining mindfulness on the plate of life. The language and sounds of traditional music echo the voices of friends, family, and community from many generations; hearing it may even cause shifts in DNA. Music has been used for thousands of years in healing ceremonies and as a digestive aid, and each country across the world has traditional music to connect the threads of life and lift the spirit. [82, 83, 84]

> *Principle 5*: Music impacts people more than any other human-made sound.

Sound purity can resonate from crystal or brass bowls, reed or bone pipes, or the human's vocal cords. The wind moving gently or fiercely through tuned wind chimes in a yard can elicit very different responses even in sleep. One can be mystical and soothing, the other harsh and alarming. The vibration of sound from many sources and rhythm or the beat has been shown to change body chemistry, altering the HPAT axis, governing the stress response. [85]

Music impacts humans beyond that of any other human-made sound and is believed by anthropologists to be a key to the advancement of archaic humans. For scientists studying early man, music and art are believed to be very important in the early modern human's ability to develop a sense of group identity and mutual trust, which resulted in a sustainable society.

> *"Music was my refuge. I could crawl into the space between the notes and curl my back to loneliness."*
>
> ~Maya Angelou

Classic listening

The power of music doesn't stop with early man; research in health science has uncovered music's capacity for reducing seizure frequency in individuals; while studying music primarily composed by Mozart. [86] Initial studies with college students reported increased IQ scores; however, this has been disproved as the results lasted only fifteen minutes. [87] Music by Mozart and Strauss has also been found to reduce blood lipid concentrations and blood pressure after twenty-five minutes. [88] In neonatal care, researchers from Tel Aviv University found that premature babies who are exposed to music by the 18th century composer, Mozart, gain weight faster and therefore become stronger. [89]

Mozart's isn't the only music being studied. Research from the University of Helsinki found listening to classical music enhanced the activity of genes involved in dopamine secretion and transport, synaptic neurotransmission, learning, and memory, as well as down-regulated genes mediating neurodegeneration. [90]

"I am an old woman now ... the buffaloes and black-tail deer are gone ... But for me, I cannot forget our old ways. Often in summer, I rise at daybreak and steal out to the cornfields: and as I hoe the corn, I sing to it, as we did when I was young."

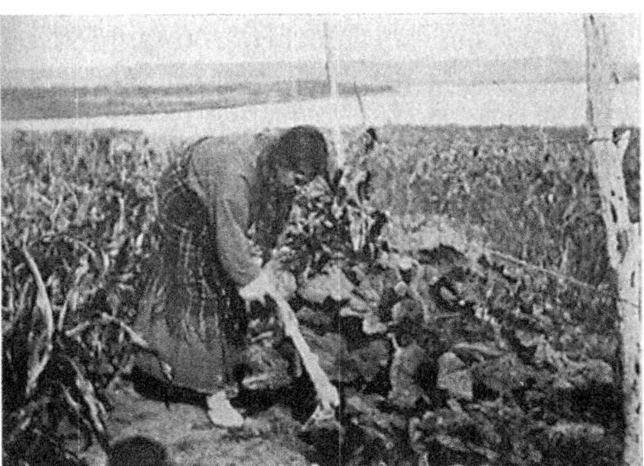

~Buffalo Bird Woman (*Maxi'diwiac)* 1839-1932

Perspective from history

When did music begin? Scientists and music historians believe humans began making music with instruments about 40,000 years ago. Tradition would suggest the first instrument was the human voice. [91, 92] Research suggests early humans' ability to use their voices to create music may have allowed man's earliest ancestors to communicate beyond that of *Neanderthals.*

Music may have been the vehicle of communication well before the invention of language, a link to establishing monogamy and the social glue needed for the emergence of the first large pre-human *Neanderthal* societies.

The desire to create a lasting image in the form of art is not new. The earliest known cave art dates to 40,000 years ago in Indonesia and is of a cow. In an article published in November 2018 in *Nature*, the scientists said that it now seemed certain that rock art emerged in Borneo at around the same time as the earliest forms of artistic expression appeared in Europe; connected to modern humans' arrival. [93]

Continued on next page

With the emergence of Homo sapiens, things changed rapidly. Researchers have found evidence that the emergence of art represented in cave paintings — and the making of figurines, whistles, and flutes out of ivory and bone — played a significant role in humans' advancement.

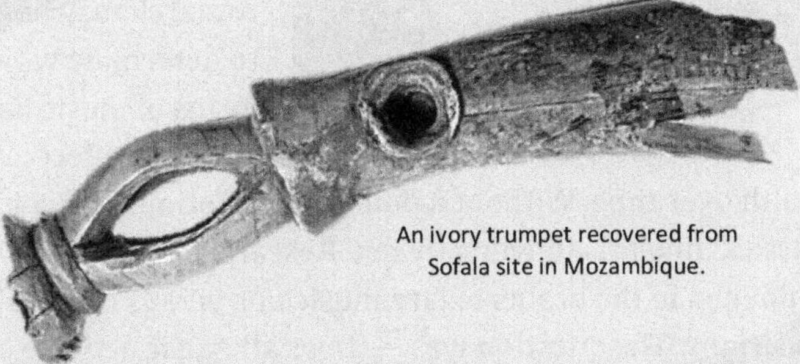

An ivory trumpet recovered from Sofala site in Mozambique.

"There is a clear musical tradition," says Nicholas Conard at the University of Tübingen in Germany, who assisted in discovering these early instruments. "In southwest Germany, we have eight flutes from three different sites." [94]

"Thus, similar cave art traditions appear to arise near-contemporaneously in the extreme west and extreme east of Eurasia," the *Nature* article said. [95] The drawings of animals in Chauvet's French cave have been dated back to approximately 33,500 to 37,000 years ago.

Visualizing music

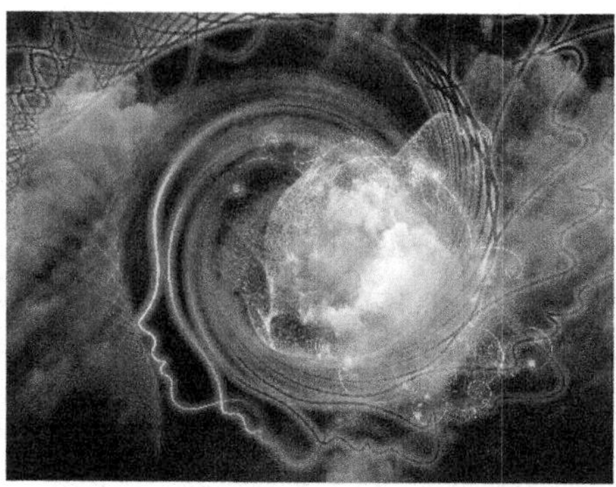

aip.scitation.org

While all may not be fans of classical music, what we listen to can and does affect our health. Musical styles and genres differ around the world; research may be able to determine which forms of music have the same effect on health over time. Without a doubt, the emotional power of classical music is universally felt. Researchers looked at what happened in the brains of jazz musicians versus classical musicians. The question was — Does all music activate the same portions of the brain? Can anyone play classical Mozart and receive benefit from it? The researchers were surprised when they found jazz pianists' brain activity differs from those of classical pianists, even when playing the same piece of music. [96]

The University of Tokyo has developed a new approach to analyzing musical structure. [97] The new system overcomes the limits of earlier research. *Recurrence plot* is a basic property of complex systems, first described mathematically in the late 19th century by French mathematician and scientist Henri Poincaré. The method developed by the Japanese team is based on the graphing technique of the recurrence plot, a two-dimensional analytical tool that visualizes the recurrences of data. [98] The study utilizing *recurrence plot* may help researchers understand the downside of sound as well.

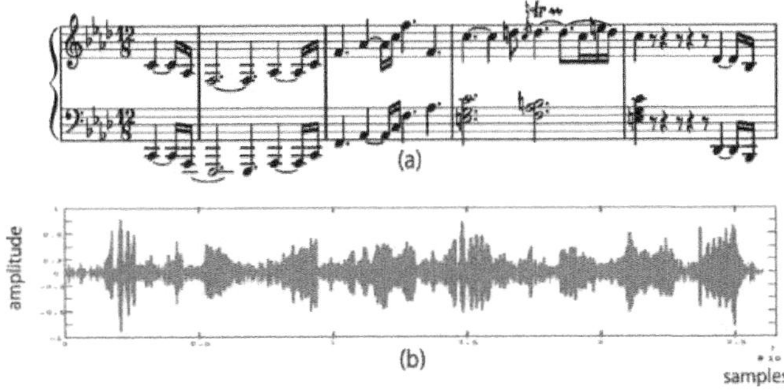

Just stop the noise

Sounds are ubiquitous, both natural and human-made alike. Sounds are perceived by humans and other living creatures as mechanical waves of pressure. Similar to light waves, the energy of sound waves is also measured in frequencies. Sounds are characterized by regular fluctuations in vibration, whereas noises contain irregular fluctuations in vibration. Noise is also a type of sound, and its classification, as such, is highly individual and subjective. The word noise, derived from the Latin *nausea*, usually connotes undesirable sounds. Sound can be described as relevant — allowing various forms of communication, warning of danger, providing solace, or entertainment in the form of songs and music. Noise, on the other hand, is often irrelevant and can range from annoying and unpleasant to downright harmful to health and well-being. [99]

The modern world is filled with noise, making it difficult to find, much less achieve, true silence. From the whir of electric fans and appliance motors to the crash and bang of garbage trucks, noises surround individuals. The sounds of contemporary life never seem to end — unless one unplugs entirely.

Environmental sounds that we refer to as noise can disturb our sleep and concentration, along with increased cardiovascular risk. Noise generated by electronics, motors, traffic, and crowds can lead to hearing loss and isolation, especially in the elderly. With increased age, noise has also been found to affect our sense of direction negatively. The scientific journal, *Nature Communications*, published a study from researchers at the German Center for Neurodegenerative Diseases (DZNE). According to their findings, the primary source of errors in determining spatial position and the cause of age-related orientation problems is described as *noisy*, causing an imprecise perception of the speed at which one is moving. [100]

Tammera found it easy to see when her elderly clients were having problems with their hearing. As they came into the office, their gait and movements seemed off-kilter, and they would be unsure on their feet. When asked if their ears were ringing or buzzing, more times than not, the answer was yes. Alarmingly, individuals with chronic tinnitus and hearing loss are more susceptible to depression, mood swings, and premature death. [101, 102]

Hearing loss isn't all about noise: In a 2018 study from Brigham and Women's Hospital, researchers found that eating a healthy diet is associated with a lower risk of acquired hearing loss in women. [103] A study published in *the*

Ear and Hearing Journal that looked at vitamin D and vitamin B_{12} insufficiencies and their connection to tinnitus and hearing loss concluded:

> There were associations between both single nutrients and dietary patterns with tinnitus and hearing difficulties. Although the size of the associations was small, universal exposure for dietary factors indicates that there may be a substantial impact of diet on levels of tinnitus and hearing difficulties in the population. [104]

Let's take a moment to think about preindustrial human ancestors and how they experienced sound. What were the loudest noises our ancestors had to deal with? What would they think of our cacophonous world today? To say they'd be startled would be perhaps an understatement. However, Nature is far from quiet. And anytime a group of people gathers, there is noise. So, although our forebears might wonder over our modern toys, and all their sounds "loud" may be relative. An average human conversation registers about 60 decibels. A loud thunderclap is about 120 decibels but lasts only a few seconds. The white male bellbird in the Amazon is the loudest bird on the planet, having a mating call that can reach 125 decibels. [105]

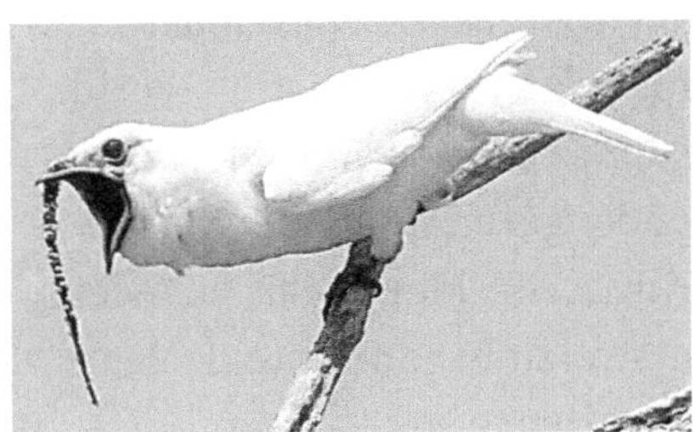

> *Principle 6*: Silence is golden.

The Sounds of Silence

No discussion of sound or music would be complete without mention of the value of silence. Great composers understand this fact and write periods of musical *rest* into their compositions. Beethoven's famous *Fifth Symphony in C Minor* begins with three eighth notes followed by a half note, with an all-important rest before the motif repeats with notes lower on the scale. The entire beginning of this iconic piece would be unrecognizable without the critical punctuating moments of silence.

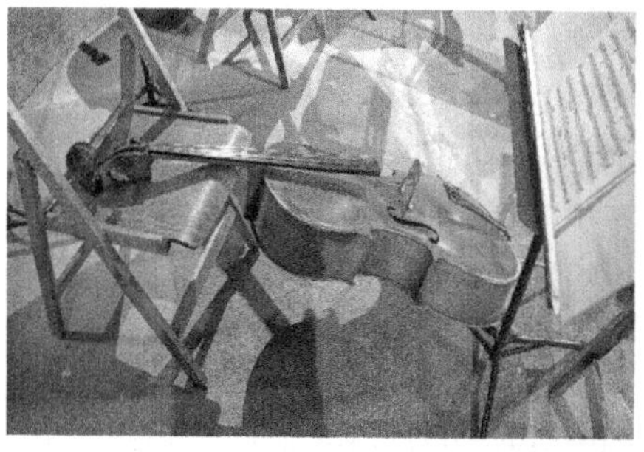

The rest periods built into music are only one example of the life-giving nourishment to be found in silence as the perfect counterpoint to the noise of existence. But silence must be consciously sought and mindfully chosen in today's overstimulating world. "In our present culture, silence is something like an endangered species, an endangered fundamental. We need it badly", says Gunilla Norris. [106] Many of us have learned to numb ourselves with distractions: things to do, learn, consume, perfect, maintain, experience, and collect.

Silence brings us back to basics, to our own selves, and our senses. Without returning to the solace of silence, we can get so far away from our true selves that we literally end up beside ourselves — living blindly day to day and acting thoughtlessly instead of mindfully.

A person does not need to withdraw from the *real* world for extended periods, nor attend a silent retreat, nor travel to an abandoned cave to cultivate the practice of silence. Small choices can be made. When things get too noisy, one can turn off the radio or TV. The relief, when unnecessary stimulation is removed, can be dramatic and amazing. Pausing to listen to and appreciate the body's wisdom is the beginning of approaching comfort with silence. Cementing the memory with deliberate breath gives the body/mind/spirit a little space to remember. Without taking more than a few moments of time, simply stopping at intervals throughout the day to feel ourselves in time and space allows us permission to be located in silence.

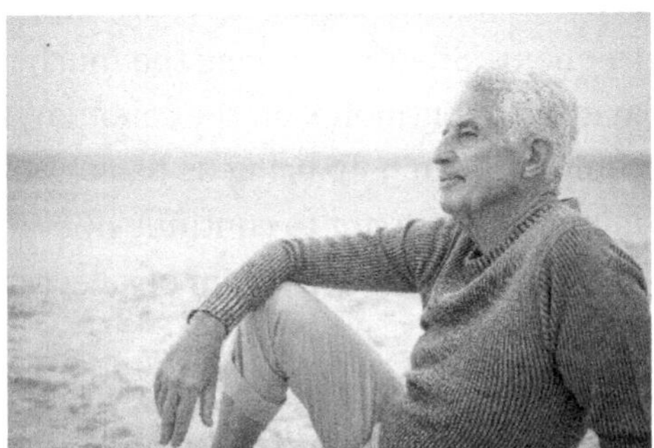

> *"Silence is the opportunity to let yourself down into mystery – to let yourself be touched by mystery. It is like the joy of music, only a thousand times deeper and greater."*
>
> ~Brother David Stendl-Rast

When practiced many times a day: before getting out of bed, before meals, before leaving for work or home, before turning on a light in the morning or shutting it off in the evening — the pauses add up. Over time, the habit of mindfully pausing, breathing, inviting, and appreciating the nourishing power of silence can help a person listen to the internal guidance that brings one back to the stillness that rests inside each of us. Nourishment encourages growth.

With small and continued efforts, anyone can grow in silent awareness of what is around them and within themselves, often becoming aware of when things are too much or too frequent. Silently noticing too much food on the plate, too many appointments on the calendar, too much time on the computer can help bring us back into balance by making a mindful choice not to continue operating on *automatic pilot*, but to listen to the wisdom of selection.

It can be challenging to set aside time for a silent meditation practice, whether with a group or alone. Most people will require training and support to achieve this worthy goal. Kathleen's many years of practice have led her to agree with author Gunilla Norris:

> When we make a place for silence, we make room for ourselves. This is simple. And it is radical .... When a space is reserved solely for mindfulness practice, the silence seems to deepen. A room devoted to silence honors and invites the unknown, the untamed, the wild, the shy, the unfathomable — that which rarely has a chance to surface within us. By making room for silence, we resist the forces of the world which tell us to live an advertised life of surface appearances instead of a

> discovered life — a life lived in contact with our senses, our feelings, our deeper thoughts, and values. [107]

After reviewing information on the effects of color, music, sound, and silence, it seems impossible for people to have sustainable health or connection to others, the environment, and community without the arts. After all, the research regarding our very long history with color and sound indicates these *seasonings* on the plate of human civilization were primary forms of nourishment moving us forward in evolution to become the people of today.

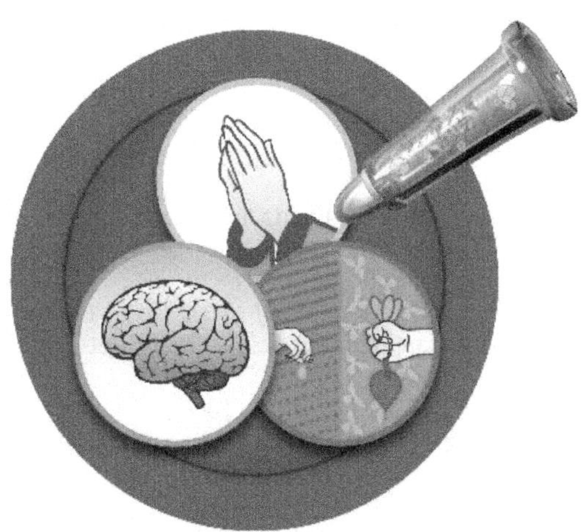

---

1. The Frequency and Wavelength of Light:
https://micro.magnet.fsu.edu/optics/lightandcolor/frequency.html
2. Sound and Music:
https://www.howmusicworks.org/103/Sound-and-Music/Amplitude-and-Frequency
3. Light, Alertness, and Performance, Lighting Research Center:
https://www.lrc.rpi.edu/programs/lighthealth/LightAlertness.asp
4. University of Liège. (2014, March 10). How light affects our brain's performance: Photic memory for executive brain responses. ScienceDaily. Retrieved August 26, 2020 from www.sciencedaily.com/releases/2014/03/140310152023.htm
5. Salk Institute. (2015, December 16). Scientists discover the function, connections of three cell types in the brain: Using genetic tools to interrogate cell types sheds light on how the brain processes visual information. ScienceDaily. Retrieved August 26, 2020 from www.sciencedaily.com/releases/2015/12/151216151943.htm
6. How do different color filters affect plant growth?
http://scienceline.ucsb.edu/getkey.php?key=3155
7. Max-Planck-Gesellschaft. (2012, January 19). Pictures of food create feelings of hunger. ScienceDaily. Retrieved August 26, 2020 from www.sciencedaily.com/releases/2012/01/120119101713.htm
8. Taste and Smell Research:
https://www.nidcd.nih.gov/about/strategic-plan/2017-2021/taste-and-smell-research
9. Dieters Beware: Pictures of Foods Increase Hunger Hormone.
https://www.medicaldaily.com/dieters-beware-pictures-foods-increase-hunger-hormone-239533
10. American Chemical Society (ACS). (2013, April 11). 'Seeing' the flavor of foods before tasting them. ScienceDaily. Retrieved August 27, 2020 from www.sciencedaily.com/releases/2013/04/130411194017.htm
11. 'Seeing' the flavor of foods before tasting them ....
https://www.sciencedaily.com/releases/2013/04/130411194017.htm
12. 6 Colors That Are Proven To Boost Sales:
Https://Www.Crazyegg.Com/Blog/Colors-Proven-To-Boost-Sales/
13. Sutton, T.M., Altarriba, J. Color Associations To Emotion And Emotion-Laden Words: A Collection Of Norms For Stimulus Construction And Selection. Behav Res 48, 686–728 (2016). Https://Doi.Org/10.3758/S13428-015-0598-8
14. The Conversation: We Can Use Colour To Communicate How We Feel – Here's How. 2018
Https://Theconversation.Com/We-Can-Use-Colour-To-Communicate-How-We-Feel-Heres-How-90157

15. Kimmerer, Robin; Braiding Sweetgrass, 2013, Milkweed Editions, page 45-46

16. The Sussex Baby Lab: https://www.sussex.ac.uk/babylab/

17. Ibid

18. A Review Of The Science Of Colorful, Plant-Based Food And Practical Strategies For "Eating The Rainbow" By Deanna Minich 2019, Journal Of Nutrition And Metabolism: Https://Www.Hindawi.Com/Journals/Jnme/2019/2125070/

19. Nutrilite Institute, America's Phytonutrient Report, Nutrilite Institute, Buena Park, CA, USA, 2018, Https://Bit.Ly/2dnlpqc.

20. The Rainbow Diet By Deanna Minich, Phd 2018 Page Xiii

21. The Chakra-Based Diet | Goop. https://goop.com/wellness/health/the-rainbow-diet/

22. www.ppt-health.com/lower/inflammation

23. www.chopracentermeditation.com

24. Symbolism Of Colors And Color Meanings Around The World By Shutterstock, 2015 Https://Www.Shutterstock.Com/Blog/Color-Symbolism-And-Meanings-Around-The-World

25. Https://Worldpopulationreview.Com/Flags/Romania/

26. Https://Martineclaessens.Com/Blog/2016/3/11/Colour-Blue-In-Romanian-Tradition

27. Our Journey With Food, 2015 First Edition, By Tammera Karr, Phd

28. Color Meanings And Their Customs: Http://Clanofdanu.Tripod.Com/Colors.Html

29. Elliot AJ. Color And Psychological Functioning: A Review Of Theoretical And Empirical Work. Front Psychol. 2015;6:368. Doi:10.3389/Fpsyg.2015.00368

30. Elliot AJ, Maier MA, Moller AC, Friedman R, Meinhardt J. Color And Psychological Functioning: The Effect Of Red On Performance Attainment. J Exp Psychol Gen. 2007;136(1):154-68. Doi:10.1037/0096-3445.136.1.154

31. Dispenza, J. (2017). Becoming Supernatural. Hay House: Ca.

32. Difference between Frequency Wavelength and Energy https://learnandbloom.wordpress.com/2018/10/17/difference-between-frequency-wavelength-and-energy/

33. Princeton University. "Spectacular Bird's-Eye View? Hummingbirds See Diverse Colors Humans Can Only Imagine: Team Trains Wild Hummingbirds To Discriminate UV Color Combinations." Sciencedaily. Sciencedaily, 15 June 2020. *Www.Sciencedaily.Com/Releases/2020/06/200615155114.Htm*

34. Candace B. Pert Quote: "To me, the rainbow was a https://quotefancy.com/quote/2247587/Candace-B-Pert-To-me-

the-rainbow-was-a-profoundly-hopeful-symbol-separating-the-the-white

35. O'Connor, Z. Colour Psychology And Colour Therapy: Caveat Emptor. Color Research & Application. 2011;36(3):229-234.

36. Azeemi STY, Rafiq HM, Ismail I, Kazmi SR, Azeemi A. The Mechanistic Basis Of Chromotherapy: Current Knowledge And Future Perspectives. Complement Ther Med. 2019;46:217-222. Doi:10.1016/J.Ctim.2019.08.025

37. Azeemi, Samina T Yousuf, And S Mohsin Raza. "A Critical Analysis Of Chromotherapy And Its Scientific Evolution." Evidence-Based Complementary And Alternative Medicine : Ecam Vol. 2,4 (2005): 481-8. Doi:10.1093/Ecam/Neh137

38. Forschungsverbund Berlin. (2019, December 19). Light pollution can suppress melatonin production in humans and animals. ScienceDaily. Retrieved September 24, 2020 from www.sciencedaily.com/releases/2019/12/191219111431.htm

39. University Of Haifa. "Blue Light Emitted By Screens Damages Our Sleep, Study Suggests." Sciencedaily. Sciencedaily, 22 August 2017. Www.Sciencedaily.Com/Releases/2017/08/170822103434.Htm

40. University Of Oxford. "Lighting Color Affects Sleep, Wakefulness: Green Light Promotes Sleep While Blue Light Delays It, Find Researchers." Sciencedaily. Sciencedaily, 8 June 2016. *Www.Sciencedaily.Com/Releases/2016/06/160608154233.Htm*

41. American Academy Of Sleep Medicine. "Light Exposure During Sleep May Increase Insulin Resistance: Chronic Overnight Light Exposure Could Have Long-Term Effects On Metabolic Function." Sciencedaily. Sciencedaily, 4 June 2018. *Www.Sciencedaily.Com/Releases/2018/06/180604172736.Htm*

42. Georgia Institute Of Technology. "Study Ties Poor Sleep To Reduced Memory Performance In Older Adults." Sciencedaily. Sciencedaily, 24 June 2019. *Www.Sciencedaily.Com/Releases/2019/06/190624111522.Htm*

43. Forschungsverbund Berlin. (2019, December 19). Light pollution can suppress melatonin production in humans and animals. ScienceDaily. Retrieved September 24, 2020 from www.sciencedaily.com/releases/2019/12/191219111431.htm

44. University Of Haifa. "Blue Light Emitted By Screens Damages Our Sleep, Study Suggests." Sciencedaily. Sciencedaily, 22 August 2017. Www.Sciencedaily.Com/Releases/2017/08/170822103434.Htm

45. Researcher Studies Green Light As Way To Relieve Migraines 2017 (Ongoing Study): Https://Ubrp.Arizona.Edu/Researcher-Studies-Green-Light-As-Way-To-Relieve-Migraines/

46. Blue Light Can Help Heal Mild Traumatic Brain Injury By Mikayla Mace University Communications Jan. 16, 2020: Https://Uanews.Arizona.Edu/Story/Blue-Light-Can-Help-Heal-Mild-Traumatic-Brain-Injury

47. PLOS Biology: PLOS Biology Is A Monthly Peer Reviewed Scientific Journal Covering All Aspects Of Biology. In Addition To Research Articles, The Journal Publishes Magazine Content Aimed To Be Accessible To A Broad Audience. Https://Journals.Plos.Org/Plosbiology/

48. PLOS. "No Blue Light, Please, I'm Tired: Light Color Determines Sleepiness Versus Arousal In Mice." Sciencedaily. Sciencedaily, 15 August 2016. *Www.Sciencedaily.Com/Releases/2016/08/160815185816.Htm*

49. Declining eyesight improved by looking at deep red light https://www.sciencedaily.com/releases/2020/06/200629120241.htm

50. University College London. (2020, June 29). Declining Eyesight Improved By Looking At Deep Red Light. Sciencedaily. Retrieved July 3, 2020 From Www.Sciencedaily.Com/Releases/2020/06/200629120241.Htm

51. American Academy Of Sleep Medicine. "Light Exposure During Sleep May Increase Insulin Resistance: Chronic Overnight Light Exposure Could Have Long-Term Effects On Metabolic Function." Sciencedaily. Sciencedaily, 4 June 2018. *Www.Sciencedaily.Com/Releases/2018/06/180604172736.Htm*

52. Permission Form. https://storage.googleapis.com/wzukusers/user-20502363/documents/ea9784edf37d4287bdc96f60d2e7172e/Permission%20Form.pdf

53. Arizona State University. "Bedtime Media Use Linked To Less Sleep In Children Who Struggle To Self-Regulate Behavior." Sciencedaily. Sciencedaily, 23 June 2020. Www.Sciencedaily.Com/Releases/2020/06/200623145328.Htm

54. American Academy Of Sleep Medicine. "Study Affirms Self-Reported Sleep Duration As A Useful Health Measure In Children: Results Show Agreement Between Sleep Measures Reported By Children And Their Parents." Sciencedaily. Sciencedaily, 14 February 2019. Www.Sciencedaily.Com/Releases/2019/02/190214093413.Htm

55. Briki, W., & Majed, L. (2019). Adaptive Effects of Seeing Green Environment on Psychophysiological Parameters When Walking or Running. Frontiers in psychology, 10, 252. https://doi.org/10.3389/fpsyg.2019.00252

56. University of Granada. (2017, November 10). Blue lighting is scientifically proven to help us relax faster than white lighting

after an argument. ScienceDaily. Retrieved September 23, 2020 from www.sciencedaily.com/releases/2017/11/171110113936.htm

57. Yellow: The Properties, Benefits And Meanings Behind The Most Powerful Colour: Https://Www.Technogym.Com/Us/Newsroom/Yellow-Benefits-Meanings-Colour/

58. https://www.disabled-world.com/disability/awareness/mood-colors.php

59. Yadav A, Gupta A. Noninvasive Red And Near-Infrared Wavelength-Induced Photobiomodulation: Promoting Impaired Cutaneous Wound Healing. Photodermatol Photoimmunol Photomed. 2017;33(1):4-13. Doi:10.1111/Phpp.12282

60. What Is Color Therapy, What Is It For, And Is It Right For Me? Https://Www.Regain.Us/Advice/Therapist/What-Is-Color-Therapy-What-Is-It-For-And-Is-It-Right-For-Me/

61. Goldenrod and Asters: My Life With Plants | Blue Mountan .... https://commons.bluemountaincenter.org/goldenrod-and-asters-my-life-with-plants/

62. Music 'releases mood-enhancing chemical in the brain' by Sonya McGilchrist, 2011: https://www.bbc.com/news/health-12135590

63. Musical chills: why they give us thrills News 2011: https://www.mcgill.ca/newsroom/channels/news/musical-chills-why-they-give-us-thrills-170538

64. Music And Customer Behavior: How Retailers Increase Sales With Music 2018. Https://Blog.Audiosocket.Com/Customer-Behavior/

65. Sensory Marketing: An Introduction 1st Edition By Bertil Hulten, 2020: ISBN-13: 978-1526423245, ISBN-10: 1526423243

66. Koithan, Mary, And Cynthia Farrell. "Indigenous Native American Healing Traditions." The Journal For Nurse Practitioners: JNP Vol. 6,6 (2010): 477-478. Doi:10.1016/J.Nurpra.2010.03.016

67. Colours And Native American Culture, 2016. Https://Www.Bergerpaints.Com/Imaginecolours/Colour-Culture/Colours-And-Native-American-Culture

68. Therapeutic Music of The Yellow Emperor's Classic Internal Medicine: http://www.windmusic.com.tw/en/pro_list.asp?LIB_ID=D&SET_NO=DX01&id=04

69. The Elements of Music: Concepts and Applications, Vol. I 2nd Edition by Ralph Turek. ISBN-13 : 978-0070654747

70. Fibonacci Numbers and the Golden Ratio https://www.math.ust.hk/~machas/fibonacci.pdf

71. Symphony of life:making music out of the human genome; Michael Zev Gordon, the Gaurdian 2010:

https://www.theguardian.com/music/2010/jun/24/dna-genome-music-michael-zev-gordon

72. "Your DNA is a Song: Scientists Use Music to Code Proteins." National Geographic 2008

73. Symphony of life:making music out of the human genome; Michael Zev Gordon, the Gaurdian 2010: https://www.theguardian.com/music/2010/jun/24/dna-genome-music-michael-zev-gordon

74. DNA Music - Healing Frequencies Music. https://www.healingfrequenciesmusic.com/dna-music/

75. Holding on to Gullah Culture by Erica R. Hendry; Smithsonian Magazine 2011: https://www.smithsonianmag.com/arts-culture/holding-on-to-gullah-culture-185296/

76. Ranky Tanky: https://www.rankytanky.com/news

77. Hilton Head Island Gullah Celebration http://gullahcelebration.com/gullah-events/hilton-head-island-gullah-celebration-opening-party

78. Edna Lewis (April 13, 1916 – February 13, 2006) was a renowned American chef, teacher, and author who helped refine the American view of Southern cooking. ... She wrote and co-wrote four books which covered Southern cooking and life in a small community of freed slaves and their descendants.

79. Edna Lewis, the grand dame of Southern cooking. http://specials.myajc.com/edna/

80. The Potlikker Papers by John T Edge, 2017, pp 147-159:

81. The History and Origins Of Traditional Irish Music; We Trace The Origins Of Our Traditional Music Back 2,000 Years. Frances Mulraney 2019: Https://Www.Irishcentral.Com/Roots/History/History-Origins-Traditional-Irish-Music

82. Restaurant Music's Effects On Your Digestion: Https://Www.Christinis.Com/Orlando-Restaurant/Restaurant-Musics-Effects-Digestion/

83. What You Need To Know About How Sound Affects Your Digestion, By Kells Mcphillips, 2019: Https://Www.Wellandgood.Com/Good-Food/How-Does-Sound-Affect-Digestion/

84. Harvard Women's Health Watch, How Music Can Help You Heal: Https://Www.Health.Harvard.Edu/Mind-And-Mood/How-Music-Can-Help-You-Heal

85. The HPA Axis Is Responsible For The Neuroendocrine Adaptation Component Of The Stress Response. This Response Is Characterized By Hypothalamic Release Of Corticotropin-Releasing Factor (CRF). When CRF Binds To CRF Receptors On The Anterior

Pituitary Gland, Adrenocorticotropic Hormone (ACTH) Is Released. ACTH Binds To Receptors On The Adrenal Cortex And Stimulates Adrenal Release Of Cortisol. Veldhuis JD, Et Al. Endocrinol Metab Clin North Am. 2013 Jun;42(2):201-25: Seeman TE, Et Al. Psychoneuroendocrinology. 2001;26(3):225

86. University Health Network. "Mozart May Reduce Seizure Frequency In People With Epilepsy." Sciencedaily. Sciencedaily, 10 June 2020. Www.Sciencedaily.Com/Releases/2020/06/200610135018.Htm

87. In 1993, In The Journal Nature, University Of California At Irvine Psychologist Frances H. Rauscher And Her Associates Reported Findings Of Enhanced Spatial Task Performance Among College Students After Exposure To Mozart's Music.

88. Deutsches Aerzteblatt International. "The Healing Powers Of Music: Mozart And Strauss For Treating Hypertension." Sciencedaily. Sciencedaily, 20 June 2016. Www.Sciencedaily.Com/Releases/2016/06/160620112512.Htm

89. American Friends Of Tel Aviv University. "Mozart Therapy: A Sonata A Day Keeps The Doctor Away." Sciencedaily. Sciencedaily, 8 January 2010. Www.Sciencedaily.Com/Releases/2010/01/100107132551.Htm

90. Helsingin Yliopisto (University Of Helsinki). "Listening To Classical Music Modulates Genes That Are Responsible For Brain Functions." Sciencedaily. Sciencedaily, 13 March 2015. Www.Sciencedaily.Com/Releases/2015/03/150313083410.Htm

91. Did Early Humans, Or Even Animals Invent Music? BBC Earth By Colin Barras 2014: Http://Www.Bbc.Com/Earth/Story/20140907-Does-Music-Pre-Date-Modern-Man

92. Tapping Into Ancient Soundscapes by Joshua Kumbani; 2020: https://www.sapiens.org/archaeology/southern-africa-instruments/?utm_source=SAPIENS.org+Subscribers&utm_campaign=43162fe26d-EMAIL_CAMPAIGN_2020_11_09&utm_medium=email&utm_term=0_18b7e41cd8-43162fe26d-227359404&ct=t()

93. Earliest Known Painting of an Animal Found in a Remote Cave. https://www.thevintagenews.com/2018/11/09/indonesian-cave/

94. Did Early Humans, Or Even Animals Invent Music? BBC Earth By Colin Barras 2014: Http://Www.Bbc.Com/Earth/Story/20140907-Does-Music-Pre-Date-Modern-Man

95. Earliest Known Painting of an Animal Found in a Remote Cave. https://www.thevintagenews.com/2018/11/09/indonesian-cave/

96. Max Planck Institute For Human Cognitive And Brain Sciences. "Miles Davis Is Not Mozart: The Brains Of Jazz And Classical Pianists Work Differently: Even When Playing The Same Piece Of Music." Sciencedaily. Sciencedaily, 16 January 2018. Www.Sciencedaily.Com/Releases/2018/01/180116123713.Htm

97. Visualizing The Emotional Power Of Music, New Way To Analyze Musical Structure Can Capture Both Local And Global Characteristics. American Institute Of Physics 2016, Https://Www.Eurekalert.Org/Pub Releases/2016-02/Aiop-Vte022316.Php

98. American Institute Of Physics. "Visualizing The Emotional Power Of Music: New Way To Analyze Musical Structure Can Capture Both Local And Global Characteristics." Sciencedaily. Sciencedaily, 23 February 2016. Www.Sciencedaily.Com/Releases/2016/02/160223132728.Htm

99. March 3, 2011 https://www.differencebetween.com/difference-between-sound-and-vs-noise

100. DZNE - German Center For Neurodegenerative Diseases. "Noise Disturbs The Brain's Compass: Identifying Causes For Troubles In Spatial Navigation." Sciencedaily. Sciencedaily, 10 June 2020. Www.Sciencedaily.Com/Releases/2020/06/200610112105.Htm

101. Columbia University's Mailman School Of Public Health. "Hearing Loss Is A Risk Factor For Premature Death." Sciencedaily. Sciencedaily, 12 December 2018. Www.Sciencedaily.Com/Releases/2018/12/181212121911.Htm

102. Sound Therapies: Https://Www.Ata.Org/Managing-Your-Tinnitus/Treatment-Options/Sound-Therapies

103 . Brigham And Women's Hospital. "Healthy Diet May Lower Risk Of Hearing Loss In Women: Patterns Of Healthy Eating May Lower Risk Of Hearing Loss By 30 Percent." Sciencedaily. Sciencedaily, 11 May 2018. Www.Sciencedaily.Com/Releases/2018/05/180511123022.Htm

104. Dawes, Piers1,2; Cruickshanks, Karen J.3; Marsden, Antonia4; Moore, David R.1,2,5; Munro, Kevin J.1,2 Relationship Between Diet, Tinnitus, And Hearing Difficulties, Ear And Hearing: March/April 2020 - Volume 41 - Issue 2 - P 289-299 Doi: 10.1097/AUD.0000000000000765

105. White bellbirds have the loudest known mating call of any bird by Sofie Bates 2019, Science News: https://www.sciencenews.org/article/white-bellbirds-have-loudest-known-mating-call-any-bird

106. Norris, G. (2004). Inviting Silence, p. 31. London: Rider.

107. Ibid. pp.49-50

Chapter Five
Time in Nature

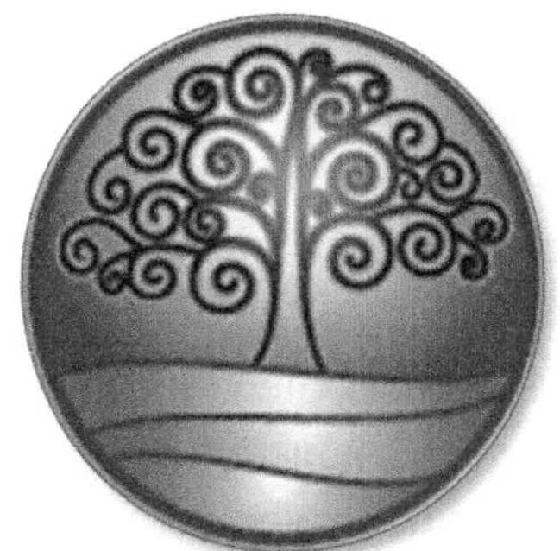

"With the varying light, sunshine, color, flora and wildlife, each gorge is a thing of beauty and delight.

For many the beauty of the gorges is the important thing. It is a beauty that changes with every shadow from a passing cloud." [1]

~ E. R. Jackman
Steens Mountain in Oregon's high desert country

What is time in Nature, and why is it important? This is a question to consider in our journey to a sustainable and mindful life. Nature is very much a form of nourishment, through the power of pheromones, lifeforms, and much more, Nature feeds humans' biochemistry, spirit, and bodies.

Some individuals have spent their entire lives in metropolitan and populated areas. A rooftop garden or city park may be as close as many come to time in Nature. While the city greenway and park are better than the total absence of any natural setting, they are a far cry from a wilderness area where time in

Nature is devoid of connectivity to the web, artificial light, and climate control.

In contrast, there are vast areas of North America where individuals and families may live more than 100 miles from the closest *town*, let alone a city. These rugged, independent souls live and work in Nature daily and are acutely aware of its cycles. When visiting the Riddle Brothers ranch at the base of Blitzen gorge in the Steens Mountain Wilderness in Oregon, an echo from the past greets one. [2] This ranch — dating from the 1880s –1987, gives a person pause to reflect on life for those who lived when times were less cluttered with electronics and cultural expectations; a sustainable life in such isolation from the outside world was not for the faint of heart nor a social butterfly. Critical and whole brain thinking in the last century led to ingenuity in building a homestead with a shower bathhouse and woven willow corrals; in a place surrounded by evidence of ancient peoples dating back over 9,000 years.

City dwellers are surrounded by a very different environment, one filled with manmade structures, chemicals, and wholly different cycles. Individuals may find themselves harried and worn from the frenzied pace of living their lives. Additionally, many people in cities are removed by several generations or more from the ways of living on the land, farm, or ranch. When those from metropolitan areas first visit wild areas, it may take them days or even weeks to calm their minds and adjust to nature's pace and quiet. The more time spent in Nature, the easier it is to focus on the subtleties from the blue butterfly on a wildflower to barometric changes signaling a thunderstorm.

> *"Poems are made by fools like me,*
> *But only God can make a tree."*
>
> ~Alfred Joyce Kilmer

The song of trees

What do you see when you look at a tree? This question may have immediately brought a rush of words to your mind, most positive, but there are some negative ones also, especially if a severe storm has placed a tree through your roof!
And while you are thinking about trees, here's another question to consider. Do plants communicate? Although not a new concept for those who come from indigenous cultures, the reality of this innate ability in the plant world may be startling to learn. In Chapter Two, we looked at how mycorrhizal fungi connect humans to animals and the environment.

Elders of the first people are helping the next generation reconnect with the stories and songs of old. These stories tell of trees communicating. According to Robin Wall Kimmerer, PhD, botanist, educator, and Citizen of the Potawatomi Nation.

> There is now compelling evidence that our elders were right — the trees are communicating to one another. They communicate via pheromones — hormone-like compounds that are carried on the air. Scientists have identified specific compounds that one tree will release when it is under the stress of

> insect attack. The downwind trees catch the drift, sensing those few molecules of alarm. This gives them time to manufacture defensive chemicals. The trees warn each other, and the invaders are repelled. The individual trees benefit, and so does the entire grove. [3]

Additionally, Dr. Kimmerer explains the connection between trees and the fungi in the soil that acts as the grocery store and the telephone service.

> The trees in a forest are often interconnected by subterranean networks of mycorrhizae, fungal strands that inhabit tree roots. The mycorrhizal symbiosis enables the fungi to forage for mineral nutrients in the soil and deliver them to the tree in exchange for carbohydrates. The mycorrhizae may form fungal bridges between individual trees to connect all the trees in a forest. These fungal networks appear to redistribute the wealth of carbohydrates from tree to tree so that all arrive at a carbon surplus at the same time. In this way, the trees all act as one because the fungi have connected them. [4]

"There is something like a mycorrhizal network that
unites us, an unseen connection of history
and family and responsibility to
both our ancestors
and our children."

~ Robin Wall Kimmerer, PhD
author of *Braiding Sweetgrass*

The basic principle of tree-ring dating—dendrochronologist matches ring patterns from living tree to living tree. The researchers, led by the University of Cambridge, used samples from more than 9000 living and dead trees to obtain a precise yearly record of summer temperatures in North America and Eurasia, dating back to the year 1 CE. [5] Once that task is accomplished, the dendrochronologist works back in time to cross date successively, providing context for examples from archaeological finds. [6]

In its many forms, the tree has held an essential role in traditional cultures all over the world. These varied cultures also have an indigenous history of trees providing medicine, food, and materials needed to live. For Tammera, the juniper and ponderosa pine trees are part of childhood memories. Stories of quaking aspen trees planted fanciful images in her mind of money trees. When looking at these three trees today, thoughts of reverence enters her mind. What have these trees witnessed throughout time? What stories do they hold?

Kathleen was told by her mother that her first word was "windy." As a baby, her home in Biloxi, Mississippi, was surrounded by towering long-needled pine trees. When the wind blew, she would toddle outside, delightedly pointing upward and repeating, *Windy*! *Windy*!! The authors' shared fascination with Nature may be the result of a lifetime living surrounded by Nature. Both claim Irish heritage and wonder if their nostalgic childhood fancies and deep feelings of reverence for trees may be part of ancestral DNA from the ancient Celts; who placed special significance on trees.

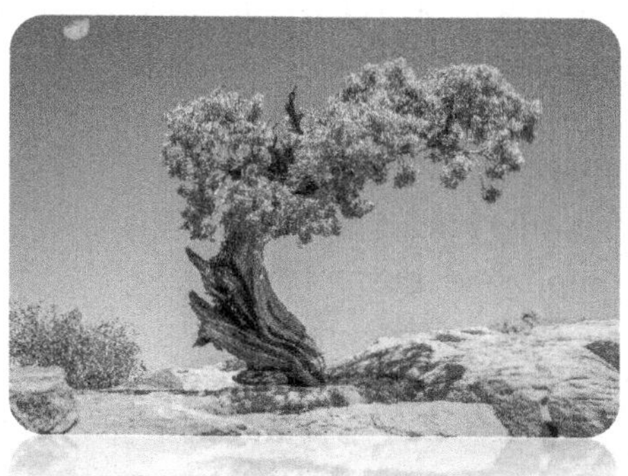
The one-seed juniper tree has deep cultural meaning for the Hopi.

Cultural reverence for trees, in particular, is by no means limited to the Celts; the Hopi peoples of the United States hold the Juniper in high regard.

With cultural origins that stretch back thousands of years in the Southwest, Hopis make use of every possible asset of their natural, mostly desert surroundings. The juniper provides Hopis the basics of warmth, shelter, tools, and food. Hopis do not cut down junipers but rather collect deadwood for winter fires and for building houses, corrals, and fences. One-Seed Juniper roots, which can stretch downward 200 feet, are carved into cradleboards, bows and arrows, and hairpieces that are used for the famous squash-blossom hairdo of Hopi maidens. [7]

> *"Just because people are living an easy life now,*
> *it hasn't always been that way.*
> *It's important to remember."*
>
> ~ Owen Numkena, a Hopi Elder

The juniper's more profound value to the Hopi lies in its powers to purify and protect. Juniper has spiritual significance as part of the sacred landscape. "It's a tree with a lot of medicine," says Bill Preston, a Hopi traditionalist from the village of Walpi. Juniper needles, boiled as a tea, are a medicine; the sap can be consumed as an intestinal cleanse. Newborns are rubbed with juniper ash, while their mothers — who may have veered toward death during childbirth — are bathed in juniper-infused water. Juniper berries ground into a paste is used to clean new mothers further. Even misbehaving youth are held to the smoke of a smoldering juniper fire to purge them of mischief.

Hopis see the juniper forests as interconnected to the entire natural world, a thread woven into the tapestry of life. Said researchers Stewart B. Koyiyumptewa, the archivist and ethnohistorian for the Hopi Tribe's Cultural Preservation Office, and anthropologist Chip Colwell. [8]

The deep connection the Hopi and many others have with trees serve as reminders of humanity's need for interaction with nature. If we are open to the idea of DNA carrying codes for health, it isn't a far leap to consider how Nature and the need to connect with it, in its many forms, is also coded into the genetic architecture of human life.

Principle 1: Learn your history, who you have come from, and the stories of your people. These things provide connection and grounding of body, mind, and spirit.

> *"For the most part, I minded not how the hours went...My days were not days of the week... nor were they minced into hours and fretted by the ticking of a clock; for I lived like the Puri Indians, of whom it is said that, 'for yesterday, today and tomorrow they have only one word; and they express the variety of meaning by pointing backward for yesterday, forward for tomorrow and overhead for the passing day.' "*
>
> ~Henry David Thoreau

Barriers of the mind

It is frighteningly easy for the human mind to work on *autopilot* without paying any conscious attention. Still, this state of affairs can end up working against an individual — even though the mind thinks it is helping. Accepting aches and pains, limiting physical health conditions and cognitive challenges, such as depression, that accompany aging as usual and customary, makes them real. The often-repeated phrase, *perception is reality* is true, indeed. Here is what it boils down to whatever a person thinks is real, in their mind, is real to them. Each person's thoughts create a reality which, as far as your mind is concerned, exists.

When you hold thoughts in your mind, they will affect how you feel and act. This is because you're being influenced by the thought, as though it is reality. Your mind is making it a reality; therefore, it must be a reality. This is how thoughts become things because you create a new reality from those thoughts. Confusing right?

> *"What we observe is not nature in itself but nature exposed to our method of questioning."* [9]
>
> ~Werner Heisenberg
> first to fathom the uncertainty inherent in quantum physics

Dr. Joe Dispenza explains it this way:

> Your thoughts and feelings come from your memories. If you think and feel a certain way, you begin to create an attitude. An attitude is a cycle of short-term thoughts and feelings experienced over and over again. Attitudes are shortened states of being. If you string a series of attitudes together, you create a belief. Beliefs are more elongated states of being and tend to become subconscious. When you add beliefs together, you create a perception. Your perceptions have everything to do with the choices you make, the behaviors you exhibit, the relationships you choose, and the realities you create. [10]

So, what is said out loud, especially repeatedly — "I'm getting older," "Just part of aging," "It isn't safe at my age," "What if something happens?" "I could fall or fail," "It won't be any fun by myself," and countless other restrictive words — ALL these beliefs can become encoded neurochemically in the brain. In essence, individuals program their brains to believe they can or can't do something as a response to their experiences, culture, family, or associations. All that is perceived at any given moment is capable of changing not only your mood but the actual physiology of the nervous, endocrine, and immune systems.

When it comes to time in Nature, it isn't about age or fitness. It is about just *being*. Being in Nature, or even viewing scenes of Nature, reduces anger, fear, and stress and the resulting neurochemicals associated with negative emotions while increasing pleasant feelings and their many beneficial biochemical responses in the body. Exposure to Nature not only makes you feel better emotionally, but it also contributes to your physical wellbeing by reducing blood pressure, heart rate, muscle tension, and the production of stress hormones. It may even reduce mortality, according to scientists Stamatakis and Mitchell. [11]

Besides, Nature helps us cope with pain. We are genetically programmed to find trees, plants, water, and other natural elements engrossing. Being mentally absorbed by nature scenes helps distracted individuals from pain and discomfort. This was demonstrated in a study of patients who underwent gallbladder surgery; post-operatively, half had a view of trees, and half had a view of a hospital wall. According to Dr. Robert Ulrich, the patients with the view of trees tolerated pain better, appeared to nurses to have fewer negative effects of surgery, and spent less time in the hospital. [12]

Rehabilitation in nature

Hundreds of disabled veterans and civilians have taken on the challenge of skiing, kayaking, fishing, horseback riding, and camping as forms of rehabilitation. According to the Veterans Health Administration (VA), recreation therapy has been part of its mission since the Civil War. Currently, over 800 Recreation Therapists and Creative Arts Therapists across the VA system help Veterans build confidence and self-esteem by focusing on strengths and by developing skills that make success possible. The VA says that centering on veteran strengths diminishes the focus on disability and emphasizes ability; increasing functioning, and restoring life quality. The Military Adaptive Sports Program (MASP) aids with healing wounded warriors by including recreation therapy and creative arts therapy interventions. Both of these therapies are an evidence-based approach to care.

> *"What we are today comes from our thoughts of yesterday, and our present thoughts build our life of tomorrow: our life is the creation of our mind."*
>
> ~*The Dhammapada* - ancient Vedic text

When you end up in the Warrior Transition Program, as I did, it's because you're very sick or very injured said Retired Army Col. Michael Malone. So, you're in a really dark place. Adaptive sports allowed me to feel competitive again and build my athletic skills. And emotionally, the program really facilitated my recovery. I got into swimming again, Malone said. "And I learned archery. I found it really meditative. It allowed me to focus on the moment, focus on the target, and just forget about my injuries and my illness.

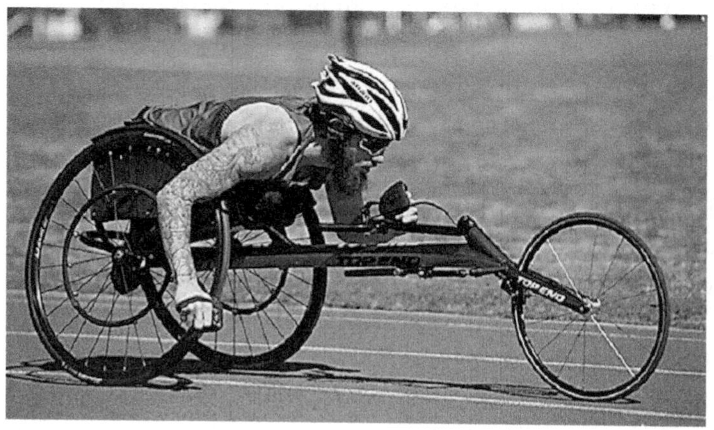

A Special Operations Forces wounded warrior competes in the Warrior Games selection camp at MacDill Air Force Base, Florida, in February. The COVID-19 pandemic forced the cancellation of the 2020 Warrior Games. (DoD Photo by Roger L. Wollenberg)

MASP is part of the Department of Defense Warrior Care Program. It provides reconditioning activities and competitive athletic opportunities for wounded, ill, and injured service members and veterans. Since the Warrior Care Office began collecting data in 2016, MASP has held more than 198 clinics, five camps, and 26 regional competitions for approximately 7,000 service members and veterans, says Sandra Mason, director of the Warrior Care Office's Recovery Coordination Program. [13]

While recovering individuals — due to age, illness, or ability — may not be able to do things at the level they once did, the unconditional acceptance of Nature renews their experience of living.

What about the role of nutrition for individuals suffering from disorders like Gulf War Illness (GWI)? Many thousands of contractors and veterans who served in the Persian Gulf from 1990 and 1991 live daily with symptoms of GWI. This multi-system illness resulted from exposure to chemical toxins such as organophosphates' (in uniforms), pesticides, and drugs intended to combat nerve gases' effects. [14] The low glutamate diet shown to reduce fibromyalgia symptoms was recommended to study participants with GWI to learn if diet could improve symptoms.

> GWI is a debilitating disorder which includes widespread pain, fatigue, headaches, cognitive dysfunction, and gastrointestinal symptoms. Veterans with GWI have a reduced quality of life as compared to veterans who do not have the illness," said American University's Associate Professor of Health Studies Kathleen Holton, who explores how food additives contribute to neurological symptoms and is a member of American University's Center for Behavioral Neuroscience. "In this study testing the low glutamate diet, the majority of veterans reported feeling better. We saw significant reductions in their overall number of symptoms and significant improvements in pain and fatigue." [15]

In the decades since Operation Desert Storm, much research has accumulated on therapies and treatments to alleviate the suffering of GWI. Understanding how completely out of balance the *whole* body/mind/spirit of affected individuals has grown. GWI is a multifactorial syndrome and responds to a wide variety of treatments and therapies, all of which endeavor to achieve the desired state of homeostasis for each individual again. Physiologically, homeostasis involves multiple dynamic body processes working in harmony to bring about a balanced equilibrium in the bodymind, ensuring stability and survival.

GWI remission can occur with an array of appropriate therapies: [16]

1) Aerobic exercise – especially outdoors
2) Cognitive behavioral therapy (CBT)
3) Yoga
4) Acupuncture
5) Holistic diet and balanced nutrition
6) Medications

Chronic invasive gastrointestinal infections have been resolved by combining nutritional therapy with antibiotics for mycoplasmas and/or antivirals, which restores the gut microbiome's natural balance, ultimately resolving multiple distressing symptoms throughout the body and mind. [17]

> *Principle 2*: Don't fall victim to "stinking thinking." Always try, even when you don't feel like it.

Seasonal changes and mood

Everything alive on Earth is subject to cyclical behavior — plants, fungi, animals (including humans), even bacteria. One example of a natural cycle is circadian rhythm, a built-in twenty-four-hour process to regulate periods of rest/sleep, hunger, and energy levels. In humans, this cycle is established in infancy. Although internally generated, it can be influenced and modified by external cues such as sunlight and temperature. A normally developed nervous system facilitates wakefulness during the daylight hours and sleep during darkness via the brain's hypothalamus activity. Hormones are the chemical messengers governing the cycle of sleeping and waking. When daylight begins to fade in the evening, melatonin production increases, causing tiredness and/or sleep. The twenty-four-hour *biological clock* plus an increase in light perception at dawn decreases melatonin, and cortisol is released to wake up the brain. [18]

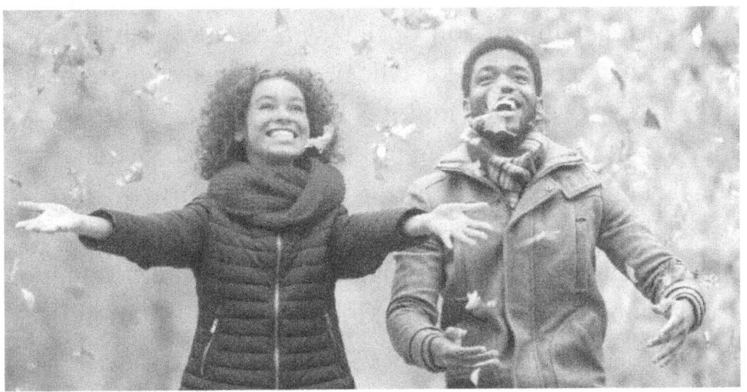

"Autumn anxiety is the tendency for people to suffer from anxiety and low mood during the autumn months. Unlike other anxiety, there often isn't an obvious external trigger, and it tends to recur annually," says Dr. Clare Morrison, medical advisor at MedExpress. Many people don't realize how common anxiety in autumn is and may not recognize it. "However, if it occurs every year, the pattern will become obvious, and one can take steps to prevent it." One of the causes is the reduction in sunlight, leading to falling levels of serotonin. This important hormone affects mood, appetite, and sleep patterns. There is also an increase in the hormone melatonin, which tends to make one feel sleepy and depressed. Less vitamin D is an effect of being exposed to less sunlight. "Lack of vitamin D has been linked with depression," said Dr. Morrison. "Other factors include behavioral changes because as the weather deteriorates, individuals become less physically active and spend less time outdoors." [19]

The best advice is to get outside in the fresh — even if bracing cold — air. If the weather is sunny, get the sun on your face. Without time in the sun, serotonin levels drop. Low serotonin levels are associated with depression and with seasonal patterns (formerly known as seasonal affective disorder or SAD). [20] Seasonal depression, or the *winter blues*, is a type of depression that occurs at a specific time each year, when the seasons change. Usually, symptoms begin in the fall and continue through the winter months. [21] Thought to be due to hormonal changes mitigated by the brain's response to decreased levels of light, treatments include: light therapy with full-spectrum light and dawn simulators, exercise to stimulate the production of endorphins that increase mood, vitamin D supplements, aromatherapy, and medications. [22, 23]

One of the many life lessons Tammera learned from spending time around cattle ranchers and farmers — no matter how you feel, the chores still have to be done. [24] This life-long habit of *just doing* and not stopping enables these hardy souls to be on horseback moving cattle off range allotments, hiking and hunting, tending the garden, cutting firewood, working in healthcare, or substitute teaching, long into their seventies, eighties, and even nineties. Nina Clark, at 92-years-old, works about thirty hours a week as a pre-admission testing nurse at Banner Del E Webb Medical Center in Sun City, Arizona. She said in a news interview, *retirement* wasn't a word in her vocabulary. [25, 26] Every day individuals need to move more than from the bed to the couch actively, and they especially need to spend time outside. [27, 28]

> *"The body will become better at whatever you do, or don't do. You don't move? The body will make you better at NOT moving. If you move, your body will allow more movement."*
>
> ~ Ido Portal

When the human body remains in an incline and inactive position for prolonged periods, brain chemistry changes occur— signaling the body to shut down, and lymphatic systems that depend on movement to function cease to work — driving inflammation markers higher. [29] Movement and time outdoors are a vital part of life for humans. [30] In less than two generations, physical activity has dropped by 20% in the U.K. and 32% in the U.S. In China, the drop is 45% in less than one generation. [31]

> *"Time is but the stream I go a-fishing in. I drink at it, but while I drink, I see the sandy bottom and detect how shallow it is. Its thin current slides away, but eternity remains."*
>
> ~ Henry David Thoreau

What is time?

A study published in 2017 in the *Journal of Environmental Psychology* titled: "Time grows on trees: The effect of nature settings on time perception" caught the authors' attention. [32] Researchers examined whether nature exposure was related to time perception. When estimating the length of time spent in nature versus an urban environment, does the subjective estimate of time duration change depending on the setting?

Answers:

- Time spent on a walk in a nature setting was overestimated compared to the actual time.
- Time spent on a walk in an urban setting was estimated accurately.
- Time felt slower in Nature than in human-made settings.
- Taking a walk in Nature (vs. urban setting) increased mood, decreased stress.
- Nature exposure can slow down time perception.

Principle 3: Time spent in Nature, especially grounding the human body to the earth, is good for body/mind/spirit

Friction and electrical charge

The modern world exposes people to a multitude of synthetic fibers in homes, clothes, and vehicles that lead to a buildup of static electricity charge in/on their bodies. We have all experienced reaching for a doorknob or reaching out a hand to touch another person and had that snap and spark of static electricity jump off of us. Modern vehicles and homes can be filled with electric motors, inverters, and circuits that move and surround individuals with electricity. These currents are often referred to as electromagnetic-frequency (EMF). The invention of electricity, followed by the switch from direct current (DC) to alternating current (AC) in homes, meant constant human exposure to currents of electricity that pulse every sixty seconds through household wiring. It is important to note that means every sixty seconds electricity is pulsing through household wiring. It is essential to note this energetic exposure has not been part of human lives for more than one hundred years and less than sixty years in North America's remote rural areas.

While grounding and earthing practices may sound like New-Age hokum to some, there is a scientifically practical side to this concept. In the case of electrical currents, grounding is necessary for power to flow correctly and safely from connection to connection. Grounding allows for an escape ramp for when the current gets too intense. Humans are bioelectrical life forms — from the electrochemically controlled heart and brain rhythms to the balance of electrolytes in the blood — electricity is literally the *spark* of life.

The modern scientific look at how grounding impacts human physiology and health began with Drs. Karol and Pawel Sokal in

Poland and Dr. Clint Ober in the United States in the 1990s. Their theory suggests: that free radicals cause inflammation and that electrons from any source neutralize free radicals. Electrons are the source of the neutralizing power of antioxidants. In a study published in 2018, researchers looked at the effects of grounding on hypertension.

> All ten patient measurements were found to improve at the end of the trial period significantly, and some, well before the end. Systolic levels decreased during this time, ranging individually from 8.6% to 22.7%, with an average decrease of 14.3%. [33]

A published study from 2004 measured cortisol levels during sleep while individuals were grounded. Measurable improvements in diurnal cortisol profiles were observed, with cortisol levels significantly reduced during night-time sleep. Subjects' 24-hour circadian cortisol profiles showed a trend toward normalization. Subjectively reported symptoms, including sleep dysfunction, pain, and stress, were reduced, or eliminated in nearly all subjects.

Conclusions: Results indicate that grounding the human body to earth (*earthing*) during sleep reduces night time cortisol levels and resynchronizes cortisol hormone secretion to be more in alignment with the natural 24-hour circadian rhythm profile. Changes were most apparent in females. Furthermore, subjective reporting indicates that grounding the human body to earth during sleep improves sleep and reduces pain and stress. [34]

Researchers in 2019 found grounding techniques significantly reduced muscle damage and improved recovery following intense exercise for athletes. [35]

Precisely what is *grounding*? It is simple if one thinks back to humans in ancient times. Humans had daily contact with the soil, and the natural fibers utilized for clothing and foot covering generated less static charge than today's modern clothing. Grounding is something gardeners do each time they put their hands in the soil; it happens when a person walks barefoot on the beach or across a lawn; it occurs when sitting on a mountain meadow rock outcropping; or when sleeping on the ground. Animals naturally lie down on the ground when they are tired, ill, or about to give birth. Grounding is nature's electrical detox, and it is available to all for no charge. (Yup, that pun was just too good to pass up!)

Electro-Magnetic Frequency (EMF) and health

How EMF energy can affect human health is still under examination. However, a growing body of data reveals some individuals are adversely affected by the continuous flow of charged energy from smart meters, cell phones, and microwave towers in urban environments. The availability to naturally discharge static electricity for individuals in metropolitan areas can be far lower than for those who work and live in more rural areas. This is only one reason why people benefit from gardening, terrace with potted plants, city parks, and time in vast areas of nature.

> *Principal 4*: Nature provides examples of cooperative relationships and interconnectedness.

Symbiotic relationships provide balance

"Today, we may know details about our family history for five or more generations, yet it only takes a small change, and that information is lost," said Dr. Elizabeth Lipski when reviewing archeological information with Tammera. The life expectancy of individuals during the paleolithic era was short compared to modern individuals. It is easy to see how knowledge can be so easily lost if there may have been only two generations alive at one time.

Lost knowledge is especially crucial for the modern understanding of Nature's cycles and influences over human health. One thing indigenous cultures try to preserve is the knowledge of Nature's symbiotic relationship with humans, which can be healing and enable harmony.

Nature is filled with patterns and cycles that take time to reacquaint oneself with. Nature also provides a treasure trove of examples of cooperative and symbiotic relationships for humans to consider and even model. Sitting on a basalt rock overlooking the Kiger Gorge at Steens Mountain, Dr. Lipski reached over and touched the lichen on the rock surface. She asked Tammera if she knew about the symbiotic nature of *lichen*. Lichen is a combination of algae and fungi that live interwoven as one. The algae use photosynthesis, water, and minerals collected by the fungi to make glucose. In turn, the fungi feed off the glucose and spread to harvest minerals from

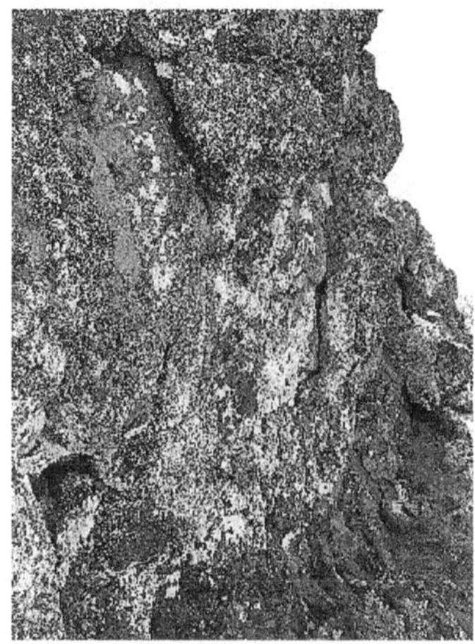

the rock surface. These two independent life forms live in adverse environments as one, but if the environment changes and survival is not so difficult, they separate and even shun the other.

> *"Lichens are a case of fungi that have discovered agriculture."*
>
> ~Trevor Goward Canadian Botanist

Not only are lichens fascinating to look at, but many contain substances that can be converted to brilliant permanent dyes. Their historical use in textiles originated thousands of years ago and came to rise in several isolated regions. [36]

Observing and accepting new perspectives are challenges presented when spending time in Nature. A part of sustainability is learning how to have and form supportive relationships, figuring out where one fits in; conversely, when to separate when conditions are no longer safe or supportive.

Time in Nature gives one a chance to reflect without all the noise and clutter that makes up the modern world. Just as trees and algae depend on their relationship with fungi to thrive, humans also need a symbiotic connection to Nature to *ground* and detox our bodies, minds, and spirits from depleting currents in the modern world. Time in Nature allows us to take that moment of pause and reset cortisol and circadian cycles so we can mindfully view the world through calm instead of chaos.

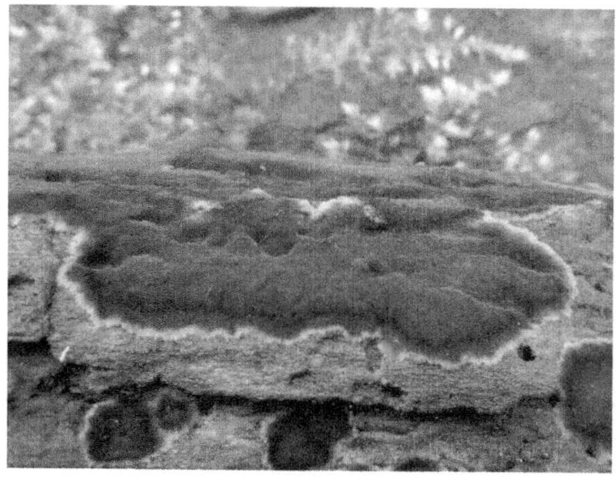

Caerulea fungus in cobalt and shades of purple is a keystone species vital to forest ecosystem health; by unlocking organic molecules that would otherwise remain inaccessible to other fauna and flora.

> *"Let Nature be thy Medicine."*
>
> ~Deanna Minich, PhD
> author of *The Rainbow Diet*

Looking for new patterns

When able to spend more than fleeting moments in nature, individuals are able to stop and take a moment to look at the tiny alpine flower, lichen, the acrobatic flight of swallows, or the gentle sway of branches in the morning breeze. These moments provide opportunities for the parasympathetic and sympathetic nervous systems to readjust. This recalibrating of the nervous system has a cascading effect on the hypothalamus, pituitary, adrenal, and thyroid axis (HPAT), which regulates hormones throughout the body. The most talked-about of these hormones is cortisol.

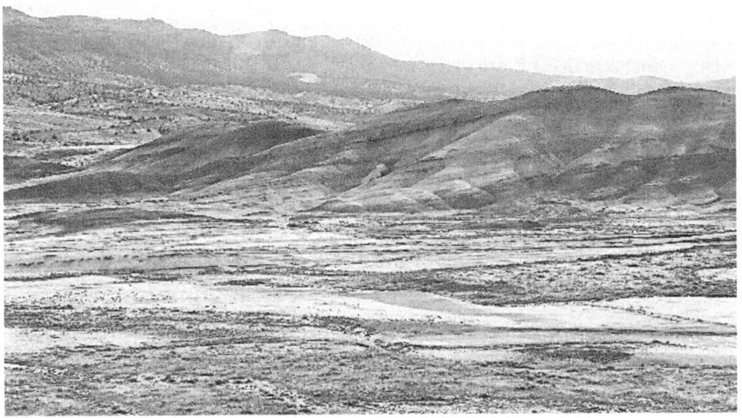

John Day Fossil Beds and Painted Hills National Monument, Oregon

Time in Nature is generating a growing body of research supporting numerous health benefits, especially in areas of chronic illnesses. Even having a simple plant in the room, or pictures of Nature can make a difference and help cancer patients feel less anxious, angry, and stressed. The best part is time in nature does not have to be limited to solitary walks or extreme exercise.

> *"The meager evidence we have for eating habits indicates, ancient peoples gathered, hunted and processed plants and animals according to their availability. Travel was vast distances governed by environmental and geological events."*
>
> ~Dennis L. Jenkins – Director of the Northern Great Basin Prehistory Project, MNCH, University of Oregon

As Tammera walked along the beach on a summer vacation, the muffled sounds of ATVs playing on the dunes caught her attention. She realized that her great-niece, nephew, and their dad love their time outside doing dune running; they laugh, tell stories, and connect as a family. [37] The same is true for Tammera's husband, son, and other family members, who each year look forward to the hunting season. She realized many years ago that it wasn't about the hunting or the meat as much as it was time in Nature and connecting with life's cycles once more. The reality is hunting or fishing does not equal killing or catching most of the time, but it does answer ancient callings for the hunt still present in human DNA; the challenge, and the success that nourishes the body/mind/spirit.

Stress activation of the hypothalamic-pituitary-adrenal (HPA) axis is a very thoroughly documented and well-characterized phenomenon. Stress regulation of the hypothalamic-pituitary-thyroid (HPT) axis, however, has received much less attention. Classically considered to play an important role in growth, differentiation, and metabolism, altered thyroid hormones have been linked to psychiatric disease, sexual behavior, and even evolution. [38, 39, 40, 41, 42]

Additionally, the time in Nature allows one to turn off the worrisome chatter of the "monkey mind" and stay in the present moment by walking or watching the goings-on for hours surrounded by the landscape's sounds. The remembered connection with traditional ways, memories of childhood, the rhythm of sun and stars; time in Nature, in all of its forms, resets our circadian rhythm, lowers blood pressure and stress hormones, increases endorphins, serotonin, and dopamine levels; adjusting our mood and improving our cognition. Nature can even boost creative problem-solving abilities, according to researchers. [43, 44, 45] Increased ability to problem solve happens when we spend time in Nature because the natural world engages our attention in a gentler way that lets one refocus their attention. The more time you spend in Nature, the more significant the benefits to creative thinking.

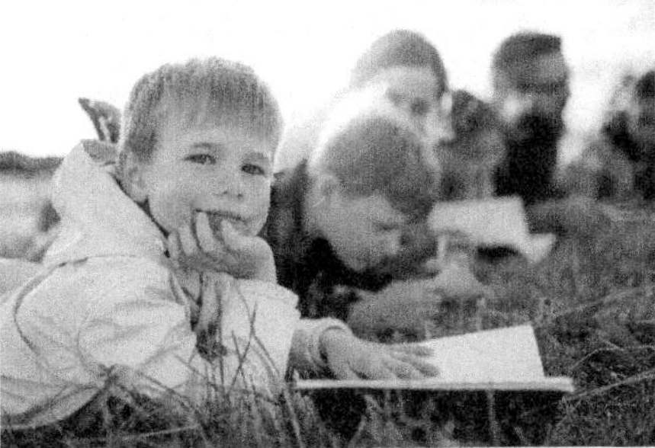

Children also need time outside. Studies show it's

not just their activity; it's the *greenness* of the outdoor space. In one study, kids with ADHD were able to concentrate better on a task after taking a walk in the park than after a walk through an urban area. [46] Like animals, children are highly sensitive to environments. The frenetic or manic energy generated by the rush of traffic, motion of crowds, and even unseen energy emitted from passersby can be contagious and unsettling for youngsters.

Tammera first became aware of Nature's cleansing power in 2002 when working in a clinic with Larry Bogart, MD. a psychiatrist who worked with veterans with post-traumatic stress-disorder (PTSD), hepatitis C, chronic health challenges, cancer, mood disorders, and addictions. Dr. Bogart required Tammera to go outside for a walk following her nutrition counseling appointments with individuals who had crystal meth addiction challenges. When Tammera asked Dr. Bogart why, he shared this rationale: the *energy* from individuals on meth was like a spiky pufferfish, and when healthcare providers spend time near this energy, it is contagious, affecting mental function and clarity. By being outside in Nature for fifteen to twenty minutes, the nervous system can reset back to a calmer state. [47]

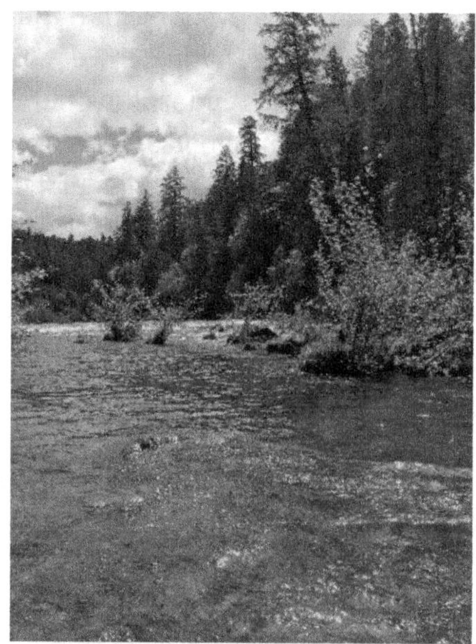

Decompress and re-balance with nature

An essential part of our time in Nature is simply having an enjoyable time, so stress hormones and life's burdens can slip away. By decompressing in Nature, our brain chemistry and stress hormones have a chance to reset; sunshine, fresh air, and movement provides necessary circulation of lymph fluids; that contribute to inflammation. [48] The lymph system is a widespread arrangement of tissues, organs, and vessels that transport lymph fluid throughout the body — it has two primary functions: balancing lymphatic fluids and producing white blood cells that fight infection. The lymph system works with blood circulation to remove chemical buildup in tissues that lead to inflammation and injury. [49] Lymph fluid circulation is vital for health. [50, 51]

Physical activity in all its forms helps maintain muscle mass and bone health in midlife, especially for women. Decreases in estrogen and progesterone production after menopause causes a decline in muscle mass. The more muscle, the denser the bones. The University of Jyvaskylan in Finland released the results of a large study of middle-aged women in 2020, showing that age-related changes in skeletal muscle are part of everyday life for women in their fifties. And that the more active a woman is, the stronger her bones will be. [52]

A study of nearly 20,000 people published in *Scientific Reports* answers the age-old question of "how much time" is needed to benefit time in nature? For the first time, researchers have established a threshold at which spending time in nature starts to be associated with good self-reported health and high self-reported well-being: 120 minutes per week. [53]

In a controlled experiment on whether nature experience would influence rumination, (repetitive thought focused on negative aspects of the self, which is a known risk factor for mental illness). Researchers found that study participants who went on a ninety-minute walk through a natural environment reported lower levels of rumination and showed reduced neural activity in an area of the brain linked to risk for mental illness compared with those who walked through an urban environment. [54]

> *"When one tugs at a single thing in nature, he finds it attached to the rest of the world."*
>
> ~John Muir

Forest bathing

Not everyone lives surrounded by deep forests and expanses of pristine Nature, like the authors of this book. Historical perspective often reminds us of the healing properties of Nature. In all its forms, Nature has a long history of providing healing compounds and medicinal plants — increases natural killer cells and offers natural deterrents to viruses. The high desert with its drying air was sought out by those with tuberculosis and asthma during the 1800s and 1900s. Even today, individuals who live in damp or high humidity areas may find a week or two in the desert does wonders for their allergies or asthma. These temporary climate changes give the immune system a chance to reset, allow inflammation levels to lower, and the respiratory system expands and recovers.

But the outdoors seems to help in other ways. Many plants put substances, including organic compounds called phytoncides, into the air that seem to boost immune function. [55]

In a study on forest bathing and cancer expression in women, thirteen healthy nurses with careers covering four to eighteen years, aged twenty-five to forty-eight, went on a three-day, two-night trip to the forest. Urine and blood samples were done at the beginning. Each subsequent day the number of natural killer (NK) cells and intracellular anti-cancer proteins in lymphocytes were measured, along with increased NK activity. The concentrations of phytoncides in the forests' atmosphere were also measured.

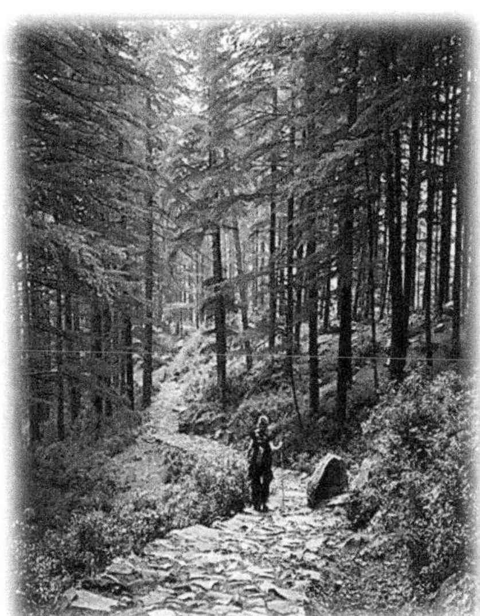

What were the findings? The forest bathing trip significantly increased NK activity and the numbers of NK, perforin, granulysin, and granzymes A/B-expressing cells; and significantly decreased the percentage of T cells and the concentrations of adrenaline and noradrenaline in the urine. Additionally, the positive effects lasted at least seven days after the forest bathing trip. Researchers are hypothesizing from the preliminary findings that phytoncides released from trees and decreased stress hormone levels may partially contribute to the increased NK activity. [56]

Trees in a city park also have beneficial effects on health, just as their deep forest relatives. A 2015 Stanford study found that when young adults spend an hour wandering through parkland, their anxiety levels and memory show improvement. [57, 58]

Forest Medicine was Born Anew: A literature review published in 2019 on forest bathing and human health provides scientific insight into Nature's healing effects.

> Humans have enjoyed forest environments for ages because of the quiet atmosphere, beautiful scenery, mild climate, pleasant aromas, and fresh, clean air. In Japan, since 2004, serial studies have been conducted to investigate the effects of forest environments on human health. We have established a new medical science called Forest Medicine. [59]

Forest Medicine is a new interdisciplinary science, belonging to alternative medicine, environmental medicine — and preventive medicine, which encompasses forest environments' effects on human health.

Shinrin-yoku, or forest bathing, is a Japanese practice that is significantly different than hiking or jogging through the woods for exercise – as is often the practice in the U.S. In Japanese, shinrin means *forest*, and yoku is a bath. Bathing in the sights, sounds, smells, tastes, and physical sensations in a forest — moving mindfully and silently among all living there — is a wholly sensual experience that profoundly affects the body/mind/spirit. One of Kathleen's favorite ways to move into the *headspace* of shinrin-yoku while in a forest is to imagine that everything, she can see is also watching her. Not just the animals and birds who can really see her with their own eyes, but the bugs and the seeds and the pine needles on the forest floor, as well as the tree trunks and their high moving leaves, and the puddles and streams and rocks and .... get the idea? Without focusing on the destination, particular speed, just wandering and being bathed in all that is freely given by the plants, wind, the sun, and the earth bridges any imaginary gap between oneself and the natural world.

The 2019 systematic literature review considered all published, randomized, controlled trials, cohort studies, and comparative studies that evaluated the forest environment's effects on changes in systolic blood pressure. A subsequent meta-analysis was performed. Twenty trials involving 732 participants were reviewed. Systolic and diastolic blood pressure of those in the forest environment was significantly lower than those in the non-forest environment. Another 2017 systematic review shows a significant effect of Shinrin-yoku on the reduction of blood pressure. [60]

The benefits of sun

As a kid, whenever she got the spring croup or crud, Tammera was tucked up in a sleeping bag for a while each day on a lawn chair in the sun. There is nothing like the warm sun on your face to nap in. Outdoors, sunshine stimulates vitamin D production in the body. Sunlight also seems to energize special cells in the immune system, called T cells, that help fight infection. And opening the lungs to fresh air improves blood pressure and detoxification capacity. The fact is, as a species, humans have spent far more time in Nature than surrounded by concrete and asphalt. Our modern environment keeps us indoors more than outside, which may play an important role in mood regulation. Sunlight and darkness activate the release of hormones in the brain. Exposure to sunlight increases the brain's release of serotonin. Serotonin is linked with a better mood and a secure feeling of calm and focus. At night, growing darkness causes the brain to release melatonin. This hormone is responsible for restorative sleep and healthy immune function.

Research published from Kings College, London, in 2020 shows improving the lifestyle of women with obesity during pregnancy could mean long-term cardiovascular benefits for their children. Researchers examined how an antenatal diet and physical activity intervention in pregnant women with obesity could positively influence the health of the women and their children three years after giving birth.

The UPBEAT trial is a randomized controlled trial which aims to improve the diet and physical activity of obese pregnant women across the UK. Three years after birth, follow-up examinations showed that the children born to the trial's intervention arm had a lower resting heart rate of -5 bpm than children treated with standard care. A higher resting heart rate in adults is associated with hypertension and

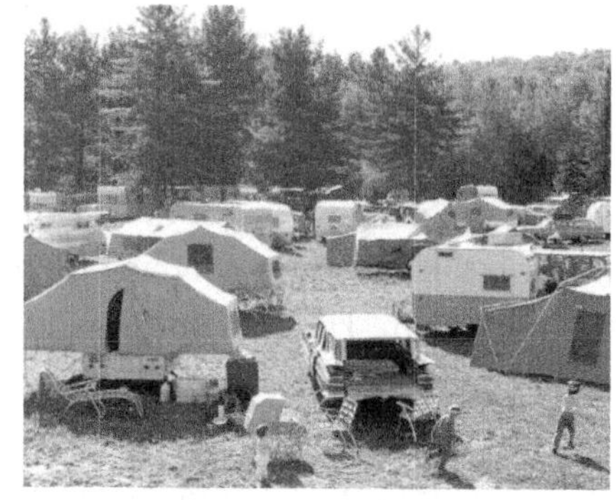

cardiovascular dysfunction. The study also showed that mothers in the intervention arm maintained a healthier diet three years after birth. [61]

When resources are limited, we look for creative solutions; often, inspiration comes from history. While reading several books on pioneer life and medicine recently, Tammera learned they talked about the sun's benefits for healing respiratory infections during outbreaks. During the 1918 Spanish influenza outbreak, nurses put infected patients out in the sun, which may have helped inactivate the influenza virus. It was believed the sun also killed bacteria, which cause lung and other infections in hospitals. During World War I, military surgeons routinely used sunlight to heal infected wounds. [62, 63, 64] They knew the sun had disinfectant properties. [65, 66, 67]

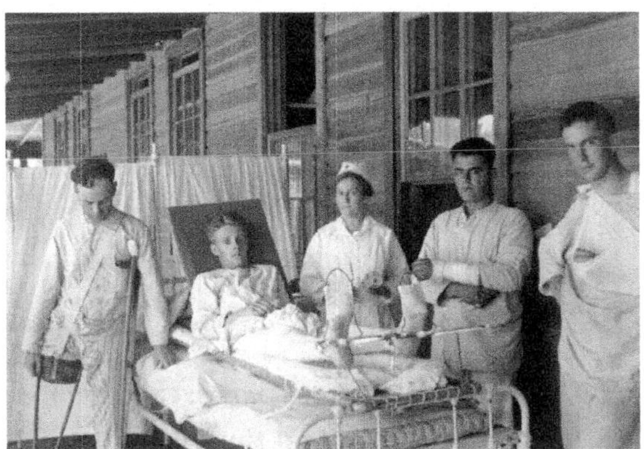

Today hospitals routinely use ultraviolet lights for disinfecting. [68] After surgery, infections are potentially fatal; current methods of fighting infections, especially drug-resistant pathogens, are hit and miss for effectiveness. Research done by David J. Brenner, PhD, out of Columbia University, looks at a narrow band of ultraviolet light as a safe and straightforward solution. Bacterial cells are ten to twenty-five times smaller than human cells, making them susceptible to the far-UVC's damaging rays. [69]

Take charge

St. Patrick's Day and many other hallmark holidays may feel like frivolous events to celebrate — but it is during times of high stress and fear that the perfect prescription is a "Lightening of the Mood with a Wee Measure of Frivolous." In truth, life goes on; most of us have deadlines, work, and responsibilities. Yet during quarantines and pandemics, we may be working from home or navigating the prickly world of board spouses and kids. The weight of events is massive, and silly celebrations lighten our feelings of isolation, fear, and boredom. It activates our immune responses and improves our brain chemistry.

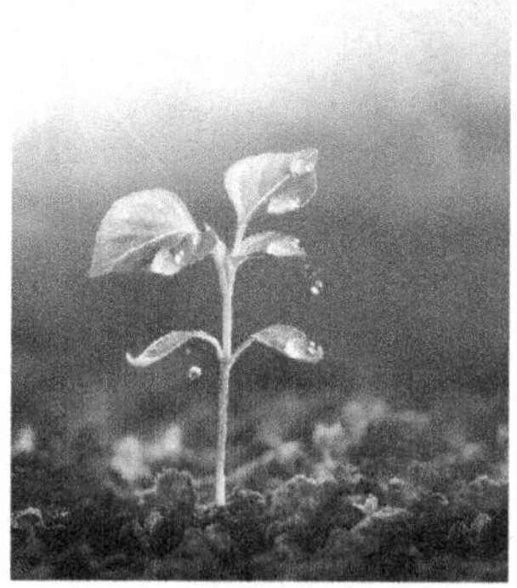

When we *put on the green*, it isn't just about the Irish. It is about new beginnings, spring, the bursting forth of new life, and those foods rich in nutrients equated with the vivid colors of greens that help us stay healthy.

Current infectious disease models are projecting the pandemic may last well into 2021. If that model is accurate, then we have every reason to order garden seeds and become proactive in taking charge of our health and supporting sustainable communities.

Principal 5: All of the natural world is cyclical.

Shifts in behavior

It turns out that there is a formula for any successful shift in behavior. This applies to everything from flossing teeth to running a marathon. The following tips can be used to create the habit of spending time in Nature and much more. Our habits are within our control to change; the first step may be as simple as a *Post It* note with the words *go outside, smile,* or today is going to be a good day." [70]

- To instill a habit, the first thing you need is motivation: Pick a behavior that you want to do rather than one you merely feel obligated to do.
- You need to be able to do it: Make the change small and straightforward at first.
- You need a personal prompt: Identify a way to trigger the behavior reliably.
- You need to celebrate your new habit so that your brain associates it with positive feelings.

Nature and traditional medicine help keep us healthy

Research shows that parks play an essential role in individuals' well-being, regardless of their social class, and that their value cannot be replaced by other venues where people meet, such as shopping centers. Patterned movement exercises such as Tai Chi and Qigong can be performed outside, often in parks, and have numerous proven health benefits.

Traditional Chinese Medicine (TCM) methods, including Qigong, have been valuable in controlling infectious diseases in China. A comprehensive health system more than 2,500 years old, TCM is associated with early Taoists and Buddhists in China who noticed energy within themselves, plants and animals, and throughout the cosmos. Based on a firm belief in the natural order of the universe and a direct correlation between the human body and Nature, TCM principles stress an ongoing search for harmony and balance within an environment of constant change. Qigong is an ancient practice involving movement and breathing techniques used to build health, heal injuries and pain, reduce stress and anxiety, and promote longevity and vitality. It is similar in appearance to Tai Chi, easier to learn, and more focused on improving health. [71]

Baduanjin qigong is one of the most common forms of Chinese Qigong. It is like a moving meditation and shares many of the same concepts as yoga. Unlike Tai Chi, which is done while standing, Qigong can be done in a sitting position. In TCM, the concept of qi (or chi) is involved in virtually every process of health and disease. Qi refers to the vital life force or energy that animates every living being in Nature. Gong means *work* or discipline. There are different types of qi: organ-specific qi relates to each human organ's function, while the more comprehensive and defensive Wei Qi is analogous to all the bodily functions that comprise the immune system in Western medicine.

In TCM, the protective *field* of Wei Qi energy both permeates and surrounds the human body, and all Qigong breathing and movements are performed within an individual's unique Wei Qi field. Human bodies can receive energy from Nature — grounding energy moves upward from the Earth, and elevating energy pours down from the sky — as well as having the capability to discharge excess or toxic energy into the earth and the immediate environment (trees). Practicing with one's feet directly on the ground and head pointed skyward utilizes Nature's supportive energies. Qigong's is a powerful mind-body integrative skill; meant to train the practitioner to regulate body, breath, and mind to bring the individual into the best state for healing and, maintain healthy functioning. [72]

> *"In every walk with nature, one receives far more than he seeks."*
>
> ~John Muir

Qigong is suitable for anyone to do inside or out: in their home, yard, park, or alpine meadow. For those with mobility challenges, especially the elderly, Qigong is made up of smooth and gentle movements that can be done from either a sitting or standing position. It can be widely applied in geriatric medicine to treat painful musculoskeletal disorders, strengthen muscle, and achieve pain relief. Qigong's mental calming effects are similar to meditation and have been found to help individuals with psychosomatic disorders as well as mood disorders and even cognitive impairment. [73, 74]

Time in Nature: a human right

The reality is much can be done to incorporate time in Nature in order to stay healthy. Start by taking a deep breath; next, throw open a few windows and air out homes. Get outside in the fresh air, no matter where that is or for how long. Go alone or with your family and friends. If the weather is sunny, get the sun on your face and arms (using sunscreen as desired). Sit or play in the sun in the yard, balcony, or porch; near an open window or along a river — the key is to get outside. An added benefit in the age of new infectious diseases, such as COVID-19; being outside in Nature easily allows maintaining a safe distance with beneficial air circulation from others.

The Center for Nature and Health is the first nature-based clinic in the U.S. to be associated with a major hospital, UCSF Beniff Children's Hospital in Oakland, CA. The clinic collaborates with the East Bay Regional Park District in a program called Stay Healthy in Nature Every Day. Participating area doctors offer nature outings for families and often join in themselves. In June 2018, the Center began billing insurance companies for patient visits that included time in Nature as part of the treatment plan. This was a breakthrough, as an increasing number of U.S. healthcare providers are now integrating time in Nature into their practice protocols.

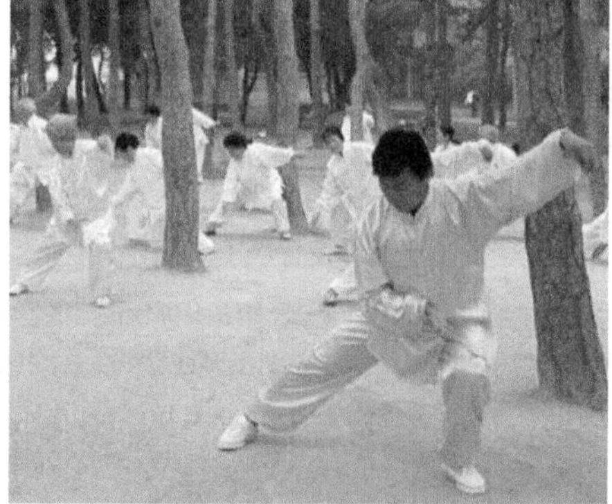

Principle 6: Just as humans have a right to the benefits of Nature, Nature has rights of its own.

Within the past decade, the body of evidence that associates time spent in natural surroundings with improvements in health and wellness and lowers mortality rates, has grown from dozens of studies to hundreds. A 2017 study published in *The Lancet Planetary Health* suggested that people who live in "green" neighborhoods live longer than those in urban settings who are farther from Nature. [75] Research shows that children who spend time in Nature have reduced attention deficit hyperactivity disorder symptoms and are less likely to be obese, myopic, or deficient in vitamin D. [76]

A growing compendium of experts —educators, researchers, and health practitioners — agree that the physical, psychological, and cognitive benefits of connection to Nature should be available to all. However, universal access to natural areas is not the reality present in the U.S. poverty-ridden neighborhoods are often areas without parks or green space and are places where parents are compelled to keep children inside due to a high incidence of violent crime.

According to a 2019 article in *Sierra* magazine, a global movement has begun, making the case that connection with Nature should be recognized as a human right. At the 2012 World Conservation Congress of the International Union for the Conservation of Nature (IUCN), the conference passed a historic resolution stating that children have a human right to experience a healthy natural world. [77] Advocates see a child-focused strategy as an excellent place to begin the long-overdue conversation about a rights-based approach to time in Nature.

The authors hope that this is only the beginning of recognizing human rights to Nature and those elements from Nature: clean water, fresh foods, and healthy soils.

> *"Nothing in Nature, besides man, thinks it exists independently."*
>
> ~Gisele Theriault,
> owner of Mindful Necessities

Each and every human being is an integral part of Nature. Although modern human civilization may believe we have succeeded in separating ourselves from Nature, all that has been done is to create alienation that affects a healthy symbiotic relationship. Man, and Nature have co-existed in harmony and can return to it once more. Advancing alongside the movement advocating for the human right to a healthy, natural world is another movement to recognize Nature's rights in itself. In 2008, Ecuador changed its constitution to give Nature "the right to exist, persist, maintain and regenerate its vital cycles." In 2017, as a result of a 140-year campaign by the Maori, the New Zealand Parliament declared that the Whanganui River has the same legal rights as a person. The third-largest river in the country, the Whanganui, became the first river in the world to be recognized as a living entity. And in 2020, the Law of the Rights of Mother Earth, which gives Nature equal rights with humans, was passed in Bolivia. [78]

Looking with a perspective of appreciation, a good case can be made for Nature and humans sharing basic needs and rights. If we support access to fundamental human rights for all, it follows that we can support access to Nature for all humans. Both humans and Nature need and deserve proper nourishment to maintain good health, growth, and resilience. Nature and humans alike appreciate protection and respect for their multifaceted and complex structures, allowing them to thrive and evolve. Just as each leaf, flower, or snowflake is unique within the natural world, each person is also wholly individual —all the while being inextricably connected to the larger whole of humankind.

The authors believe that spending time in Nature is fundamental to good health. How much of a dose is needed? A 2019 study found that a minimum of 120 minutes a week spent in parks, woodlands, or beaches promotes physical and mental health for people of all ages, abilities, genders, and economic levels. [79] It is worth considering what can be done to facilitate providing at least two weekly hours outdoors for everyone. Following the flowing patterns on our empty plate illustrates the beauty and complexity of interconnectedness. If ways can be found to support the interconnectedness of human rights and Nature's rights, we return to the role of caretaker of the Earth. And in so doing, sustain ourselves.

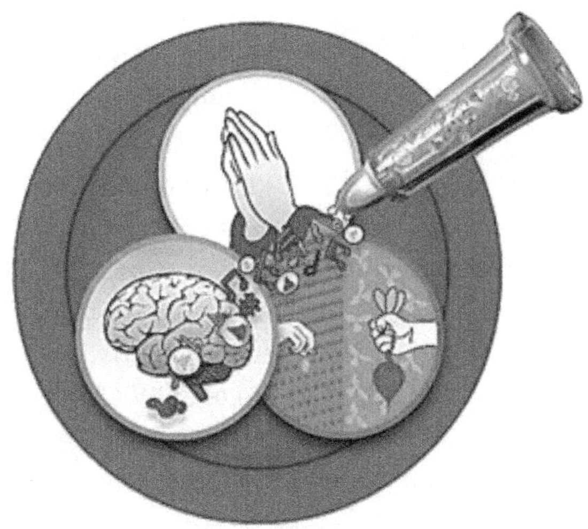

Perspective through history

When we use the lens of history, we can see humankind has spent most of its time in Nature, governed by the ebb and flow of the cycles and patterns of seasons, animals, and the environment; rather than being ruled by technology. The large cities of antiquity were not interwoven with electric currents, artificial light, and synthetic fibers that are found all over the world in metropolitan areas today.

Archeological evidence from Dirty Shame Shelter near the headwaters of the Owyhee mountains in Eastern Oregon [80, 81] tells the story of a population that hunted, gathered, cooked, and engaged in tool making for thousands of years.

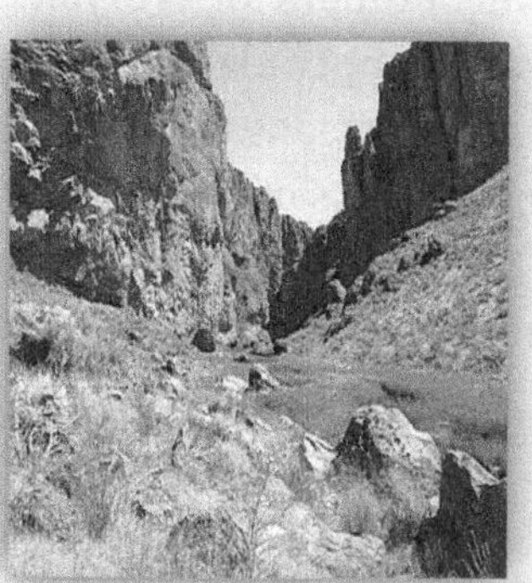

Dirty Shame Rock shelter: Courtesy U.S. Department of the Interior

What happened that changed the pattern? A volcanic eruption of Mount Saint Helens in western Washington sent clouds of ash approximately four hundred miles east, burying the landscape and rock shelter. [82] Scientists approximate an occupation gap of 3,000–5,000 years between inhabitation of the rock shelter due to volcanic eruptions. [83, 84, 85]

---

1. Edwin Russell Jackman was an American agricultural expert from Oregon. He helped form the Oregon seed growers' League and the Oregon wheat League. In 1964, he joined Reub Long to write the Oregon Desert, which is still a very popular book forty years after its original publication. Jackman's professional papers and photograph collection are maintained in the Oregon State University Archives.
2. Riddle Brothers Ranch Historical Site, Steens Mountain Wilderness, Harney County Oregon.
3. Kimmerer, Robin, Braiding Sweetgrass 2013, Milkweed Editions page 20
4. Ibid Kimmer, Robin
5. University of Cambridge. (2020, September 28). The testimony of trees: How volcanic eruptions shaped 2000 years of world history. ScienceDaily. Retrieved September 29, 2020 from www.sciencedaily.com/releases/2020/09/200928090500.htm
6. How Archaeologists Uncover History With Trees by Stephen E. Nash, Sapiens Anthropollgy Magazine, 2017: https://www.sapiens.org/column/curiosities/tree-ring-dating-mesa-verde/
7. Sapiens Anthropology Magazine 2017, The Struggle to Protect a Tree at the Heart of Hopi Culture by Stewart B. Koyiyumptewa and Chip Colwell: https://www.sapiens.org/culture/hopi-juniper-tree-mining/
8. Ibid
9. How Much Can We Know? Scientific American Special Edition Fall 2020 page 110
10. You Are the Placebo: Making Your Mind Matter by Joe Dispenza 2014, Hay House
11. How does time in nature impact wellbeing: https://www.takingcharge.csh.umn.edu/how-does-nature-impact-our-wellbeing
12. What is Happening in Healthcare Settings Today? https://www.takingcharge.csh.umn.edu/explore-healing-practices/healing-environment/what-happening-healthcare-settings-today
13. Health.mil, Military Adaptive Sports Program aids with healing our Wounded Warriors: https://health.mil/News/Articles/2020/07/07/Military-Adaptive-Sports-Program-aids-with-healing-our-Wounded-Warriors
14. www.healthquality.va.gov./guidelines/MR/cmi/VADoDCMICPGPatientSummary2014.pdf
15. American University. (2020, August 31). Research shows how a diet change might help US veterans with Gulf War illness.

ScienceDaily. Retrieved September 1, 2020 from www.sciencedaily.com/releases/2020/08/200831112333.htm

16. https://www.sciencedaily.com/terms/circadian_rhythm.htm

17. Seth, R.K. et al (2019) Gut DNA Virome Diversity and its Association with Host Bacteria Regulate Inflammatory Phenotype and Neuronal Immunotoxicity in Experimental Gulf War Illness. Viruses, 11/910:968 Doi: 10.3390/v11100968

18. https://www.sciencedaily.com/terms/circadian_rhythm.htm

19. Autumn Anxiety: Why You May Feel More Stressed This Season by Cathy Cassata 2019, Healthline: https://www.healthline.com/health-news/autumn-anxiety

20. . https://www.mhanational.org/conditions/seasonal-affective-disorder-sad

21. What Are the Benefits of Sunlight?: https://www.healthline.com/health/depression/benefits-sunlight

22. https://healthprep.com/conditions/7-surefire-ways-to-beat-seasonal-affective-disorder-and-cure-the-winter-blues/14/?utm_source=bing&utm_medium=search&utm_campaign=328752041&utm_content=1146791188588169&utm_term=seasonal+affective+disorder

23. Müller E, Pröller P, Ferreira-Briza F, Aglas L, Stöggl T. Effectiveness of Grounded Sleeping on Recovery After Intensive Eccentric Muscle Loading. Front Physiol. 2019;10:35. Published 2019 Jan 28. doi:10.3389/fphys.2019.00035

24. Global Environmental Change Volume 23, Issue 5, October 2013, Pages 992-1000, Happiness Is Greater In Natural Environments: Https://Www.Sciencedirect.Com/Science/Article/Abs/Pii/S0959378013000575

25. 92-year-old nurse still in the workforce; has no plans of retirement, 2019: https://www.fox2detroit.com/news/92-year-old-nurse-still-in-the-workforce-has-no-plans-of-retirement

26. Pride, passion, experience and expertise: older nurses have been helping to stem the nursing shortage, but a crisis looms: https://blog.nurserecruiter.com/pride-passion-experience-older-nurses-nursing-shortage/

27. University of East Anglia. (2018, July 6). It's official -- spending time outside is good for you. ScienceDaily. Retrieved September 27, 2020 from www.sciencedaily.com/releases/2018/07/180706102842.htm

28. How Exercise Affects Circulation (And Vice Versa). Discover How Your Circulatory System Can Support Athletic Performance — And Also Benefit From Optimal Fitness. By Laine Bergeson Becco, FMCHC, 2017: Https://Experiencelife.Com/Article/How-Exercise-Affects-Circulation-And-Vice-Versa/

29. Interacting With Nature Improves Cognition And Affect For Individuals With Depression 2012: Journal Of Affective Disorders. Volume 140, Issue 3, November 2012, Pages 300-305: Https://Www.Sciencedirect.Com/Science/Article/Abs/Pii/S0165032712002005

30. Ecopsychology: How Immersion in Nature Benefits Your Health by Jim Robbins 2020: https://e360.yale.edu/features/ecopsychology-how-immersion-in-nature-benefits-your-health

31. Designed to Move Report: http://tafisa.org/newsletter

32. Time grows on trees: The effect of nature settings on time perception: https://www.sciencedirect.com/science/article/abs/pii/S0272494417301081

33. Elkin, Howard K., Winter, Angela, Grounding Patients With Hypertension Improves Blood Pressure: A Case History Series Study; Alternative Therapies, Nov/Dec 2018, Vol. 24 NO. 6; https://earthinginstitute.net/research/

34. Ghaly M, Teplitz D. The biologic effects of grounding the human body during sleep as measured by cortisol levels and subjective reporting of sleep, pain, and stress. J Altern Complement Med. 2004;10(5):767-776. doi:10.1089/acm.2004.10.767

35. Müller E, Pröller P, Ferreira-Briza F, Aglas L, Stöggl T. Effectiveness of Grounded Sleeping on Recovery After Intensive Eccentric Muscle Loading. Front Physiol. 2019;10:35. Published 2019 Jan 28. doi:10.3389/fphys.2019.00035

36. Getting Started with Lichen Dyes 2012 by Alissa Allen

37. Global Environmental Change Volume 23, Issue 5, October 2013, Pages 992-1000, Happiness Is Greater In Natural Environments: Https://Www.Sciencedirect.Com/Science/Article/Abs/Pii/S0959378013000575

38. Baumgartner A: Thyroxine and the treatment of affective disorders: An overview of the results of basic and clinical research. Int J Neuropsychopharmacol 2000; 3: 149–165.

39. Joffe R, Segal Z, Singer W: Changes in thyroid hormone levels following response to cognitive
therapy for major depression. Am J Psychiatry 1996; 153: 411–413.

40. Dellovade T, Zhu YS, Krey L, Pfaff D: Thyroid hormone and estrogen interact to regulate behavior. Proc Natl Acad Sci USA 1996; 93: 12581–12586.

41. Crockford S: Thyroid rhythm phenotypes and hominid evolution: A new paradigm implicates pulsatile hormone secretion in speciation and adaptation changes. Comp Biochem Physiol A Mol Integr Physiol 2003; 135: 105–129.

42. https://www.researchgate.net/publication/7723683_Relation_between_the_Hypothalamic-Pituitary-Thyroid_HPT_Axis_and_the_Hypothalamic-Pituitary-Adrenal_HPA_Axis_during_Repeated_Stress

43. Landscape And Urban Planning Volume 138, June 2015, Pages 41-50 The Benefits Of Nature Experience: Improved Affect And Cognition By Gregory N.Bratman, Gretchen C.Daily, Benjamin J.Levy, James J.Gross 2015, Https://Www.Sciencedirect.Com/Science/Article/Pii/S0169204615000286

44. Kim, Gwang-Won Et Al. "Functional Neuroanatomy Associated With Natural And Urban Scenic Views In The Human Brain: 3.0T Functional MR Imaging." Korean Journal Of Radiology Vol. 11,5 (2010): 507-13. Doi:10.3348/Kjr.2010.11.5.507

45. Interacting With Nature Improves Cognition And Affect For Individuals With Depression 2012: Journal Of Affective Disorders. Volume 140, Issue 3, November 2012, Pages 300-305: Https://Www.Sciencedirect.Com/Science/Article/Abs/Pii/S0165032712002005

46. Health Benefits Of Getting Outside: Https://Www.Webmd.Com/Balance/Ss/Slideshow-Health-Benefits-Nature

47. Larry Bogart, M.D. Passed Away Following Complications From A Bicycle Injury In 2009 In Roseburg Oregon.

48. How Exercise Affects Circulation (And Vice Versa). Discover How Your Circulatory System Can Support Athletic Performance — And Also Benefit From Optimal Fitness. By Laine Bergeson Becco, FMCHC, 2017: Https://Experiencelife.Com/Article/How-Exercise-Affects-Circulation-And-Vice-Versa/

49. Schwager, Simon, And Michael Detmar. "Inflammation And Lymphatic Function." Frontiers In Immunology Vol. 10 308. 26 Feb. 2019, Doi:10.3389/Fimmu.2019.00308

50. Encyclopaedia Britannica, Lymphatic System: Https://Www.Britannica.Com/Science/Lymphatic-System

51. What Are The Benefits Of Sunlight? By Rachel Nall, RN, BSN, CCRN, 2019: Https://Www.Healthline.Com/Health/Depression/Benefits-Sunlight

52. University Of Jyväskylä - Jyväskylän Yliopisto. "Physical Activity In All Of Its Forms May Help Maintain Muscle Mass In Midlife: Hormonal Changes During Menopause Decrease Muscle Mass, But Physical Activity Might Slow The Decrement." Sciencedaily. Sciencedaily, 8 June 2020. Www.Sciencedaily.Com/Releases/2020/06/200608104727.Htm

53. White, M.P., Alcock, I., Grellier, J. Et Al. Spending At Least 120 Minutes A Week In Nature Is Associated With Good Health And Wellbeing. Sci Rep 9, 7730 (2019). Https://Doi.Org/10.1038/S41598-019-44097-3

54. Nature Reduces Rumination And Sgpfc Activation, Gregory N. Bratman, J. Paul Hamilton, Kevin S. Hahn, Gretchen C. Daily, James J. Gross, Proceedings Of The National Academy Of Sciences Jul 2015, 112 (28) 8567-8572; DOI: 10.1073/Pnas.1510459112

55. Https://Www.Webmd.Com/Balance/Ss/Slideshow-Health-Benefits-Nature

56. Li Q, Morimoto K, Kobayashi M, Et Al. A Forest Bathing Trip Increases Human Natural Killer Activity And Expression Of Anti-Cancer Proteins In Female Subjects. J Biol Regul Homeost Agents. 2008;22(1):45-55.

57. Study Finds Living Near Trees Comes With 6 Surprising Health Benefits by Robert Locke: https://www.lifehack.org/323241/study-finds-living-near-trees-comes-with-6-surprising-health-benefits

58. USDA Forest Service - Pacific Northwest Research Station. (2013, January 16). Tree and human health may be linked. ScienceDaily. Retrieved October 3, 2020 from www.sciencedaily.com/releases/2013/01/130116163823.htm

59. Li Q. Effets Des Forêts Et Des Bains De Forêt (Shinrin-Yoku) Sur La Santé Humaine : Une Revue De La Littérature [Effect Of Forest Bathing (Shinrin-Yoku) On Human Health: A Review Of The Literature]. Sante Publique. 2019;S1(HS):135-143. Doi:10.3917/Spub.190.0135

60. Ideno Y, Hayashi K, Abe Y, Et Al. Blood Pressure-Lowering Effect Of Shinrin-Yoku (Forest Bathing): A Systematic Review And Meta-Analysis. BMC Complement Altern Med. 2017;17(1):409. Published 2017 Aug 16. Doi:10.1186/S12906-017-1912-Z

61. King's College London. (2020, September 11). Healthy diet and exercise during pregnancy could lead to healthier children. ScienceDaily. Retrieved October 10, 2020 from www.sciencedaily.com/releases/2020/09/200911110804.htm

62. Coronavirus And The Sun: A Lesson From The 1918 Influenza Pandemic By Richard Hobday 2020. Https://Medium.Com/@Ra.Hobday/Coronavirus-And-The-Sun-A-Lesson-From-The-1918-Influenza-Pandemic-509151dc8065

63. Hobday RA And Cason JW. The Open-Air Treatment Of Pandemic Influenza. Am J Public Health 2009;99 Suppl 2:S236–42. Doi:10.2105/AJPH.2008.134627.

64. Anon. Weapons Against Influenza. Am J Public Health 1918 Oct;8(10):787–8. Doi: 10.2105/Ajph.8.10.787.

65. Hobday RA. The Open-Air Factor And Infection Control. J Hosp Infect 2019;103:E23-E24 Doi.Org/10.1016/J.Jhin.2019.04.003.

66. Schuit M, Gardner S, Wood S Et Al. The Influence Of Simulated Sunlight On The Inactivation Of Influenza Virus In Aerosols. J Infect Dis 2020 Jan 14;221(3):372–378. Doi: 10.1093/Infdis/Jiz582.

67. Hobday RA, Dancer SJ. Roles Of Sunlight And Natural Ventilation For Controlling Infection: Historical And Current Perspectives. J Hosp Infect 2013;84:271–282. Doi: 10.1016/J.Jhin.2013.04.011.

68. Could A New Ultraviolet Technology Fight The Spread Of Coronavirus? By Carla Cantor, Columbia University 2020: Https://News.Columbia.Edu/Ultraviolet-Technology-Virus-Covid-19-UV-Light

69. Medical News Today Specific UV Light Kills MRSA Without Damaging Human Tissue By Tim Newman 2016. Https://Www.Medicalnewstoday.Com/Articles/310818

70. Tiny Habits by B. J. Fogg

71. Feng, F. Et Al. (2020). Qigong For The Prevention, Treatment, And Rehabilitation Of COVID-19 Infection In Older Adults. The American Journal Of Geriatric Psychiatry. Https://Doi.Org/10.1016/J.Jagp.2020.05.012. Https://Www.Sciencedirect.Com/Science/Article/Pii/S1064748120303419?Via%3Dihub

72. Fontaine, K. (2019) Complementary and Alternative Therapies for Nursing Practice, 5thEd. Pearson: Upper Saddle River, NJ

73. Feng, F. Et Al. (2020). Qigong For The Prevention, Treatment, And Rehabilitation Of COVID-19 Infection In Older Adults. The American Journal Of Geriatric Psychiatry. Https://Doi.Org/10.1016/J.Jagp.2020.05.012. Https://Www.Sciencedirect.Com/Science/Article/Pii/S1064748120303419?Via%3Dihub

74. Using Qigong To Manage COVID-19 In Older Adults By Dr. Liji Thomas, MD 2020: Https://Www.News-Medical.Net/News/20200525/Using-Qigong-To-Manage-COVID-19-In-Older-Adults.Aspx

75. Crouse, D. et al. (2017). Urban Greeness and Mortality in Canada's Largest Cities: A National Cohort Study, The Lancet Planetary HealthDoi:https://doi.org/10.1016/52542-5196(17)30118-3

76. What Are The Benefits Of Sunlight? By Rachel Nall, RN, BSN, CCRN, 2019: Https://Www.Healthline.Com/Health/Depression/Benefits-Sunlight

77. Crouse, D. et al. (2017). Urban Greeness and Mortality in Canada's Largest Cities: A National Cohort Study, The Lancet Planetary Health Doi:https://doi.org/10.1016/52542-5196(17)30118-3

78. Louv, R. (May/June, 2019) Outdoors for All, Sierra, pp. 27-35, 52.

79. Louv, R. (Oct/Nov, 2020) Growing Outdoors, National Wildlife, p. 28

80. The Oregon Desert By ER Jackman And RA Long, 1964ISBN#: 087004-074X

81. Paleoethnobotanical Evidence Of Early Formative Period Diet In Coastal Oaxaca, Mexico, Author Links Open Overlay Paneléloibérubéa Guy Davidheppbshantimorell-Harta

82. Antelope creek, which flows past the shelter to empty into the owyhee river several miles downstream, created a narrow but long and moist canyon bottom environment that provided sunflower and goosefoot seeds, prickly pear cactus pads, sego lily bulbs, wild onions, and fruits of the wild rose and cherry. The creek supplied freshwater crayfish, mussels, and chubs, while its bottoms and the adjacent basalt plateau uplands offered nutritious insects, including ants and termites; small game, including pocket gophers, field mice, cottontails, jackrabbits, and marmots; and large game, including antelope, mule deer, bighorn sheep, and bison. All these species were attested in the archaeological deposits.

83. Oregon Archaeologists Discover 15,000-Year-Old Knife By Amelia Templeton, 2015: Https://Www.Opb.Org/News/Article/Oregon-Archaeologists-Discover-15000-Year-Old-Knife/

84. The British Lower Palaeolithic Of The Early Middle Pleistocene: Https://Www.Sciencedirect.Com/Science/Article/Abs/Pii/S0277379110000582

85. Early Human Evolution In The Western Palaearctic: Ecological Scenarios: Https://Www.Sciencedirect.Com/Science/Article/Abs/Pii/S0277379111000941

Chapter Six
Sweet Rewards

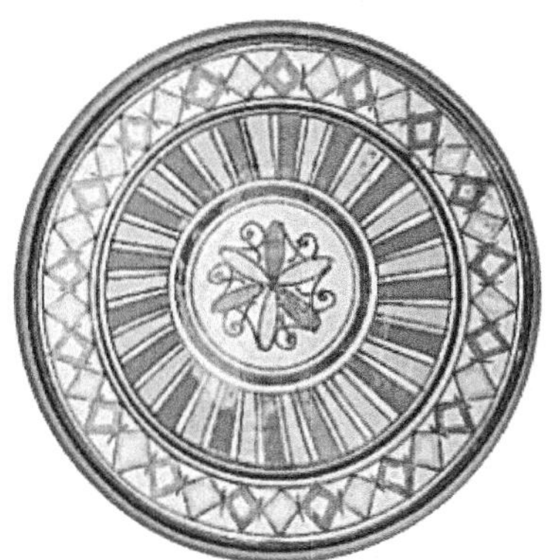

"Every human society we know about cares for their sick, injured, and infirm, going at least as far back as our Neanderthal cousins. Human communities do so using the knowledge and expertise available to them at the time, and the faith they hold dear."

~ Stephen E. Nash,
historian of science and an archaeologist at the Denver Museum of Nature & Science

The human capacity to care for others is immense. According to Margaret Mead, what separates humans from animals is the caring for the old, injured, infirm, and children. Archaeologists have found the human effort and care taken with loved ones dates back to man's earliest known origins. Even children the world over exhibit altruistic behavior, sometimes before they can talk. They clearly demonstrate caring for animals and others. "It turns out that concern for others is bred in the bone, endemic and hard-wired. We become human beings by caring for our being — physical and mental, developing relationships and connections, working together, and helping one another." [1] Like Kathleen, some know from their earliest memories that caring for others is their life's work. Nurses and many others in healthcare appear to spend more of their life caring for the chronically ill, elderly, and injured than the average person. But throughout history, caring for individuals was not limited to healthcare. Each day thousands of ministers, teachers, and family members *care* for others, preserve connection and work together. When a grandmother makes the favorite cookies or dishes for her family, she is expressing love and caring through her time, skill, and willingness. She, in turn, receives care, a sense of connection, and value from her family. In the simplest terms, this is *reciprocity*, which we will look at in the pages ahead.

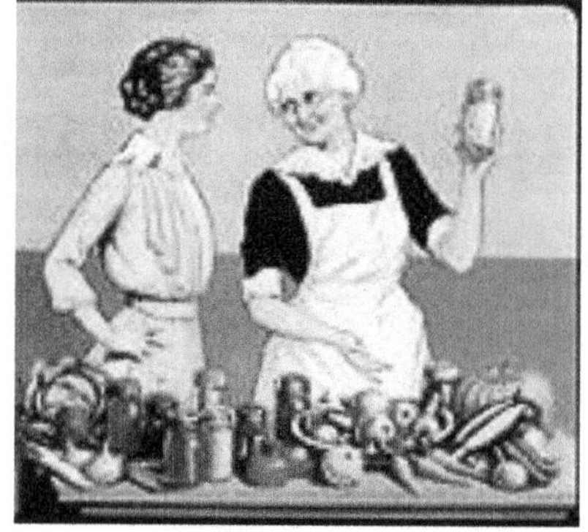

> *Principle 1*: We become human beings by caring for and helping one another.

While researching this final chapter, Tammera found information on the depth of compassion healers of old offered their community members. Instinctively we know every human society cares for the sick, injured, and infirm. Traditional communities do so using the accumulated knowledge and expertise available, passed down from generation to generation — master craftsman to apprentice, healer to intern — at the relevant time, and supported by the faith they hold sacred. In traditional cultures, the elderly retain a place of purpose and importance as keepers of culture and history.

> *Once or twice a year, the abbot at the San Francisco Zen Center, Tenshin Reb Anderson, speaks with the hospice volunteers on caring.*
> *He said simply, 'Stay close and do nothing.'*
> *That's how we try to practice at the Zen Hospice Project. We stay close and do nothing.*
> *We sit still and listen to the stories.*
>
> *~Frank Ostaseski*

The inclusion of historical tidbits in this book has allowed for an adjustment in *perspective*. Perspective allows us to view the world in full-on color versus shades of gray. History enables an opportunity to see the connection and ripple effect of consequences; good and bad. The award-winning book *The Giver* by Lois Lowry offered a peek into a monochromatic society, which appears to be utopian but is revealed as dystopian as the story progresses. Society has taken away pain and strife by converting to *Sameness*; a plan that has also eradicated emotional depth, individuality, color, and creativity from their lives. *The Giver* carries all the memories for the community; preserving them for times when they must be drawn upon — and the wisdom gained from history to aid in the community's decision making. The book's story is also about a journey from being part of sameness into entering the world full of life, color, sound, change. And yes, disharmony and messiness. As the Frank Sinatra song lyrics go — "That's Life!"

Our memories, genetics, diverse foods, and communities — while messy, add the seasoning to life, which, in the authors' opinions, make it all worth it. These elements make it possible for us to care for ourselves, others, and our unique culture and communities — just like trees do when signaling threat or regulating carbohydrate distribution — our connection to the past, present, and future preserves and nourishes the life of our species.

When we use our life's experiences with the lens of perspective, it directly affects our ability to be nourished, nurtured, and feel — pain and joy. These feelings provide intention and motivation, desire to learn, and develop skills and challenge deeply held beliefs. Our memories, history, and culture provide perspective and context and allow one to be connected, comfortable, and motivated with "intention" in the journey with others, ourselves, and the world.

> *If we keep our attention focused on the present, we can be sure of one thing: whatever we are attending to in this moment will change, giving us the opportunity to practice accepting whatever it is that will emerge in the next moment.*
> *Clearly, there is wisdom in cultivating acceptance.*
>
> ~Jon Kabat-Zinn

Be bold and evaluate deeply held beliefs

During the writing of *Empty Plate,* a colleague remarked on the *bold statements* being made. This gave us a *moment of pause* that then transitioned into *intention* and *motivation* to continue challenging *deeply held beliefs* on nutrition, sustainability, and the interconnectedness of mindfulness.

Often refreshing the memory with definitions of what words like *intention* mean, opens our thoughts to broader possibilities or understanding. Words can have more than one meaning, and it is easy to misplace some definitions due to cultural changes or trends. *Intention* is one such word that has meanings other than prayer or determination — like to act in a set way: New Year's resolutions are one example.

Principle 2: Be bold and evaluate deeply held beliefs.

Intention, perspective, and reciprocity are three ingredients that build *homeostasis or balance* in daily lives that grow *resiliency* and *regeneration* of individuals' spirits and health.

"Community does not necessarily mean living face-to-face with others; rather, it means never losing the awareness that we are connected to each other."

~Parker Palmer

Perspective

The word perspective has a Latin root meaning "look through" or "perceive," and all the meanings of perspective have something to do with looking.[2] *Perspective* involves a particular attitude toward something; it is an individual way of regarding something — or everything — and is continually influenced by beliefs and experiences. Perspective is paramount regarding nutrition science, traditional foods, and how they can nourish life in multiple ways. A personal perspective is how individuals see something, with a mental point of view reflecting the state of their ideas. This unique individual perspective, especially regarding food, may be filled with biases or acceptance. Perspective is pliable and can change. It can be refreshed or grow stale; shrink or expand as an individual is exposed to new thoughts, feelings, and ideas over time.

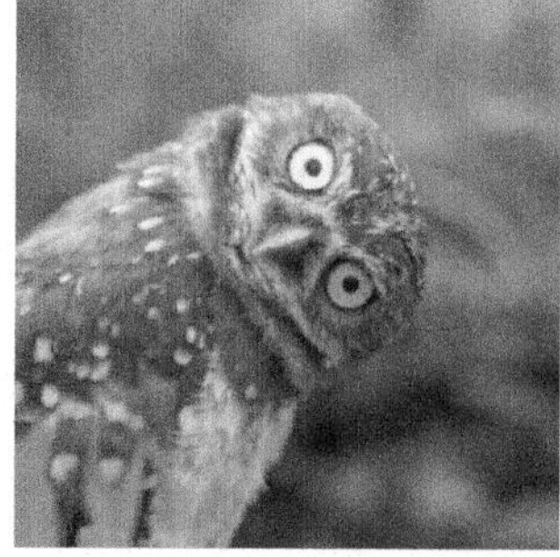

> *Principle 3*: Perspective is an individual's way of looking at things and is continually influenced by beliefs and experiences.

We have seen deeply held scientific, medical, nutritional, and cultural beliefs challenged and ultimately debunked or expanded throughout history. Great scientific minds have always challenged deeply held beliefs by pure *intention*, *motivation*, and *change*. Thor Heyerdahl, Margaret Mead, Linus

Pauling, Stephen Hawking, Greta Thunberg, Bill Schindler, David Zava, and Terry Wahls are only a few of the great minds challenging, educating, and expanding our understanding in this modern age. They follow Galileo's footsteps in their intention and fortitude in being bold and challenging former deeply held *scientific* perspectives.

Science is no less stodgy and resistant to change today than in Galileo's' day. The fall 2020 Special Collector's Edition of *Scientific American* is a perfect example. The cover reads: *Truth vs. Lies*. Hmmmm, words like "anti-science thinking," "misinformation," "bias," and "conspiracy" fill the cover page. However, the final article promises *hope*. Marcelo Gleiser writes, "*How Much Can We Know*?"

> Just think of biology before and after the microscope or gene sequencing, or of astronomy before and after the telescope, or of particle physics before and after colliders or fast electronics. Now, as in the 17th century, the theories we build and the worldviews we construct change as our tools of exploration transform. This trend is the trademark of science.
>
> What we observe is not nature in itself, but nature exposed to our method of questioning," wrote German physicist Werner Heisenberg, who was the first to fathom the uncertainty inherent in quantum physics.
>
> To those who think of science as a direct path to the truth about the world — there are clear unknowable's in science—reasonable questions that, unless currently accepted laws of nature are violated, we cannot find answers to. [3] Science isn't about truth it is about asking better questions.

Perspective in the first word of the introduction to this book, and in it, the authors have endeavored to share not only their own but to introduce various other perspectives from the past and present. In creating *Empty Plate,* we sought more than providing research findings and evidence-based information. We wanted readers to walk here and there in the shoes of our ancestors.

Meaningful communication depends on developing some shared perspective, which may lead to mutual understanding. The common wisdom of not being able to understand a person until one has "walked a mile in his/her shoes" illustrates a way to gain a sense of a shared perspective. This applies to all the concepts on diet, sustainability, and mindfulness presented in this book.

During the process of filling the empty plate, we wanted to surprise and captivate, to present ideas both old and new in a fresh and contemporary way, with the intent of stimulating new perspectives and practices aimed at health, well-being, and wholeness.

Intention

In 2004, Kathleen lost both parents within the same month. The accompanying shock and grief caused her to change her job and set her on a new holistic pathway of inquiry. She read *The Seven Spiritual Laws of Yoga* by Drs. Deepak Chopra and David Simon. These "laws" were based on Dr. Chopra's 1994 book titled *The Seven Spiritual Laws of Success*, which explored how the laws of nature apply to the human experience; "principles through which the unmanifest becomes manifest." [4] Law number five is the Law of Intention and Desire, which is based on understanding the quantum field of energy. The science of quantum physics is the science of infinite possibilities; at its heart is the premise that everything on the planet is made of energy and information. English physicist Dr. David Bohm called the realm of the quantum "the implicate order of Nature where everything is connected." [5]

> *Shaped a little like a loaf of French country bread, our brain is a crowded chemistry lab, bustling with nonstop neural conversations.*
>
> ~Diane Ackerman

Humans experience the quantum field subjectively via thoughts, feelings, memories, needs, desires, expectations, fantasies, and beliefs. Objectively, people share the same quantum field as their physical bodies, along with all that is in the physical world. This influence is activated by two qualities of consciousness: attention and intention. Drs. Chopra and Simon say it elegantly, "Attention enlivens, while intention transforms." [6] According to ancient yogic principles, the energy of clear intention has organizing power and can catalyze energy and information and transformation into new forms.

> *Principle 4*: Attention enlivens, while intention transforms.

This capacity has been studied in-depth by the pioneering work of the HeartMath Institute (HMI). Since 1991, HMI has researched and developed reliable, scientifically based tools to help people strengthen the connection between their hearts and minds, and to deepen their connection with the hearts of others. Dr. Joe Dispenza writes about neuroscience and quantum physics in his books, *You Are the Placebo* and *Becoming Supernatural.*

> So the quantum model, which states that all possibilities exist within this moment, gives us permission to choose a new future and observe it into reality — that means there's a lot of potential out there that you and I might be missing. Where you place your attention is where you place your energy — as a result, you're affecting matter with your attention and observation. [7]

When the intention is clear, temporarily losing the way does not derail the journey. Course corrections are always possible, using the strong rudder of intention as a guide. If one were to ask Kathleen to name the single most important thing learned on her holistic journey, the answer would be this:

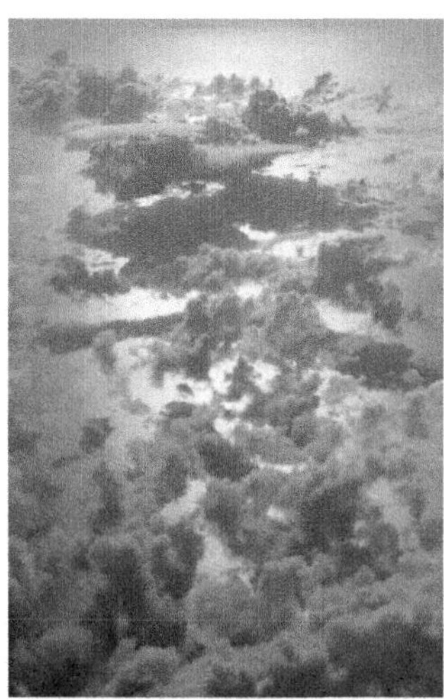

"Intention is the most powerful force on the planet. Nothing of human making has ever happened that did not begin with intention."

intention

1) *a: what one intends to do or bring about*
   b: the object for which a prayer, mass, or pious act is offered
2) *a determination to act in a certain way: resolve*
3) *intentions plural: purpose with respect to marriage*
4) *import, significance*
5) *a process or manner of healing of incised wounds*
6) *concept especially: a concept considered as the product of attention directed to an object of knowledge*

Merriam Webster Dictionary third edition

Balance/Homeostasis

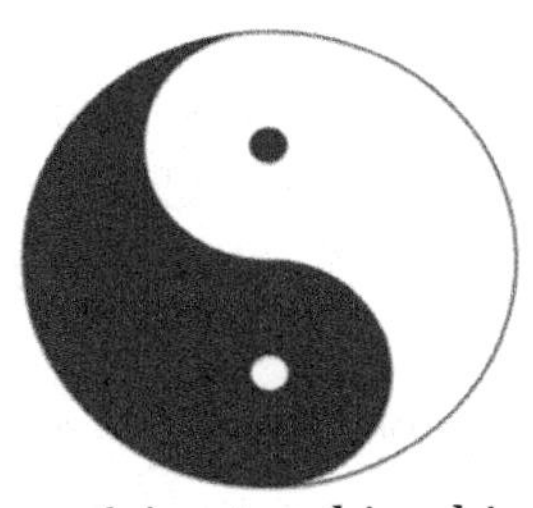

A story about the young man who would later become the Buddha illustrates the nature of balance. According to Buddhist legend, Siddartha was sitting in meditation along a riverbank one day and overheard a musician teaching his student. The musician said about his instrument," If you tighten the string too much, it will snap; but if you leave it too loose, it won't play." Siddartha realized that the same principle — the balance of opposite values — applied to much of life. This important insight later became incorporated into Buddhist teachings and is known as "the middle way."

While we can operate in an imbalanced state, and often do, it is never the ideal. The brain is so adaptable, however, that it runs on what Drs. Chopra and Tanzi call "dual control." [8] Most body processes run perfectly fine on automatic pilot, but if one instructs the brain to run in a certain way — like reaching for that fifth piece of pizza, going without sleep, putting off time in Nature or other health-sustaining practices — then *will* and *desire* take over, and one's balance can easily be lost. Regaining it involves the effort to restore alignment, which reinstates congruence between one's values and the forces, influences, and elements in everyday life.

Mindfulness can raise awareness of individual choices and behavioral patterns; it gives the brain a foundation for change.

In physiologic terms, a state of balanced equilibrium is called homeostasis. There is nothing static about the term, however. *Homeostasis* is an always dynamic interplay of opposing processes in the human body to ensure its stability and survival. Homeostasis is the way a balanced body wants to go. Every cell has been superbly engineered to stay in balance — which is why cells typically do not store energy. They only have enough *food* to last a few seconds. In the body's overall homeostatic state, every cell counts on being nourished continuously.

Principle 5: Homeostasis is a dynamic interplay of opposing processes that generate the ability to maintain a relatively stable internal state despite changes in the outside world.

Physiologist Walter Cannon coined the term *homeostasis* in the 1920s, expanding on the work of physiologist Claude Bernard. In the 1870s, Bernard described how complex organisms must maintain balance in their internal environment, or *milieu intérieur*, in order to lead a *free and independent life* in the world beyond. Cannon honed the concept and introduced homeostasis to popular audiences through his book, *The Wisdom of the Body* (The British Medical Journal, 1932).

Homeostasis is the ability to maintain a relatively stable internal state that persists despite changes in the world outside.

All living organisms, from plants to nature to humans, must regulate their internal environment to process energy and ultimately survive. [9]

The ability to maintain a *relatively stable state* ... there is power in this small phrase; a power that can help us understand nature's resilience — to *persist* despite *manifest destiny* or the current condition of health fed and surrounded by poor nutrition as well as impact to the natural environment through industrial practices. [10]

The brain is the source of all bodily functions, and the mind is inextricably tied to both body and brain. What each individual strives to perfect is bringing their brain into balance. A balanced brain uses its ability to bring everything else into balance —hormones, habits, behavior, cravings, and desires. The *balance* between autonomic (involuntary) and sympathetic (voluntary) nervous system control lies at the fulcrum of *homeostasis*. Once the brain is in balance, it will naturally tend to preserve this state. [11] A meditation/prayer practice can help restore balance to the mind through periods of conscious rest and to the body through relaxation, accompanied by all of its related physiologic changes.

When the body is in a homeostatic state, relative equilibrium exists among all body systems that work in harmony, and minimal amounts of energy are wasted. This balance is required to maintain equanimity: the quality of being composed, calm, even-tempered, and emotionally stable, particularly in times of high stress.

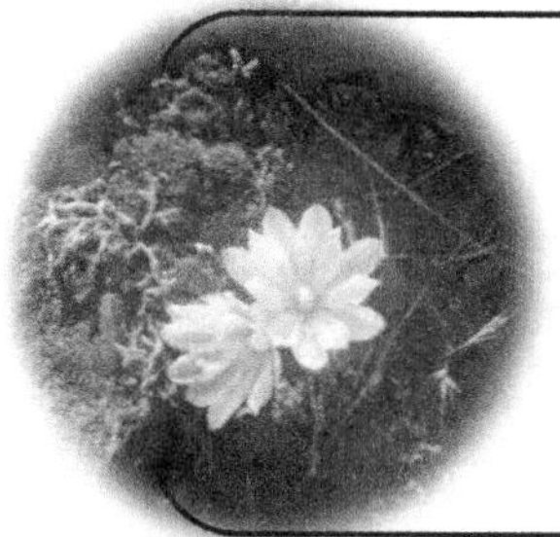

Nature tops the list of potent tranquilizers and stress reducers. The mere sound of moving water has been shown to lower blood pressure.

~Patch Adams

Reciprocity

> reciprocity
> *1: the quality or state of being reciprocal: mutual dependence, action, or influence*
> *2: a mutual exchange of privileges specifically: a recognition by one of two countries or institutions of the validity of licenses or privileges granted by the other*
> Webster's College Dictionary third edition

This principle pits practices of competition against those of cooperation. When viewed through a Darwinian lens, all species living on Earth contain separate individuals — whether persons, animals, or plants — and can be seen as *competing for a spot* in the struggle to survive. The opposite view would be to see the natural world and humanity as connected, interdependent communities that all work better when cooperating for the benefit of all concerned.

Discussing this principle in the book *Drawdown*: *The Most Comprehensive Plan Ever Proposed to Reverse Global Warming*, plant biologist Janine Benyus tells of her observations of plants that actively help one another grow in harsh environments.

> It's counterintuitive to imagine plants growing closer together in the face of scarcity when our competition bias and our economic theories tell us they should do otherwise. For years, careful researchers tried to explain this [plant behavior] as an anomaly. Now we know that it's not just one plant helping another; complex exchanges of goodness — are playing out above and below ground in

extraordinary ways — The practice of reciprocity will require a more nuanced understanding of how ecosystems work. [12]

For almost two centuries, a single-minded focus on competition has led to the view of all life forms as consumers and competitors, including humanity. For those living in America, the term *Manifest Destiny* became part of history lessons, continuing the belief of *if you want it, take it.* However, advances in human genome science have revealed there is a cooperation mechanism among species known as *gene transfer.* Living organisms integrate their cellular communities by *sharing* genes. [13, 14] One of the best examples of this phenomenon is the human microbiome. Hundreds of trillions of microbes, mostly residing in our guts, are necessary for our survival — and they outnumber human cells in the body by ten times. [15]

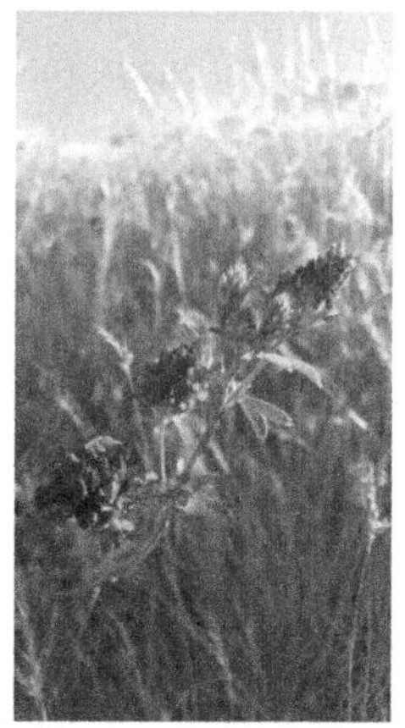

It is high time to move beyond Darwinian thinking that stresses individuals' importance and move towards recognizing the ubiquity of sharing and community within the *whole of life.* Perhaps then we can resume our role as nurturers helping in the story of healing.

Principle 6: Humanity and the natural world are interdependent, connected communities that work best when cooperating for the benefit of all.

Adapting to change

The coming on of fall and the trees kaleidoscopic colors are all a part of how Nature shows how necessary adapting is. Without a trees' ability to collect and store the summer's sunshine in the form of carbohydrates, we might never know the delight in maple sugar leaves as holiday treats. How dull and boring fall would be without the fire and glow of maple, aspen, willow and countless other deciduous trees.

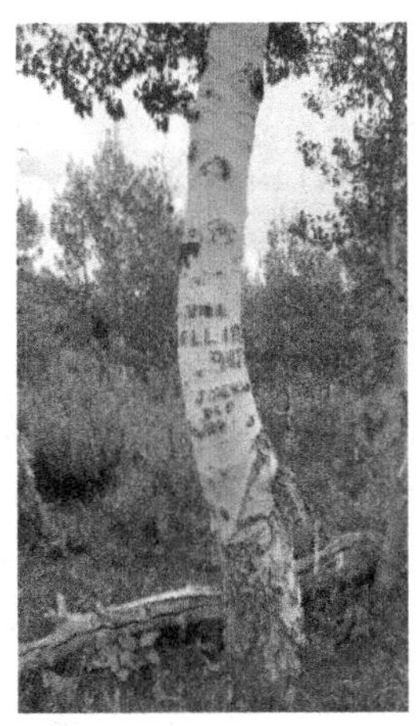

Change can leave life-long marks. As Tammera walked among the changing aspens, she noticed the scars left by individuals branding the trees as location markers. These scars have not altered the life cycle, growth, or course of seasonal change for these high elevation trees. These permanent marks add to the story of the tree and the area — one reads 1910, another 1992 — some are legible names, others are patterns whose meaning has been lost. Not all the scars are from human hands. Deer and elk have used these trees to rub the velvet from antlers, and woodpeckers have left their mark as they opened the bark to draw the tree's sap to attract insects for food.

Change can bring beautiful and miraculous opportunities and knowledge into one's life. Change also means death and rebirth; the journey doesn't end with one person; as the Human Genome Research shows, it is the beginning of human adaptation — the future.

> *"We delight in the beauty of the butterfly, but rarely admit the changes it has gone through to achieve that beauty."*
>
> ~Maya Angelou

The pandemic year of 2020 was a giant roller coaster of change, not just for those in the United States but the entire world. So very much of what took place was out of people's control and comprehension, relentlessly sapping their resiliency and reserves of energy. In any town or country, the heavy weight of uncertainty, loss, and frustration was visible when viewing individuals walking along streets, in stores, and neighborhoods. Heads and shoulders bowed, feet plodding all too closely — resembling a crowd scene in zombie movies — it was the reality of the day. Anger, fear, sorrow, loss, depression, frustration are the words many will associate with 2020; how can we regain our balance, hope, and energy when negative words have supplanted all others in our thoughts?

> *Principle 7*: The only constant in life is change.

A mindful pause can stop the noise and craziness in our heads even for a few moments. Look at the magic of Nature — even if all one can do is direct their focus on a leaf or golden blade of grass — an individual can begin to feel calmer and the intentional shift to mindfulness results. This doesn't mean all is *utopian* and *Disney World.* There will still be sorrow, moments of anger, disruption of work schedules and private lives, or feelings of being overwhelmed — but the moment of pause can help regain a little *resiliency, energy,* and *perspective* — allowing for moving forward.

Remember that environment is not solely that of the Natural World; it is also the internal environment; that comprises one's innermost being — sometimes called the soul. It is important to remember we are a part of Nature, our environment. That means we have the innate ability gifted by the *Divine* to gain *relatively stable states* that persist, grow, change, nourish, and flourish. As humans, we can thrive on adversity or allow adversity to paralyze and weaken us.

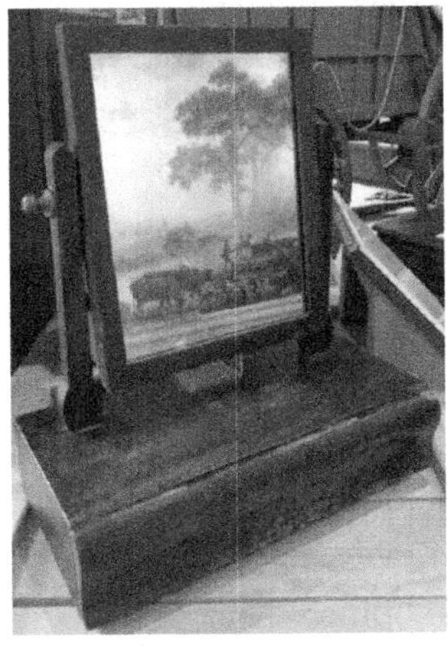

Artifact found on the Oregon Trail – Mirror is reflecting the image of a painting on the opposite wall.
Oregon Trail Interpretive Center, Baker, Oregon

Looking at history, one can find countless examples where individuals passed through difficult to harrowing events and became influencers for advancement, industry, exploration, literature, and even government. They embraced *change*, modified it to their needs, and gained insight and strength from it. Mastering change can provide the courage to lift heads, straighten shoulders, and walk through life with purpose and power.

"Today, we have gathered, and when we look upon the faces around us, we see that the cycles of life continue. We have been given the duty to live in balance and harmony with each other and all living things. So now, let us bring our minds together as one as we give greetings and thanks to each other as People. Now our Minds are One."

~ Thanksgiving address of the Haudenosaunee Confederacy Onondaga Nation [16]

Resilience

Resilience is your ability to bounce back after difficulties. It has been called *grit* or toughness, and it has everything to do with your reserves. Health reserves help you bounce back

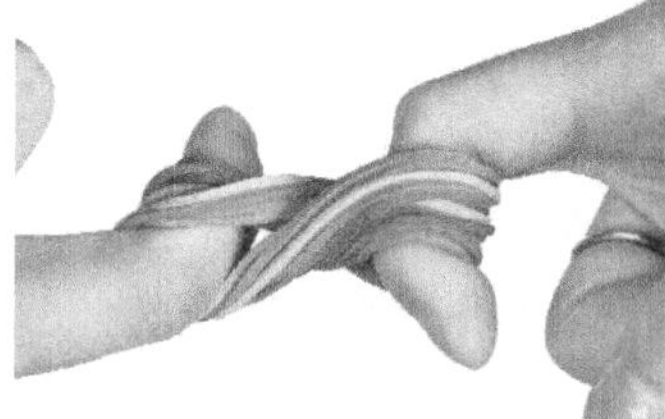

physically. Financial reserves help you bounce back economically. Information reserves help you build your systems and best practices. And, perhaps most important, self-esteem reserves help you rebuild your will. Will is connected to hope and faith. It has a significant influence over where we put our energy. It's essential for our survival and long-term success in life." Christopher Van Buren, author of *Noble Artist* at The HeartMath Institute; defines resilience as "the capacity to prepare for, recover from, and adapt in the face of stress, adversity, trauma or challenge." [17]

I've learned that you can tell a lot about a person by the way he/she handles these three things: a rainy day, lost luggage, and tangled Christmas tree lights.

~Maya Angelou

How resilient are you?

When individuals are faced with something new, they either embrace it or they freeze up, shy away, or experience anxiety. Not everyone is a daredevil or turns into a *fainting goat* over change. [18] Most transition into the *new normal*, or so they think. How one responds or reacts to change is a gauge of resiliency. *Resiliency* is a measure of how well-nourished we are in our lives. The better the nutrition received from food, life choices, and mindfulness, the better individuals, can face the multitude of changes tossed at them by life. This is especially apparent in the elderly. Researchers have found that adaptability and resiliency decline with age. Resiliency is also viewed as a marker for age-related cognitive degeneration. [19]

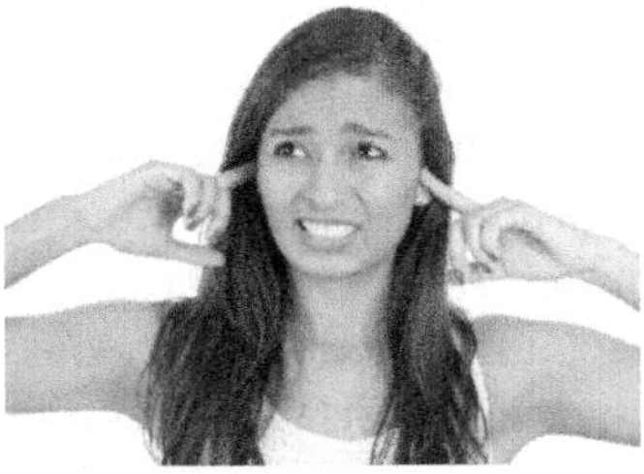

Principle 8: Resiliency is a measure of reserves.

The push to study cognitive reserve in more depth across the scientific disciplines was born out of recommendations from the Cognitive Aging Summit III in 2017.

> According to Peter Rapp, senior investigator in the Neurocognitive Aging Section of the NIA, 'cognitive reserve is what makes some older adults cognitively resilient' — whether and how people with high cognitive reserve simply age more slowly than their peers — whose thinking and memory are impacted by neuropathology, genetic, environmental or life experience protective factors. [20]

The authors of *Empty Plate,* like millions of others, found resiliency waning by the end of 2020; never-ending challenges and a faltering sense of normalcy began to affect their lifestyle choices. While standard American snack foods and candies rarely entered their diets — *sacks of sadness* — became daily lunches for Tammera's husband while working on forest fires. [21] Ease of access to *junk* foods, varying degrees of stress, poor sleep, and increasing uncertainty led to subtle brain chemistry changes, which resulted in increased cravings for refined sugars, flour, and salt in many people. Digestive issues resurfaced for some. Mounting stress increased blood pressure for others. It was no real surprise to the authors to learn that — counter to their hopes of improved diets due to newfound pandemics eating habits, with meals cooked at home — instead, the result was the snack food industry's projected record sales during 2020. [22, 23, 24]

How can we hope to gain sustainable health and move forward into resilient and regenerated health of body and mind? First, recognizing that if individuals continue to feed themselves with empty calories — they will fail in the pursuit of health. Next, accept that health is not made up of simple chemical compounds or calorie consumption.

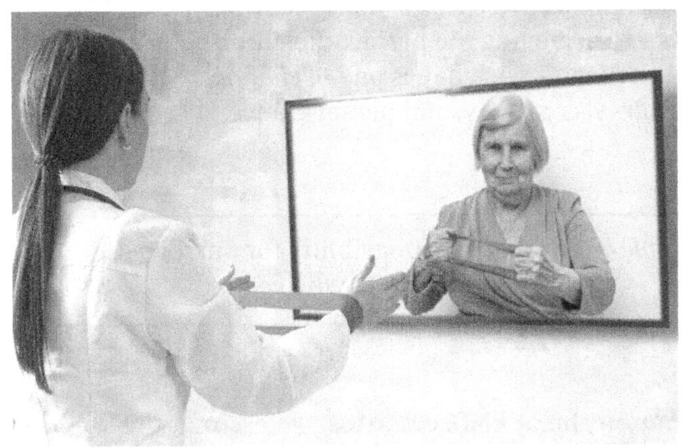

Health is a complex synergistic dance of nourishing foods, lifestyle, connections, and interaction with the world around us.

How does one regain resiliency after trying times, loss, frustration, and global uncertainty? It isn't with caffeine, energy drinks, online shopping, or indulgent behavior. Just as the authors have spoken in detail on nourishing a *holistic* approach for mind, body, and spirit, we have also provided the principles to achieving *homeostasis* in lifestyle.

PRACTICE! The old saying from childhood comes to mind – "if at first, you don't succeed, try, try again." And "Don't give up too easily; persistence pays off in the end." These little verses can be traced back to American educator, Thomas H. Palmer and English novelist Frederick Maryat (1792–1848). When it comes to falling off the wagon of a *healthy diet* (remember back to Chapter Two - all that the words diet means?), one can find themselves sitting in the weeds on the side of the road, needing time to shake the dust from their clothes. Before being able to stand once more and resume the journey. We need to gain our balance. [25] There is no right or only one way to achieving the perfect diet, lifestyle, or health plan — each day is one of *change*, adaptability, creativity, and perseverance.

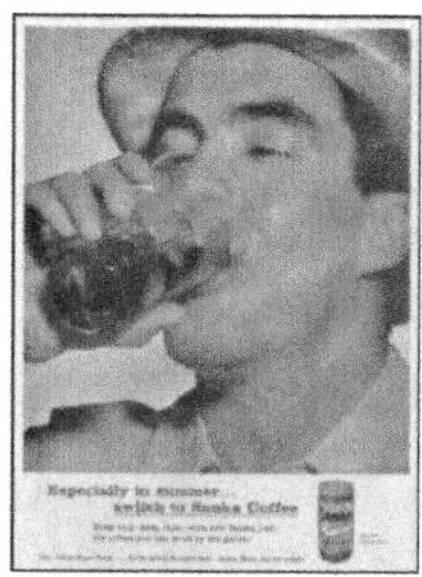

Life Magazine 1959

Principle 9: We share responsibility for ourselves, others, and the world we live in.

Shahram Heshmat Ph.D. emeritus professor at the University of Illinois and founder of the Science of Choice, explains how eight aspects of choice and lifestyle — similar to those found to have the most significant influence on longevity in the *Blue Zone* research — affect resiliency. The following is an excerpt from the article *The 8 Key Elements of Resilience*, which offers sound information. [26, 27]

- *Pursuing a meaningful goal*

Resilient individuals find a calling and dedicate themselves to what gives life purpose. Pursuing a meaningful purpose may involve stress and pain in the short run, but it brings meaning over the long run. People with a sense of purpose feel less anxiety and stress. [28, 29]

- *Challenge assumptions/deeply held beliefs*

Resilience requires creativity and flexibility. Traditional beliefs should be examined in the light of new experiences and ideas. Creativity requires one to consider many perspectives to avoid being imprisoned by one's habitual thoughts. In the aftermath of major life struggles, where fundamental assumptions are seriously confronted, it can lead to positive psychological change. [30]

- *Cognitive flexibility*

Resilient people tend to be flexible in their way of thinking and responding to stress. An important component of cognitive flexibility is accepting the reality of our situation, even if that situation is frightening or painful. Acceptance is a key ingredient in the ability to tolerate highly stressful situations. Avoidance and denial are the most common counterproductive coping strategies that can help people temporarily, but it ultimately stands in the way of growth. [31]

- *Growth through suffering*

Resilient people generally meet failure head-on and use it as an opportunity to learn and grow. Thus, we can view any experience of emotional pain as an opportunity that will strengthen our ability to better deal with any future pain. However, when we medicate away our suffering, we miss the opportunity to grow. [32]

- *Acting despite the fear*

Courage is an important aspect of positive psychology that allows one to overcome personal limitations and pursue a full life. Courage is not a matter of feeling no fear. Courage is acting despite fear. [33]

- *Emotion regulation*

One of the basic principles of Stoicism. [34] Much, if not all, of our thinking is up to us. We can liberate ourselves from destructive emotions such as anger and hatred by developing a capacity to choose how to interpret the situation. Our ability to manage the flow of thought and the capacity to visualize the future contribute to happiness.

➢ *The feeling of agency*

The sense of agency refers to the capacity of individuals to act independently and shape their life circumstances. By exerting free will, the person expands his options and freedom. When feeling free and self-determined, we generally flourish. Believing that things are beyond our control is a recipe for helplessness.

➢ *Social support*

Resilient individuals draw strength from their social networks. They also provide social support to others. When you have strong social support, you don't have to use as many of your own personal resources to cope with adversity. Those relationships give you a profound sense of emotional security and the feeling that someone has your back no matter what. [35]

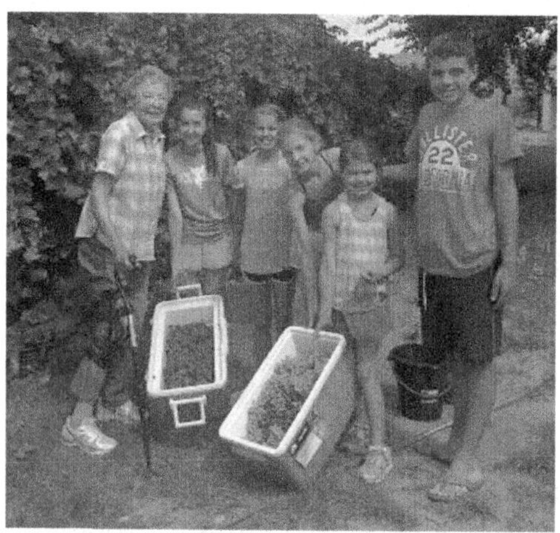

Betty Sits age 94, harvesting concord grapes, with her great grandchildren. (Sitz Ranch 2017)

Perspective from history

In 1917, archaeologist Earl Morris excavated the burial of a young woman in Room 139 at Aztec Ruins, a national monument located just outside Aztec, New Mexico. [36] This seventeen to twenty-year-old woman had experienced a severe injury, resulting in her death over 800 years ago. Archaeologist Erin Baxter of the Denver Museum of Nature & Science showed x-ray photos of the 5-foot-5-inch tall woman's skeleton to several emergency room physicians, orthopedists, and the like, who offered the following scenario. [37, 38]

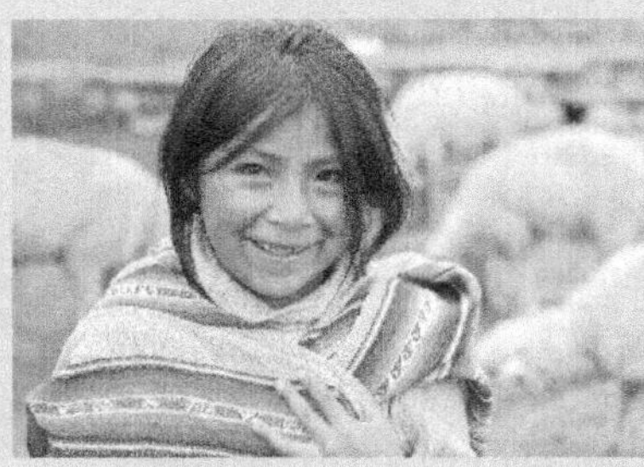

The young woman fell or was pushed, probably from a significant height. She landed on the palm of her left hand with a force of about 400 pounds per square inch. The violence of that event caused both bones of her forearm (the left ulna and radius) to break completely.

A smaller but still tremendous amount of force then impacted her midsection and lower back, creating a vertical crack in her lower lumbar vertebrae and sacrum. Her left hip then caved outward, dislocating the ball joint. Secondary internal injuries would have led to bruised and possibly ruptured intestines, bladder, and kidneys.

Continues on the next page

Whoever attended to this injured woman didn't just engage in palliative care to ensure she was comfortable until she died. Care for the injured has been increasingly reported in archaeology findings over the last twenty years, from Kennewick Man and the Spirit Cave Man of Paleo-Americans to today's traditional indigenous healing. Puebloan culture from eight centuries ago obviously supported skilled healers, one of which set six wooden splints to stabilize the bones of the young woman's left forearm, presumably in the hope that the arm might heal somewhat and retain some functionality. Evidence of a staph infection around the splints indicates she remained alive and well cared for — at least for a time.

These findings would have been highly controversial when Earl Morris argued this was the first evidence of pre-Columbian surgery in the Americas. It is equally astounding today. This young woman and her culture illustrate how remarkable, brave, and tough ancient peoples were.

Hope

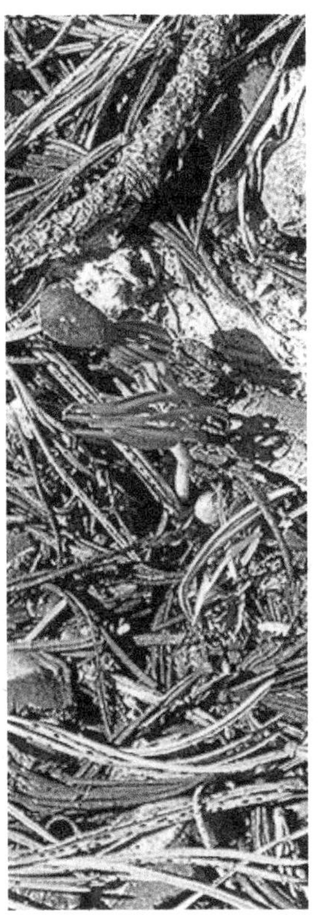

In the fall of 2020, Tammera found herself walking through an area of the forest that had been engulfed in flames only two weeks prior. At first, she only saw the blackened remains of lodgepole pine. Then, as she narrowed her vision, she saw the ground was covered in areas with unaffected clumps of grass, wild strawberry leaves, and clusters of huckleberry and manzanita. In the areas where the ground, at first glance, appeared black, she now saw the thousands of pine tree seeds scattered by the wind. Lodgepole and knobcone pine trees depend on fire to release their seeds from the cone, kill pine beetles, and stimulate new growth of the forest microbiome that converts carbon into nourishment for seeds and young trees. This intricate cycle of life brings hope, wonder, and calm.

> *"Hope is the thing with feathers that perches in the soul – And sings the tune without words — and never stops..."*
>
> ~ Emily Dickinson

Man has been actively managing nature from the beginning. As Robin Wall Kimmerer shares in *Braiding Sweetgrass*, harmony can happen between man and nature. It does not have to be *all or nothing* in humankind's interactions with the environment — the environment that resides within us and that which surrounds us.

To become an active participator in harmony with nature, to plant that seed of hope - first individuals may need to *clean house*, get rid of the overgrowth and congestion to establish homeostasis within themselves. As we reach the end of this book, and the empty plate has filled with information on food, sustainability, and mindfulness — the seed of hope has planted itself in each reader's mind.

What kind of world do we want to leave to our children, those who are growing up right now? What needs do they have of us, and what needs does the Earth have of us?

These are questions asked by Pope Francis on May 24, 2015, in his second encyclical letter, *"Laudato Si,"* about the global environment. [39] It is subtitled *On Care for Our Common Home.* [40]

"Laudato si', mi' Signore" means *Praise be to You, my Lord* in Latin; the first words of a beautiful canticle written by the Catholic Saint Francis of Assisi, in which he reminds individuals the common home of earth is like a sister with whom we share life, as well as a beautiful mother who opens her arms to us.

Pope Francis says,

> Many things have to change course, but it is we human beings above all who need to change. We lack an awareness

of our common origin, of our mutual belonging, and of a future that is shared with everyone. We must regain the conviction that we need one another, that we have a shared responsibility for others and the world, and that being good and decent are worth it.

I go among trees and sit still.
All my stirring becomes quiet
around me like circles on water.
My tasks lie in their places where
I left them, asleep like cattle.

Then what I am afraid of comes.
I live for a while in its sight.
What I fear in it leaves it,
and the fear of it leaves me.
It sings, and I hear its song.

After days of labor,
mute in my consternation,
I hear my song at last,
and I sing it. As we sing,
the day turns, the trees move.

~Wendell Berry

Joy

Spending time in Nature, holding a newborn baby, witnessing the sunrise or sunset, playing with a puppy, consciously returning to a perspective of awe and appreciation for whatever is yours at the moment, witnessing or just reading about the power of the human spirit — all of these can bring joy. Joy resonates deep within our being; it nourishes resiliency and adaptability. Joy is not "happiness" and should not be viewed in the same manner.

> joy (noun)
> a. the emotion evoked by well-being, success, or good fortune or by the prospect of possessing what one desires
>
> Merriam-Webster Dictionary third edition

Happiness and joy are often interchanged in describing positive emotions. However, happiness and joy do not mean the same as pleasure and satisfaction. Often in the pursuit of happiness, individuals fill empty areas of their lives with those things that give pleasure and satisfaction but fail to bring *contentment* or joy. [41] The reward pathway uses dopamine to communicate between neurons in the ventral tegmental area (VTA). Through the generation

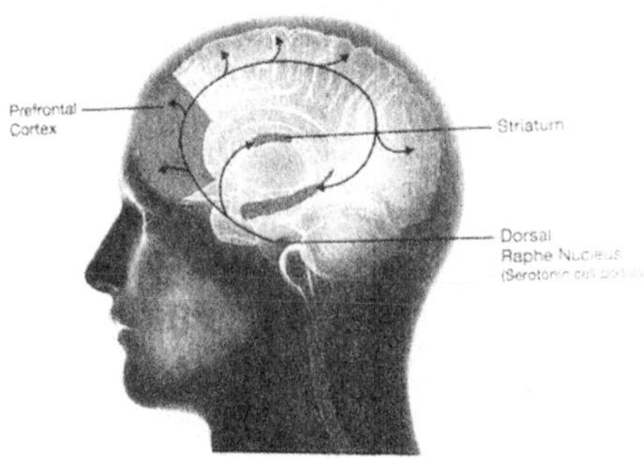

of dopamine receptors of the nucleus accumbens (NA), the feelings of motivation from learning and rewards results. [42] The contentment pathways use serotonin to communicate with neurons of the dorsal raphe nucleus and the cerebral cortex where the brain interprets impulses as "good" or "bad." [43] Joy is infused in the interdependent web of life. It is fruit ripening, bees pollinating, humans journeying. It is life-sustaining itself, moment to moment, over eons. When we feel this quality of joy, we recognize that life sustains and nourishes us; and that we are a part of the whole of life. [44]

Principle 10: Happiness is fleeting; joy is integral.

Vedic wisdom teaches that the core of human expression is *Ananda*, which means love, bliss, and unconditional joy. This philosophy teaches we were all born content as an expression of the deep, undiminishable radiance of love. *Ananda* is a joy that does not come and go. It is not dependent on conditions in the world or our lives. It was not coming and going from us at birth, and it is not now. Joy is a pure and simple delight in being alive!

"Gratefulness brings joy to my life. How could I find joy in what I take for granted?
The moment I stop 'taking for granted' there is no end to the surprises I find."

~Brother David Steindl-Rast

Regeneration/Renewal

Regeneration is not limited to the politically polarized and contested climate change topics and global warming. Regeneration happens on the cellular level, and it happens as we move beyond sustainable health into restored health. This applies to the natural world and that of our human selves. As the authors have shown in earlier chapters, sustainable health is only part of our goal; once sustainability is reached, the next logical step is to move forward and to *step up* to the next level, instead of hanging out in one place.

With the focus on regeneration and renewal of health, a natural progression occurs — an awakening to the possibilities as individuals begin to see improvement, more energy, mobility, and cognitive function. Soon the progression moves to those dear to us, then the little piece of earth a community share, and so on.

> *Principle 11*: Regeneration follows a natural process towards restoration and renewal.

An example of how each small change individuals make toward the mindful practices of food, sustainability, regeneration, and a holistic lifestyle is illustrated in the 2017 worldwide compendium — *Drawdown*: *The Most Comprehensive Plan Ever Proposed to Reverse Global Warming*, edited by Paul Hawken. In it, 100 strategies are proposed to decrease the carbon dioxide content in the Earth's atmosphere and minimize environmental changes in upcoming decades. The strategies are delineated by number according to the gigatons of carbon dioxide removed, their cost, and the savings generated if adopted. Number eleven in the ranking is regeneration. [45]

> The purpose of regenerative agriculture is to continually improve and regenerate the health of the soil by restoring its carbon content, which in turn improves plant nutrition, health, and productivity. ... Regenerative agriculture increases organic matter, fertility, texture, water retention, and the existence of trillions of organisms that convey health and protection to the roots and the plants themselves.

The quality of food is intrinsically linked with both the land itself and farming practices. *If you do not provide your body with real quality foods as nourishment, it becomes obese, diseased, and disabled.* [46] *If a farmer does not provide nourishment to the soil, it becomes depleted, infertile, deadened, and diseased.* These common-sense ideas underlie regenerative practices regardless of the discussion being about human, animal, or planetary health.

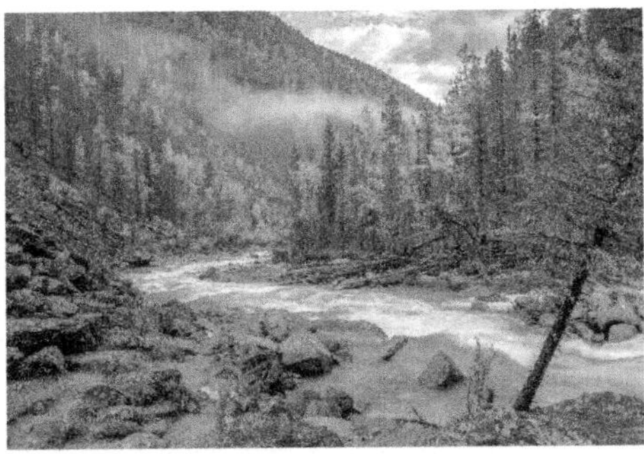

> *"When you do things from your soul, you feel a river moving in you, a joy."*
>
> ~Rumi, b.1207

Wholeness

Over the last few years, the words *holistic/wholistic* and *wholism* have been batted about like a badminton shuttlecock. These words have deep meaning and value. In our marketed pursuit of health In the U.S., *holistic* has been denigrated by underwear ads, vampire movies, and marketing campaigns. The authors are saying, *Enough*! — let's remind readers of how important these concepts are and why they matter in nutrition and nursing.

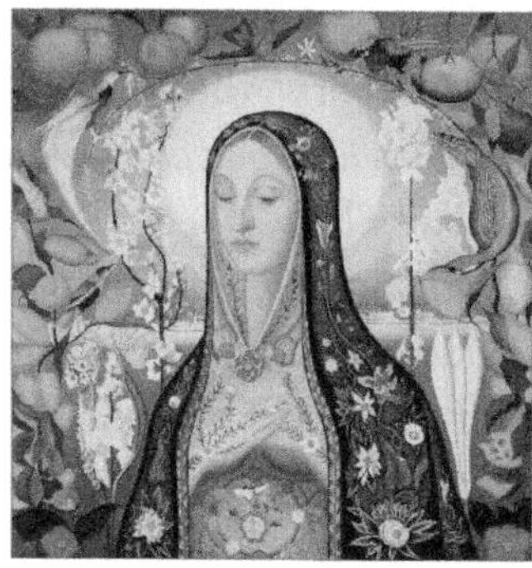

Holistic care dates to our beginnings — the combining of care, healing, ceremonial foods, and spiritual beliefs have long been interwoven — connecting individuals to their culture, community, and the natural world. Great minds and sages such as Hildegard von Bingen in the 10th century utilized holistic care elements daily in their communities. As she gained practical skills in diagnosis, prognosis, and treatment, this ancient mystic and physician combined nature, music and verse into *spiritual healing.* [47] She has been considered by many in Europe to be the founder of *scientific natural history* in Germany. [48] By cutting crucial threads from the complex tapestry of many elements and shrinking our present healthcare to a reductionist perspective, much is lost.

It is the height of hubris to believe one perspective has all the answers or that our modern intellect is superior to that of countless people who have come before us. *We do not know what we do not know*, and until better tools of science are available to find better answers – a *wholistic* approach to health care opens the window to the realm of possibilities. *Remember, Science does not have all the answers*. The knowledge of herbs, power of intention and prayer, the necessity of time in nature, and connection with culture and community — all possess healing energy. As science continues to look for better answers, the *truth* of traditional approaches gains credibility.

holistic
Philosophy
characterized by comprehension of the parts of something as intimately interconnected and explicable only by reference to the whole.

wholistic
Medicine
characterized by the treatment of the whole person, taking into account mental and social factors, rather than just the symptoms of a disease.

Merriam Websters Dictionary third edition

Our greatest challenge is accepting the fact that these traditional healing methods are effective without being viewed through the reductionist lens and recognizing their priceless value as gifts to humanity, now as then.

Principle 12: Wholeness is the manifestation of right relationship at multiple levels of the mind-body-spirit-environment-energy system.

Celebration

a personal note to you, the reader

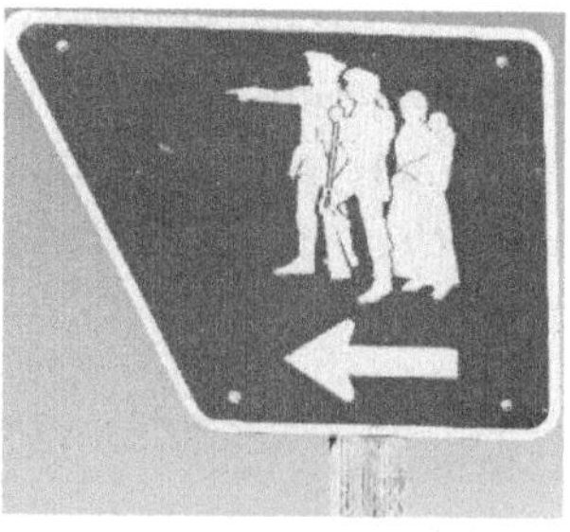

When Lewis and Clark traveled to the Pacific Ocean across the vast North American continent in 1804, they were uncertain what they would find or if they would survive the journey. There were times their path seemed to falter, wander, circle back, or even dead-end, requiring backtracking. Some days went with ease; others seemed to never end, as the challenges became insurmountable. Theirs can be viewed as an unsuccessful attempt, a monumental waste of resources, or it could be viewed as exploring the unknown from a different perspective.

Today we know the Lewis and Clark party was made up of diverse and skilled individuals – each member was valued, necessary, depended on their companions, and had a purpose. They were astute observers of nature and the indigenous populations they met. And those they met along the way provided knowledge, respite, and companionship to soothe the fatigue. While moving forward as a party, individuals also broke into smaller groups; to follow land contours, water routes, wildlife, and Indian trails; mapping the terrain as time would allow. These early side trips of exploration made it easier for those who came west after them.

Some individuals can keep to the straight and narrow path with a herculean feat of mental control. The reality for many is different. We are more like the explorers of old, following rabbit trails to see how far they go or what is on the other side of a hill. There are times we step backward two paces for every one forward, stumble, fall, or sit on the ground with our head in our hands.

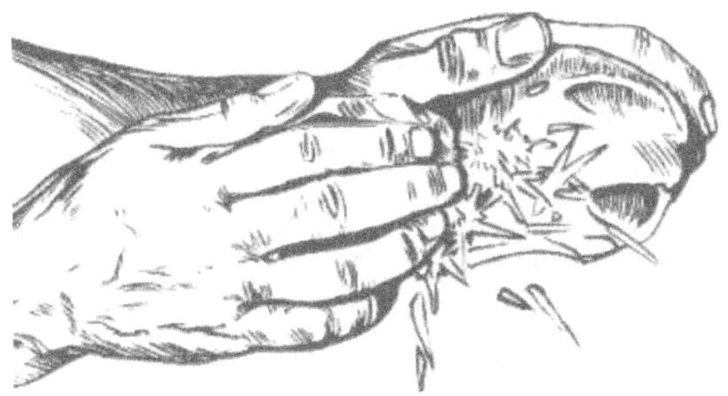

It takes a lot of hitting a flint to rock to make sparks before a flame emerges. Each attempt brings a flicker of light.

Each backward step leads to discovery. Without seemingly disjointed travels, we wouldn't have filled in the blank areas in our map of life. Know that each path taken will gift us with opportunities, experiences, new people, and stories. The map of *your* life may well be filled with dead ends, short excursions, and cross-continent adventures. But without these little setbacks, fatigue, and skinned egos, you miss out on a lot of growth and understanding about who you are. **All** adds to your story, exploration of inner-self, acceptance, and ability to throw your arms open wide to life. Otherwise, we miss out on the chance to *celebrate* what we have gained, experienced, and added to our lives, to the lives of others, and the world that is home.

Principle 13: Even backward steps or going off the track can lead to discovery.

The authors have challenged preconceived notions and judgments about food, water, mindfulness, sustainability, and holistic health. *Empty Plate* is a guidebook on viewing life, food, and health through *new perspectives* — these perspectives are fluid. They are meant to change throughout each individual's journey. Every journey is what you make of it — each day and how we greet it, move through and end it; all is determined by our choices and how we respond. Neale Donald Walsch says,

> The deepest secret is that life is not a process of discovery but a process of creation. You are not discovering yourself but creating yourself anew.

Let's review what was said earlier in this final chapter about Intention: *"Intention is the most powerful force on the planet. Nothing of human making has ever happened that did not begin with intention."*

We are only victims of circumstances if we allow it — life with all its warts is meant to be celebrated. The highest holistic viewpoint is about embracing every experience from the perspective of expanding, growing, and evolving. What keeps life going? Life itself. When we celebrate life — not only do we honor those who have come before us and will follow after us — the action connects individuals, even if they are not in the same place. Celebration floods our brains with endorphins and actively changes brain chemistry, cell regulation, resiliency, and longevity. Celebration provides an event that takes us out of the *normal* or *rut* of daily life; it changes our perspective, motivation, and adds joy.

Celebration could turn out to be our most potent holistic health tool; when we place our trust in its value as the best expression of joy in being alive.

Principle 14: Celebrate life!

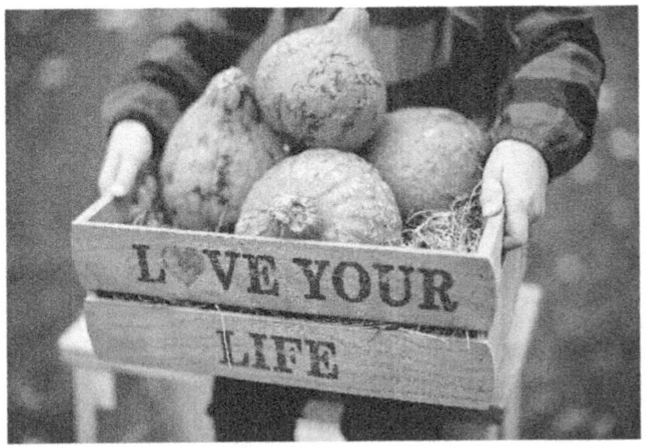

Here is to the feast that makes
our empty plate full — let's celebrate!

Arms Open Wide

As the seasons change, the trees show us how.
How to change with gusto, grace, and ease.
How to dance on the wind and float in the breeze.
How to accept change and how to celebrate.

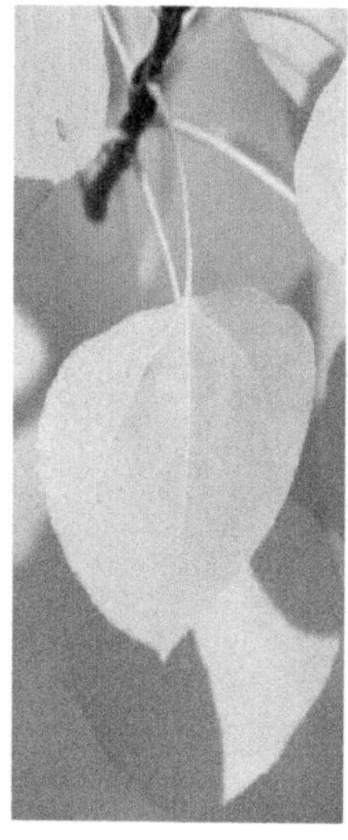

As I watch the golden coins of the aspen, I
see them one at a time turn loose from
the limb, throw their arms open wide, and
dance on the air.

These golden coins know not where they
will land.
Will it be the soft grass, the curve of a log,
or the surface of a lake or stream?

It doesn't matter to the tree or the coin
that it tosses from its purse of life.

With arms open wide, change is accepted,
embraced as a dear friend
and welcomed into the journey of life.

~ Tammera Karr

---

1. Hawken, P. (2017). Drawdown: The Most Comprehensive Plan Ever Proposed to Reverse Global Warming., p. 217 Penguin Random House: NY
2. www.vocabulary.com/dictionary/perspective
3. Scientific American fall 2020 Special Edition page 110
4. Chopra, D. & Simon, D. (2004). The Seven Spiritual Laws of Yoga, Wiley and Sons: NJ. Page 49.
5. Bohm, D. (2002). Wholeness and the Implicate Order. Volume 135. Routledge:NY
6. Chopra and Simon, The Seven Spiritual Laws of Yoga, p.64
7. Dispenza, J. (2014) You Are the Placebo. Hay House: CA. p. 184
8. Ibid. p.96
9. What Is Homeostasis? By Nicoletta Lanese July 15, 2019: https://www.livescience.com/65938-homeostasis.html
10. Manifest Destiny, a phrase coined in 1845, is the idea that the United States is destined—by God, its advocates believed—to expand its dominion and spread democracy and capitalism across the entire North American continent. The philosophy drove 19th-century U.S. territorial expansion and was used to justify the forced removal of Native Americans and other groups from their homes. The rapid expansion of the United States intensified the issue of slavery as new states were added to the Union, leading to the outbreak of the Civil War.
11. Chopra, D. & Tanzi, R. (2012) Super Brain.
12. Hawken, P. Drawdown, pp. 212-215
13 Nitz, et al.(2004). Heritable Integration of kDNA Minicircle Sequences from Tripanosoma cruzi into the Avian Genome: Insights into Human Chagas Disease. Cell 118, pp.175-186.
14. Dutta, C. & Pan, A. (2002). Horizontal Gene Transfer and Bacterial Diversity. Journal of Biosciences (Bangalore) 27 (1 Supplement 1) pp.27-33
15. Saey, T. (2013) Year in Review: Your Body is Mostly Microbes. Science News, 184
16. Words Before All Else: Greetings to the Natural World, https://danceforallpeople.com/haudenosaunee-thanksgiving-address/
17. McCraty, R. & Atkinson, M. (2012). Resilience Training Program Reduces Physiological and Psychological Stress in Police Officers. Global Advances in Health and Medicine, Vol 1, No.5, pp.44-66
18. The Myotonic or Tennessee Fainting is an American breed of meat goat. It is characterized by myotonia congenita, a hereditary condition which may cause it to stiffen or fall over when startled. It may also be known as the Fainting, Falling , Stiff-legged or Nervous goat, or as the Tennessee Wooden Leg.

---

19. Scientists Seek To Discover Why Some Minds Resist The Damage That Comes With Old Age by Robin Seaton Jefferson, 2019, Columbia University Neurology Department: https://www.columbianeurology.org/scientists-seek-discover-why-some-minds-resist-damage-comes-old-age

20. Scientists Seek To Discover Why Some Minds Resist The Damage That Comes With Old Age by Robin Seaton Jefferson, 2019, Columbia University Neurology Department: https://www.columbianeurology.org/scientists-seek-discover-why-some-minds-resist-damage-comes-old-age

21. Michael Karr coined this phrase when presented with his daily pre-packaged, industrial-ultra-processed lunch from fire camp food cateres. Historically fire fighters could count on traditionally prepaired hearty meals – covid-19 restrictions left fire crews poorly nurrished by ultra-processed foods.

22. Snack Foods market worldwide is projected to grow by US$217.2 Billion: https://www.globenewswire.com/news-release/2020/05/21/2036781/0/en/Snack-Foods-market-worldwide-is-projected-to-grow-by-US-217-2-Billion.html

23 Permissible indulgences and refrigerated snacks poised for growth in 2020: https://www.bakingbusiness.com/articles/51202-permissible-indulgences-and-refrigerated-snacks-poised-for-growth-in-2020

24 Snack Foods Market 2020 Global Industry Trends, Competitors Strategy, Key Players Profile, Size, Share, Growth, Segments, Regional Analysis, Review, Statistics and Growth Forecast to 2025: https://www.marketwatch.com/press-release/snack-foods-market-2020-global-industry-trends-competitors-strategy-key-players-profile-size-share-growth-segments-regional-analysis-review-statistics-and-growth-forecast-to-2025-2020-08-29

25. The Phrase Finder: https://www.phrases.org.uk/bulletin_board/5/messages/266.html

26. https://www.bluezones.com/2018/08/secret-to-longer-life-is-low-tech/

27. The 8 Key Elements of Resilience, A roadmap for developing mental resilience skills, by Shahram Heshmat Ph.D.,2020: https://www.psychologytoday.com/us/blog/science-choice/202005/the-8-key-elements-resilience

28. Hagerty BB (2016), Life Reimagined. Riverhead books.

29. Lyubomirsky, S. (2013).The myths of happiness: What should make you happy, but doesn't, what shouldn't make you happy, but does.New York: Penguin Press.

30. Robertson, Donald (2019), How to Think Like a Roman Emperor: The Stoic Philosophy of Marcus Aurelius, St. Martin's Press.

31. Solomon, Robert C. (2007). True to Our Feelings: What Our Emotions Are Really Telling Us. Oxford University Press, USA

---

32. Antifragile, Nassim Taleb (2012)

33. Seligman, Martin E. P. (2011). Flourish: A Visionary New Understanding of Happiness and Well-being. New York: Free Press.

34. Southwick, S. M., & Charney, D. S. (2018). Resilience: The science of mastering life's greatest challenges. 2nd edition. New York: Cambridge University Press.

35. Tedeschi RG, Calhoun LG (2004), Posttraumatic growth: conceptual foundations and empirical evidence. Psych Inquiry, 15(1-18).

36. Earl Halstead Morris, born June 24, 1889, is famous for his contributions and dedication to the field of archaeology, particularly at Aztec Ruins National Monument.

37. Two Surgeries, 800 years apart by Stephene E. Nash, 2020: https://www.sapiens.org/column/curiosities/ancient-surgery/

38. https://www.crowcanyon.org/index.php/lister-fellowship/53-about-us/lister-fellowship-recipients/384-erin-baxter

39. www.vatican.va/content/francesco/en/encyclicals/document

40. www.thejesuitpost.org/2015/06/an-overview-of-Laudato-si/

41. The Hacking of the American Mind by Robert H. Lustig, MD, MSL: 2017 Avery ISBN: 9781101982594, page 8

42. Ibid Lustig, page 29

43. Ibid Lustig, page 30

44. Marsh, S. (2015). Hunger, Hope and Healing. Shambala: Boston.

45. Hawken, P. (2017) Drawdown. P.54

46. Pollan, M. "Why Bother?" Essay in NY Times Magazine. 5/20/2008

47. Sweet, V. (1999). "Hildegard of Bingen and the greening of medieval medicine." Bulletin of the History of Medicine, 73(3), pp. 381–403. Project MUSE, doi:10.1353/bhm.1999.0140

48. Jöckle, Clemens (2003). Encyclopedia of Saints. Konecky & Konecky. p. 204.

Principles for a Sustainable and Mindful Journey

Chapter One

Principle 1: To achieve sustainable health, which allowing oneself us to enjoy our lives fully, we need to consume nutrient-dense whole food prepared in traditional ways.

Principle 2: If we are following merely the course of least resistance with food and behavioral choices in our lifestyle, our good health and well-being will not be sustainable.

Principle 3: If we fail to view our diet, health, and lifestyle through the lens of mindfulness, all that is most precious in our life will not be sustainable.

Principle 4: No one can care more than you - it is vital individuals play an active, responsible role in their health.

Principle 5: Use a quality water filter for all drinking and cooking water to reduce toxins.

Principle 6: Buy as much food as possible from local sources, especially fresh produce and meats.

Principle 7: Fruits and veggies are Mother Nature's fast foods - most of them are highly portable and can be eaten with minimal processing or preparation.

Principle 8: Celebrate your heritage by eating foods once a week from your origins as a gift to your DNA.

Chapter Two

Principle 1: Lasting lifestyle and health changes require allowing one to be empowered; small changes can take up to eight weeks to become sustainable.

Principle 2: A strict-one diet approach may not work for everyone, even if they are in the same family.

Principle 3: Connection with community and culture combined with a sense of value and purpose contribute to health as much or more than foods consumed.

Principle 4: The most proactive thing we can do for our health is cut 300 calories daily from industrial processed foods and add 300 calories of locally produced vegetables.

Principle 5: Planning ahead for the manageable "what ifs," adds a level of freedom from fear and worry - allowing for more enjoyable adventures in life.

Principle 6: Select glass, low toxin/HM ceramic, metal, wood, bamboo, and paper over plastic or vintage dishware.

Principle 7: Eat those foods from your personal genetics that make your DNA sing.

Principle 8: Diets should be based on individual needs, not agendas, politics, philosophy, or dogma. One size does not fit all.

Chapter Three

Principle 1: Mindfulness is not about paying more attention but involves paying attention differently.

Principle 2: Mindfulness practice encourages an individual to become a compassionate and non-judgmental observer of oneself.

Principle 3: Being aware of the breath takes attention and creates mental space.

Principle 4: Behavioral choices can support or compromise innate cellular intelligence.

Chapter Four

Principle 1: Color and Sound take us on a journey into the world of frequencies.

Principle 2: Celebrate your history by including music, art, and creative pursuits that resonate with your DNA and culture.

Principle 3: Color has definitive and measurable effects on the mind, body, and spirit.

Principle 4: Sound is an organizing force of nature.

Principle 5: Music impacts people more than any other human-made sound.

Principle 6: Silence is golden.

Chapter Five

Principle 1: Learn your history, who you have come from, and the stories of your people. These things provide connection and grounding of body, mind, and spirit.

Principle 2: Don't fall victim to "stinking thinking." Always try, even when you don't feel like it.

Principle 3: Time spent in Nature, especially grounding the human body to the earth, is good for body/mind/spirit

Principal 4: Nature provides examples of cooperative relationships and interconnectedness.

Principal 5: All of the natural world is cyclical.

Principle 6: Just as humans have a right to the benefits of Nature, Nature has rights of its own.

Chapter Six

Principle 1: We become human beings by caring for and helping one another.

Principle 2: Be bold and evaluate deeply held beliefs.

Principle 3: Perspective is an individual's way of looking at things and is continually influenced by beliefs and experiences.

Principle 4: Attention enlivens, while intention transforms.

Principle 5: Homeostasis is a dynamic interplay of opposing processes that generates the ability to maintain a relatively stable internal state despite changes in the outside world.

Principle 6: Humanity and the natural world are interdependent connected communities that work best when cooperating for the benefit of all.

Principle 7: The only constant in life is change.

Principle 8: Resiliency is a measure of reserves.

Principle 9: We share responsibility for ourselves, others, and the world we live in.

Principle 10: Happiness is fleeting, joy is integral.

Principle 11: Regeneration follows a natural process towards restoration and renewal.

Principle 12: Wholeness is the manifestation of right relationship at multiple levels of the mind-body-spirit-environment-energy system.

Principle 13: Even backward steps or going off the track can lead to discovery.

Principle 14: Celebrate life!

References

Arbesman, A. (2013). *Half-Life of Facts.* New York: Current.

Archibald, A. (2019). *The Genomic Kitchen.*

Ballantyne, S. P. (2017). *Paleo Principles: The Science Behind the Paleo Template, Step-by-Step Guides, Meal Plans, and 200+ Healthy & Delicious Recipes for Real Life.* Canada: Victory Belt Publishing.

Brown, G. (2018). *Dirt to Soil.* White River Junction: Chelsea Green Publishing.

Chokoisky, S. (2015). *Sex, Love, and Dharma: Ancient Wisdom for Modern Relationships.* Rochester: Destiny Books.

Chopra, D. M. (2018). *The Healing Self: A Revolutionary New Plan to Supercharge Your Immunity and Stay Well for Life.* New York: Harmony.

Civitello, L. (2011). *Cuisine & Culture 3rd edition.* Hoboken: Wiley.

Coelho, P. (1994). *The Alchemist.* New York: Harper One.

Collingham, L. (2012). *The Taste of War and the Battle for Food.* New York: Penguin Press.

Dietert, R. (2016). *The Human Super - Organism.* New York: Dutton.

Dukes, G. H. (2016). *A Short History of Eating.* London: London Press.

Edelstein, S. (2014). *Food Science and Ecological Approach.* Burlington: Jones and Bartlett Learning.

Edge, J. T. (2017). *The Potlikker Papers, a food history of the modern south.* New York: Penguin Press.

Fernandez, A. F. (2002). *Near a Thousand Tables, a history of food.* New York: Free- Press.

Fishman, C. (2011). *The Big Thirst.* New York: Simon and Schuster.

Fitzgerald, K. N. (2016). *Methylation Diet & Lifestyle.* Medford: www.drkarafitzgerald.com.

Flandrin, J. L. (1996). *FOOD a culinary history from antiquity to the present.* New York: Columbia University Press.

Fogg, B. J. (2019). *Tiny Habits: The Small Changes That Change Everything.* New York: Houghton Mifflin Harcourt.

Gaby, A. R. (2017). *Nutritional Medicine Second Edition.* Concord: Fritz Perlberg Publishing.

Gazzaley, A. (2016). *The Distracted Mind: Ancient Brains in a High-Tech World.* Cambridge: MIT Press.

Gittleman, A. L. (2010). *Zapped.* New York: Harper One.

Gladwell, M. (2002). *The Tipping Point.* New York: Little Brown and Company.

Gladwell, M. (2005). *Blink.* New York: Little Brown and Company.

Harari, Y. N. (2018). *Sapiens: A Brief History of Humankind.* New York: Harper Perennial.

Harmer, B. R. (1938). *Text-Book of the Principles and Practice of Nursing.* New York: Columbia University, MacMillan Company.

Hawken, P. (2010). *The Ecology of Commerce Revised Edition: A Declaration of Sustainability.* New York: Harper Business; Revised edition.

Hawken, P. L. (2000, 2010). *Natural Capitalism.* New York: Routledge.

Hay, W. H. (1929). *Health via Food.* East Aurora: Sun-Diet Press.

Hesterman, O. B. (2011). *Fair Food.* New York: Public Affairs.

Issued by the Medical Department of the General Conference of the Seventh-day Adventists. (1921). *Home Nursing a comprehensive series of lessons on hygiene and the practical care of the sick.* Washington, D.C.: Review and Herald Publishing Association.

Jenkins, M. (2017). *Food Fight.* New York: Avery.

Jensen, B. A. (1990). *Empty Harvest.* New York: Avery.

Kalanithi, P. (2016). *When Breath Becomes Air.* New York: Penguin Random House.

Karr, T. J. (2015). *Our Journey with Food.* Bozeman: Summerland.

Kirschmann, J. (2007). *Nutrition Almanac 6th edition.* New York: McGraw Hill.

Krimsky, S., Gruber, J. (2014). *The GMO Deception.* New York: Skyhorse Publishing.

Lama, D. (2009). *For the Benefit of All Beings.* Boulder: Shambhala.

Lipton, B. H. (2016). *The Biology of Belief 10th Anniversary Edition: Unleashing the Power of Consciousness, Matter & Miracles.* Hay House Inc.

Lovegren, S. (2005). *Fashionable Foods, Seven Decades of Food Fads.* Chicago: The University of Chicago Press.

Lustig, R. H. (2017). *The Hacking of the American Mind.* New York: Avery.

Mahan, K. (2017). *Krauses's Food & The Nutrition Care Process, 14th edition.* St. Louis: Elsevier.

Masaru, E. (2005). *The Hidden Messages in Water.* Hillsboro: Beyond Words Publishing.

Minger, D. (2013). *Death by Food Pyramid.* Malibu: Primal Blueprint Publishing.

Minich, D. P. (2018). *The Rainbow Diet.* Newburyport: Conari Press.

Moss, M. (2013). *Salt Sugar Fat.* New York: Random House.

Nestle, M. (2018). *Unsavory Truth How Food Companies Skew the Science of What We Eat.* New York: Basic Books.

Owsley, D. W. (2014). *Kennewick Man: The Scientific Investigation of an Ancient American Skeleton.* Washington, DC: Smithsonian.

Perlmutter, D. M. (2015). *Brain Maker.* New York: Little Brown and Company.

Perlmutter, D. P. (2020). *Brain Wash.* New York: Little, Brown Spark.

Provenza, F. (2018). *Nourishment.* London: Chelsea Green Publishing.

Rodgers, D. R. (2020). *Sacred Cow: The Case for (Better) Meat: Why Well-Raised Meat Is Good for You and Good for the Planet.* New York: BenBella Books.

Rost, A. (2016). *Natural Healing Wisdom and Know-How.* New York: Black Dog.

Roth, B. (2018). *Strength in Stillness: The Power of Transcendental Meditation.* New York: Simon & Schuster.

Scott-Dixon, K. P. (2017). *Genetics: The Universe Within.* Precision Nutrition.

Sherman, S. (2017). *The Sioux Chef's Indigenous Kitchen.* Minneapolis: University of Minnesota Press.

Shimer, P. (2004). *Healing Secrets of the Native Americans.* New York: Black Dog.

Sinclair, D. (2019). *Lifespan.* London: Thomson Press.

Snodgrass, M. E. (2004). *Encyclopedia of Kitchen History.* New York: Fitzroy Dearborn.

Standage, T. (2009). *An Edible History of Humanity.* New York: Walker & Company.

Strehlow, W. P. (1988). *Hildegard of Bingen's Medicine.* Rochester: Bear and Company.

Tannerhill, R. (1988). *Food in History.* New York: Three Rivers Press.

Teicholz, N. (2014). *The Big Fat Surprise.* New York: Simon & Schuster.

Tennant, J. (2013). *Healing Voltage, The Handbook.* Tennant.

Wahls, T. M. (2020). *The Wahls Protocol A Radical New Way to Treat All Chronic Autoimmune Conditions Using Paleo Principles.* New York: Avery.

Wall Kimmerer, R. (2015). *Braiding Sweetgrass.* Minneapolis: Milkweed Editions.

Wilson, B. (2019). *The Way We Eat Now.* New York: Basic Books.

Wilson, G. (1917). *Buffalo Bird Woman's Garden.* St. Paul: Minnesota Historical Society.

Wohlleben, P. (2016). *The Hidden Life of Trees.* Vancouver, BC: Greystone Books.

Wrangham, R. (2009). *Catching Fire How Cooking Made Us Human.* Philadelphia: Basic Books.

Acknowledgments

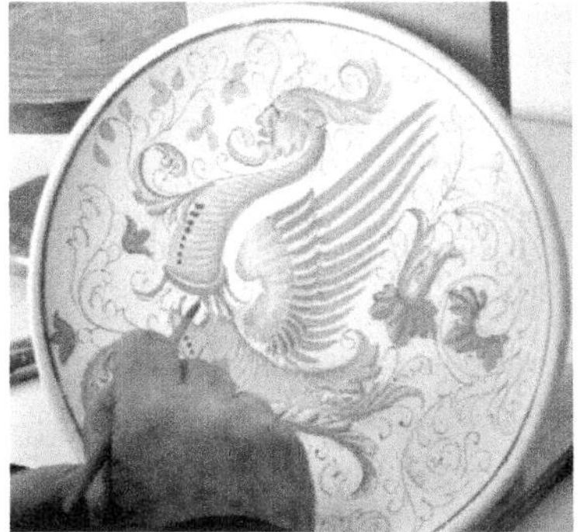

We would be remiss not to mention all those who made this book possible through their mentoring, steadfast support and dedication. We thank them for their commitment, involvement, and inspiration. Their hands and hearts have helped form and fill Empty Plate.

~Michael Karr, for his love, loyalty, dedication, support, countless hours learning how to make formatting work, proofreading, researching, and providing feedback and encouragement.

~Rick Bell, the man who has rescued Kathleen many many times from life's little disasters — especially when computers are involved — not only for exceptional tech support but for his never-ending unconditional love.

~ Veda L. Ardrus, EdD., RN, MSN, HN-BC®, an award-winning holistic nurse and master teacher.

~ Davidji, for teaching mantra and inspiring Kathleen to teach meditation.

~Deepak Chopra, MD, whose wise teachings introduced Kathleen to Ayurveda's ancient science and modern of holism.

~Sara Cimino, RN, PhD, who was a sterling example of professionalism in nursing. Even after her death, she continues to inspire and challenge Kathleen to do more for others.

~ Chris Dennen, PhD, has patiently explained meditation, mindfulness, and many other thoughts, broadening understanding and openness to life's patterns.

~ Elizabeth Lipski, PhD, shared her expertise in digestive health, microbiome, and virome science. Her generosity as a professor, mentor, and friend provided encouragement and guidance in Empty Plate's formation.

~Helen Manock, PhD, for her brilliant individualism while teaching the importance of spirituality and values.

~Deanna Minich, PhD, who continues to illustrate the vibrancy and color of nutrition.

~ Joanna K. Rowe, PhD, for her significant contributions to nursing literature and education and her confidence in a new faculty member as a professional writer.

~ Crystal Shepard, BS, provided literary feedback and support regarding soil, mycorrhizal, and wildlife ecology.

~Susan Taylor, PhD, for her unique program, which teaches the science of meditation and how to teach meditation to others.

~Terry Wahls, MD, for her determination and generosity.

~ James Wilson ND, DC, PhD who has inspired, mentored, and educated.

~Miriam Zacharias, who encouraged digging deeper and pairing history with science.

~ To all our students and clients who keep us eager to celebrate and learn from each other.

~All the Holistic Nutritionists and National Association of Nutrition Professionals are trailblazers, clinicians, researchers, educators, and visionaries on healing with the first medicine - FOOD.

~All the Nurses who have held us high on their shoulders: Kelly Alandt, RN, Lorrie Amitrano, FNP-C; Christina Dynamite, RN,-BC, BSN, NC-BC, Mary Hagood, FNP-C; Marina Ormes, RN, HN-BC (ret): Jean Thomsen, RN, Cordann Anderson, RN, BSN, CCMHP, QTTT: Breeze Powel-Spivey, RN, and Deonne Wright, RN, HN-BC®

Index

C

D

E

F

G

H

I

J

K

L

O

P

T

U

About the Authors

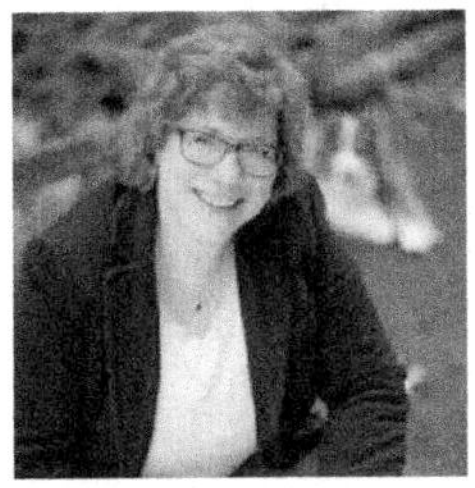

TAMMERA J. KARR, Ph.D., BCHN®, CGP, CNW®, with 20-plus years of clinical experience, is an author, educator, food historian, and researcher. Passionate about nutrition as the key to stopping many modern illnesses, Tammera first-authored *Our Journey with Food* in 2015 and the expanded second edition in 2018. *Our Journey with Food Cookery Book* followed and adds to the story filling in many gaps in food knowledge for health. Believing "Traditional Foods" is all about community, Tammera went on to create *Our Journey with Food* Online Education in 2020; This course, while initially created for nurses eager to use food as medicine, is equally suitable for anyone wanting to return to traditional food and health models. This program inspired the expansion of key concepts of Holistic Nutrition in the book co-authored with Holistic Nurse Kathleen Bell, *Empty Plate: Food ~Sustainability~Mindfulness.*

Tammera has served on the boards of the National Association of Nutrition Professionals (NANP), Oregon Holistic Nurses Association (ONHA), and is currently a special advisor for ONHA and serves on the American Naturopathic Certification Board (ANCB). Tammera is the primary instructor for *HN4UOnline.Ed* at https://yourwholenutrition.com/online-education/ and provides more information through her online Blog at https://yourwholenutrition.com/blog/

A Native of Oregon, Tammera enjoys the challenge of nutrition research, food history, traditional food preservation: canning, drying and fermenting, traditional whole food cooking. Tammera and her family have lived in remote areas of Oregon for over fifty years; being prepared for the unexpected is second nature. She resides at a remote Ranger Station in Central Southern Oregon and explores nature and history with her husband, Michael.

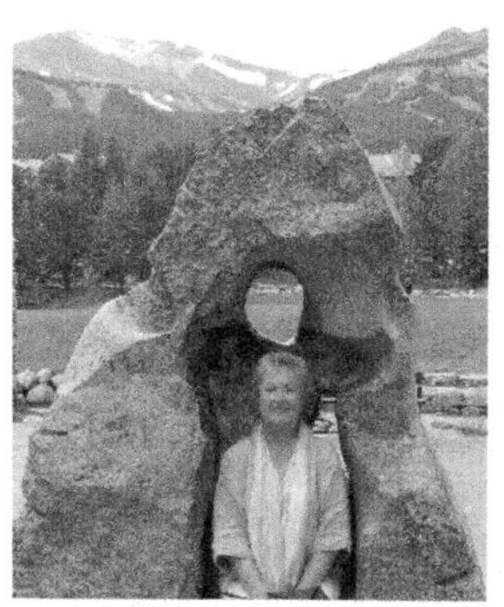

KATHLEEN BELL, RN, MSN, CNM, AHN-BC, MSI-BC; Kathleen's nursing career of nearly 50 years encompasses maternal–child nursing, Nurse-Midwifery, education, integrative health, and holism. She has held many national certifications and is a retired Certified Nurse Midwife (CNM), Advanced Holistic Nurse (AHN-BC), and Certified Meditation Specialist (CMS1-BC). She trained in Primordial Sound Meditation and Ayurvedic principles for health/dietary practices with the Chopra Center and was certified to teach meditation by The Center for Meditation Science. In 2020 she completed second degree Usui Reiki practitioner certification.

Retired from full-time academia — having taught nursing and midwifery at undergraduate and graduate levels in Utah, Oregon, Washington, and abroad — Kathleen is one of six holistic nursing faculty teaching the Integrative Healing Arts Program for the American Holistic Nurses Association (AHNA). She served on the Board of Directors with the Center for Meditation Science and a special advisor to the National Association of Nutrition Professionals' BOD.

An AHNA member since 2010, Kathleen chaired their annual conference in Portland, OR in 2014. She has also served as an advisor to the BOD of the Oregon Holistic Nurses Association since 2013. Kathleen writes, researches, and frequently presents on topics related to maternal-child/women's health, nursing and consumer education, meditation/mindfulness, integrative health, and holism. Kathleen offers consultation on holistic wellness practices and works with individuals and groups to develop their meditation practice under the business name of Northern Light: Illuminating the Path to Wholeness.

Additional Resources

Tools

- ***Berkley Water Filters***
  https://theberkey.com/

- ***FlashFish***
  Personal Power Supply
  https://www.flashfishtech.com/

- ***Hot Logic***
  Personal Oven/Food Warmer
  https://hotlogic.com/

- ***JetBoil Flash***
  Personal Cook System
  https://www.jetboil.com/explore/the-flash-cooking-system

- ***New Wave Enviro 10 Stage Plus Water Filter***
  https://www.newwaveenviro.com/products/10-stage-water-filter/

- ***Oko*** personal water filter
  https://okoh2o.com/

- **Patriot Power Cell**
  Solar backup-Pocket Sized chargers
  https://4patriots.com/collections/survival-gear/products/patriot-power-cell-four-packs

- ***Sawyer*** personal water filter
  https://sawyer.com/products/sawyer-personal-water-bottle-filter/

Training/Information

- ***Beginnings***: A quarterly magazine published by AHNA
  https://www.ahna.org/Home/Publications

- ***Chopra Foundation***
  https://www.choprafoundation.org
  Chopra Global
  https://www.chopra.com

- **Joe Dispenza, D.C.**
  www.drjoedispenza.com

- ***The Institute for Functional Medicine***
  505 S. 336th Street, Suite 600
  Federal Way, WA 98003
  Tel: 1.800.228.0622
  https://www.ifm.org/about/

- ***Journal of Holistic Nursing*** – a publication of AHNA
  https://www.ahna.org/Home/Publications

- ***LabSmarts*** makes functional blood chemistry analysis simple for practitioners. Efficient time saver, highlighting root cause faster, making you more effective. LabSmarts does not use diagnostic terms, so non-licensed healthcare practitioners of all types can feel safe using it and sharing the results with their clients/patients. www.labsmarts.com

- ***Dr. Vasant Lad***
  www.ayureveda.com

- ***Bruce Lipton***
  www.brucelipton.com

- ***Mindful magazine***
  https://www.mindful.org/magazine

- ***Dr. Terry Wahls***
  The Wahls Protocol Health Practitioner Certification
  https://terrywahls.com/certification/
  General Information
  https://terrywahls.com/

- ***ZRT***
  8605 SW Creekside Pl,
  Beaverton, OR 97008
  https://www.zrtlab.com/

Organizations

- ***American Holistic Nurses Association*** (AHNA)
  2900 SW Plass Court
  Topeka, KS 66611-1980
  https://www.ahna.org

  AHNA Chapter of Portland, Oregon
  https://sites.google.com/site/ahnaoregonchapter

- ***American Naturopathic Certification Board***
  https://ancb.net/

- ***Environmental Working Group***
  https://www.ewg.org/
  Oregon Holistic Nurses Association

- ***HeartMath Institute***
  14700 W Park Avenue
  Boulder Creek, CA 95006 (831) 338-8500
  www.heartmath.org

- ***Institute of Noetic Sciences*** (IONS)
  101 San Antonio Road Petaluma, CA 94952
  (707) 775-3500 info@noetic.org

- ***National Association of Nutrition Professionals***
  Setting the Standards for Holistic Nutrition
  https://www.nanp.org/

- ***Oregon Holistic Nurses Association (OHNA)***
  1081 SE Christie Place
  Grant's Pass, OR 97526
  https://www.oregonholisticnurses.org

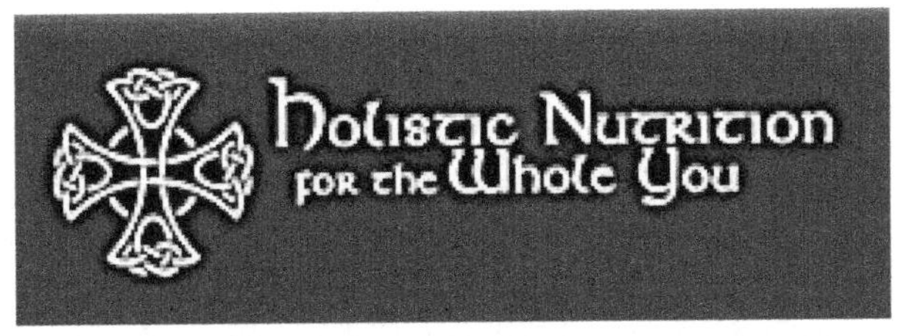

Get Your Full-Color E-Books Today

@ YourWholeNutrition.com

Print Editions available through Amazon.Com &

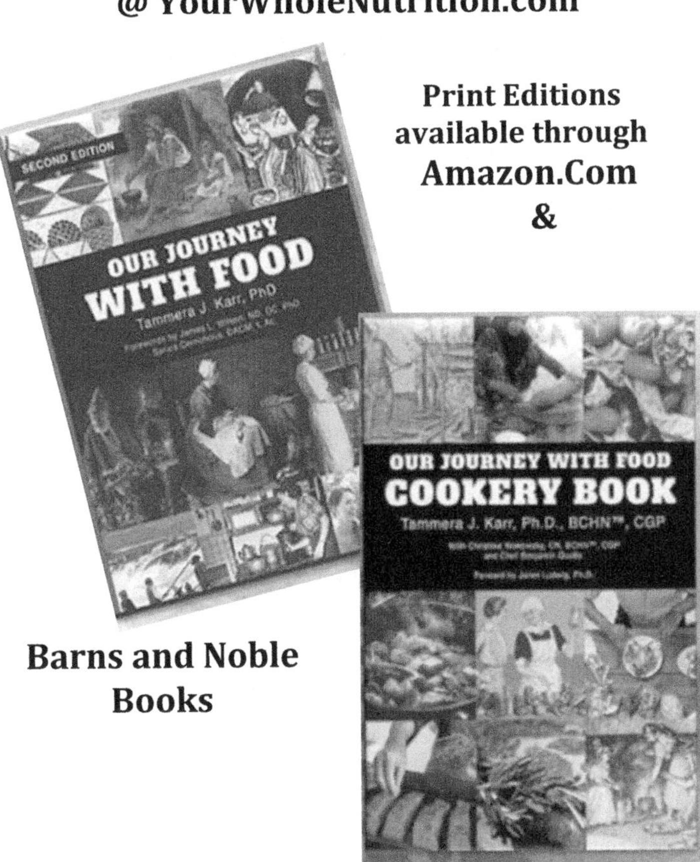

Barns and Noble Books

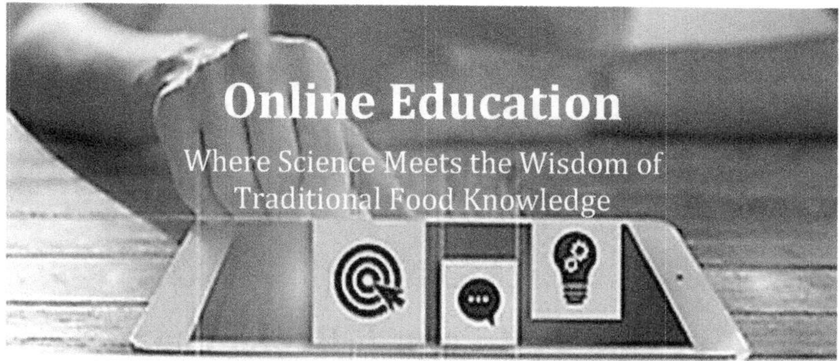

HN4U Our Journey with Food @ Yourwholenutrition.com

Who is this program for?

This course, while initially created for nurses eager to use food as medicine, is also suitable for anyone motivated to learn how to create delicious meals with health-promoting qualities.

Evidence-Based

Why You Want to Take This Program

Food and Health

There is a growing body of science supporting traditional food choices for sustainable health.

- Self-Paced Course with Instructor Access
- 12 Evidence-Based Presentations
- Over 20 Videos with Downloadable Tools
- 3 Exams to Test Knowledge
- Scientific and Historical Citations
- Group Interaction, Recommended Reading, Activities, Support, Tips, and Tools
- 25 credit-hour Certificate of Completion*

This Course Will Cover:

- Nutrition Foundations
- Sustainability in Food Choices for Health
- Mindfulness in Food Selection and Lifestyle

Made in the USA
Middletown, DE
17 November 2020

24302525R00229